Bennett's Cardiac Arrhythmias

Bennett's Cardiac Arrhythmias
Practical Notes on Interpretation and Treatment

8th Edition

David H. Bennett, MD FRCP

Senior Consultant Cardiologist
University Hospital of South Manchester
Manchester, UK

WILEY-BLACKWELL

A John Wiley & Sons, Ltd., Publication

This edition first published 2013 © 2013 by John Wiley & Sons, Ltd.

Wiley-Blackwell is an imprint of John Wiley & Sons, formed by the merger of Wiley's global Scientific, Technical and Medical business with Blackwell Publishing.

Registered office
John Wiley & Sons, Ltd, The Atrium, Southern Gate, Chichester, West Sussex,
PO19 8SQ, UK

Editorial offices
9600 Garsington Road, Oxford, OX4 2DQ, UK
The Atrium, Southern Gate, Chichester, West Sussex, PO19 8SQ, UK
111 River Street, Hoboken, NJ 07030-5774, USA

For details of our global editorial offices, for customer services and for information about how to apply for permission to reuse the copyright material in this book please see our website at www.wiley.com/wiley-blackwell

Library of Congress Cataloging-in-Publication Data

Bennett, David H.
Bennett's cardiac arrhythmias : practical notes on interpretation and treatment / David H. Bennett. – 8th ed.
    p. ; cm.
  Cardiac arrhythmias
  Rev. ed. of. Cardiac arrhythmias / David H. Bennett. 7th ed., 2006.
  Includes bibliographical references and index.
  ISBN 978-0-470-67493-2 (pbk. : alk. paper)
I. Bennett, David H. Cardiac arrhythmias. II. Title. III. Title: Cardiac arrhythmias.
  [DNLM: 1. Arrhythmias, Cardiac–diagnosis. 2. Arrhythmias, Cardiac–therapy. WG 330]
  616.1'28–dc23

                                        2012021105

A catalogue record for this book is available from the British Library.

Wiley also publishes its books in a variety of electronic formats. Some content that appears in print may not be available in electronic books.

Cover image courtesy of the author
Cover design by Andrew Magee Design Ltd

Set in 9/12pt Palatino by SPi Publishers Services, Pondicherry, India

1 2013

Contents

Contents

Preface

There are several large textbooks which comprehensively cover the field of cardiac arrhythmias with thorough referencing of scientific papers. This book does not attempt to replicate these texts. The purpose of this eighth edition (the first edition was published in 1981, and there have been translations into five other languages) remains the same as that of its predecessors: to provide a concise, up-to-date, practical guide to the diagnosis, investigation and management of the main cardiac arrhythmias, with particular emphasis on the problems commonly faced in practice.

In order to be proficient in the interpretation of arrhythmias it is necessary to study a range of examples of each rhythm disturbance. For this reason, it has always been a purpose of this book to present a large number of electrocardiograms so that the reader can gain experience in ECG interpretation and can test him- or herself out, and thereby gain confidence, during the reading of the book. In this edition there are many new electrocardiograms, and the quiz section has been revised and enlarged to provide a challenge to those who may be familiar with previous editions.

The book has been written with junior hospital doctors in mind. They receive little formal training in the management of cardiac arrhythmias and yet, because prompt action is often required, the onus of diagnosis and treatment usually falls on them. It should also be of interest to medical students, who themselves will soon be responsible for dealing with arrhythmias, to nurses working in coronary and intensive care units, to cardiac technicians/ physiologists, whose responsibilities nowadays include a major input into arrhythmia management, and to physicians who want a brief review of the practical aspects of cardiac arrhythmias. In recent years there has been a trend to sub-specialisation in cardiology. Whatever the sub-specialty, cardiac arrhythmias will frequently be encountered. An appreciation of the significance and management of cardiac arrhythmias is required of all who treat patients with cardiac disease.

I am most grateful to my technical, medical and nursing colleagues for their help, and to the staff of my new publisher at Wiley-Blackwell for their expertise.

The title of this edition, *Bennett's Cardiac Arrhythmias*, was chosen by the publisher to indicate that the author has described the major disturbances of heart rhythm, not, at least to date, that the author has experienced all of them!

The book is dedicated to my family, Irene, Samantha and Sally.

David H. Bennett, MD FRCP
Senior Consultant Cardiologist
University Hospital of South Manchester
Manchester, UK

Notes

The electrocardiograms in this book have been recorded at the conventional paper speed of 25 mm/s, unless otherwise indicated. At this speed, each large square represents 0.2 s and each small square represents 0.04 s. Heart rate (beats/minute) can therefore be calculated by dividing the number of large squares between two consecutive complexes into 300, or by dividing the number of small squares between two complexes into 1500.

A single ECG 'rhythm strip' may be inadequate for diagnosis. Scrutiny of several ECG leads, preferably recorded simultaneously, may be necessary. For example, atrial activity is often the key to diagnosis but may not be clearly shown in all ECG leads: it is often best seen in leads II and V1. Frequently, a '12-lead ECG' will provide much more information than a rhythm strip.

An ECG recorded during an arrhythmia that is of diagnostic importance should always be safely stored in the patient's notes. This guideline, which may be very important to the long-term management of a patient, is often ignored, particularly on intensive and coronary care units!

1 Sinus Rhythm

The sinus node lies at the junction of the superior vena cava and right atrium. Atrial activation travels inferiorly from the sinus node to the atrioventricular (AV) node, resulting in a positive P wave in the inferior ECG leads, II, III and aVF. If the QRS complex is preceded by a P wave that is not positive in the inferior leads then the rhythm is other than sinus rhythm. The sinus node impulse is conducted relatively slowly via the AV node to reach the His–Purkinje system, which then conducts very rapidly to activate the ventricular myocardium.

Normal sinus rhythm is characterised by a rate of 60–100 beats/min; PR interval 0.12–0.21 s; QRS duration ≤0.10 s; QTc ≤0.44 s.

ECG characteristics

The sinus node initiates the electrical impulse that activates atrial and then ventricular myocardium during each normal heartbeat. Sinus node activity itself does not register on the electrocardiogram (ECG).

P wave

Atrial activity, the P wave, is usually apparent in most ECG leads (Figure 1.1). However, occasionally the P wave in some leads is not visible or is of low amplitude, and it may be necessary to inspect all leads of the ECG to establish that there is sinus rhythm (Figure 1.2).

The sinus node lies at the junction of the superior vena cava and right atrium. *Atrial activation therefore spreads from the sinus node in an inferior direction* (i.e. towards the feet) to the atrioventricular (AV) junction. The P wave, therefore, is upright in those leads that are directed to the inferior surface of the heart (i.e. II, III and aVF), and is inverted in aVR, which faces the superior heart surface (Figure 1.1). If a P wave does not have these characteristics then, even though a P wave precedes each ventricular complex, the sinus node has not activated the atria and the rhythm is abnormal (Figure 1.3).

PR interval

The AV node is the only electrical connection between atria and ventricles: the mitral-tricuspid valve ring that separates the atria from the ventricles is fibrous and cannot

Bennett's Cardiac Arrhythmias: Practical Notes on Interpretation and Treatment, Eighth Edition. David H. Bennett.
© 2013 John Wiley & Sons, Ltd. Published 2013 by John Wiley & Sons, Ltd.

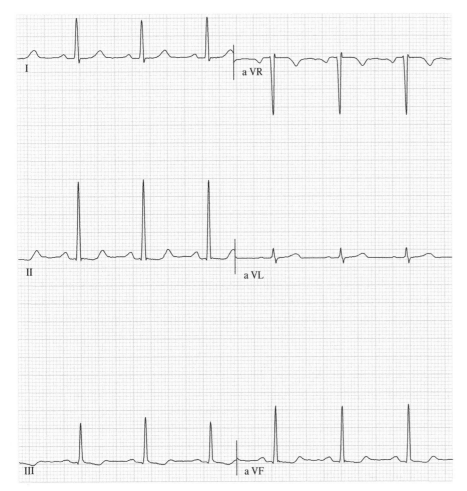

Figure 1.1 Sinus rhythm. Atrial activity is clearly seen in the limb leads.

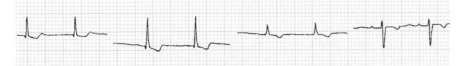

Figure 1.2 Sinus rhythm with low-amplitude P waves (leads I, II, III and V1). Atrial activity is only clearly seen in V1.

conduct electrical impulses. The AV node conducts relatively slowly, thereby delaying conduction of the atrial impulse to the ventricles. Conduction through the AV node does not register on the ECG. The PR interval, which is measured from the onset of the P wave to the onset of the ventricular complex, indicates the time taken for an atrial impulse to reach the ventricles. The normal PR interval ranges from 0.12 to 0.21 s. It should shorten during sinus tachycardia.

QRS complex

After traversing the AV node, the activating impulse reaches the bundle of His, which divides into the right and left bundle branches. The bundle of His, the bundle branches and their ramifications, the Purkinje fibres, constitute the 'specialised intraventricular conducting system' which facilitates very rapid conduction of the impulse through the ventricular myocardium. Ventricular activation (i.e. depolarisation) is represented by the QRS complex, which is normally no greater than 0.10 s in

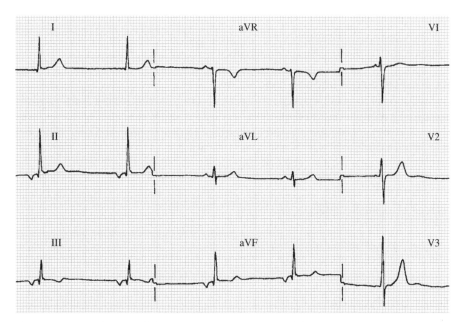

Figure 1.3 Junctional not sinus rhythm: a P wave precedes each QRS complex but is superiorly directed: i.e. it is negative in leads II, III and aVF.

duration. The amplitude of the QRS complex is larger than that of the P wave because the mass of the ventricles is much greater than that of the atria.

T wave

The T wave is the result of the electrical recovery of ventricular myocardium prior to the next heartbeat, i.e. repolarisation. Sometimes, a low-amplitude wave can be seen following the T wave, termed a U wave. It is thought to result from repolarisation of the Purkinje fibres and is usually seen in leads V2–4.

The QT interval, which is measured from the onset of the QRS complex to the end of the T wave, represents the duration of ventricular activation plus recovery. The QT interval normally shortens with increasing heart rate, partly due to the increase in rate itself and partly due to the increase in sympathetic nervous system activity related to sinus tachycardia. When measuring the QT interval it is necessary to correct the measured interval for heart rate. The corrected QT interval (QTc) is calculated by selecting the ECG lead showing the longest QT interval, and then dividing the square root of the cycle length into the measured QT interval. For example, a patient with a

---

ECG characteristics of normal sinus rhythm

P wave
    Precedes each QRS complex
    Upright in leads III, aVF
    Inverted in lead aVR

PR interval
    Duration 0.12–0.21 s

QRS complex
    Duration ≤0.10 s

QTc interval
    Duration ≤0.42 s (men), ≤0.44 s (women)

measured QT interval of 0.40 s at a heart rate of 60 beats/min has a cycle length of 1.0 s and therefore also has a QTc of 0.40 s. QT prolongation and a prominent U wave are seen in certain hereditary and acquired conditions.

Relative speeds of impulse conduction

Appreciation of the relative speeds of impulse conduction through the heart – slowest through the AV node, fastest through the specialised intraventricular conducting system and at an intermediate rate through ordinary working myocardium – is important in understanding the mechanisms of a number of arrhythmias as well as generation of the normal P-QRS complex.

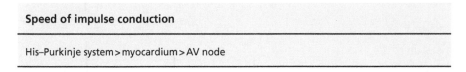

Speed of impulse conduction
His–Purkinje system > myocardium > AV node

Sinus bradycardia

Sinus bradycardia is sinus rhythm at a rate less then 60 beats/min (Figure 1.4). It may be physiological, as in athletes or during sleep, or it may result from acute myocardial infarction, sick sinus syndrome or from drugs such as beta-adrenoceptor blocking drugs (beta-blockers). Non-cardiac disorders such as hypothyroidism, jaundice and raised intracranial pressure can also cause sinus bradycardia.

Atropine, isoprenaline or pacing can be used to increase the rate but are only necessary when sinus bradycardia causes symptoms or marked hypotension, or leads to tachyarrhythmia.

Sinus tachycardia

Sinus tachycardia is defined as sinus rhythm at a rate greater than 100 beats/min (Figure 1.5). Exercise, anxiety or any disorder that increases sympathetic nervous system activity may cause sinus tachycardia.

Occasionally, sinus tachycardia can be inappropriate. Hyperthyroidism is a possible cause. However, often no cause is found. Young females are most commonly affected. Fast rates are usually persistent and there is an exaggerated response to exercise with rates increasing rapidly almost immediately exertion begins. Rarely, inappropriate sinus tachycardia is due to a primary disorder of the sinus node (sinus node re-entry).

Since sinus tachycardia is usually a physiological response, there is rarely a need for specific treatment. However, if sinus tachycardia is inappropriate, the rate may be slowed by a beta-blocker, or by ivabradine, which is a selective inhibitor of sinus node function.

At rest, the sinus node rate is seldom above 100 beats/min unless the patient is very ill. If there is apparent sinus tachycardia at rest alternative rhythms such as atrial tachycardia or atrial flutter should be considered.

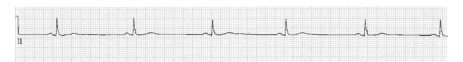

Figure 1.4 Sinus bradycardia (lead II): rate 34 beats/min.

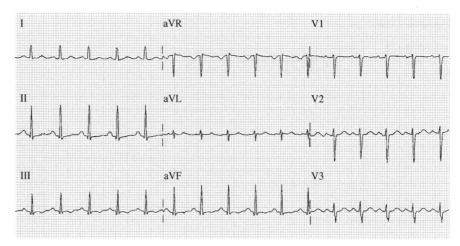

Figure 1.5 Sinus tachycardia during exercise. The rate is 136 beats/min.

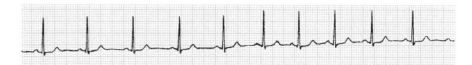

Figure 1.6 Sinus arrhythmia.

Sinus arrhythmia

In sinus arrhythmia, which is of no pathological significance, there are alternating periods of slowing and increasing sinus node rate. Usually the rate increases during inspiration (Figure 1.6). Sinus arrhythmia is most commonly seen in the young.

2 Ectopic Beats

The terms ectopic beat, extrasystole and premature contraction are, for practical purposes, synonymous. They refer to an impulse originating from the atria, atrioventricular (AV) junction or ventricles that arises prematurely in the cardiac cycle.

Usually the AV junction and bundle branches will conduct an atrial ectopic to the ventricles normally, resulting in a narrow QRS complex. The prematurity of an atrial ectopic beat is such that the P wave may be superimposed on the preceding T wave.

The impulse of a ventricular ectopic beat is not conducted through the ventricles via the rapidly conducting His–Purkinje system. The resultant complexes are therefore broad (>0.12s) and bizarre in shape, and will not be preceded by a premature P wave. Ventricular ectopic beats are often idiopathic but when caused by cardiac disease are associated with an increased cardiovascular mortality that will not be reduced by antiarrhythmic drugs.

Prematurity

The terms ectopic beat, extrasystole and premature contraction are, for practical purposes, synonymous. They refer to an impulse originating from the atria, AV junction (i.e. the AV node together with the bundle of His) or ventricles that arises prematurely in the cardiac cycle (Figures 2.1–2.3).

By definition, an ectopic beat must arise earlier in the cardiac cycle than the next normally timed beat would be expected. Thus the interval between the ectopic beat and the preceding beat, i.e. the coupling interval, is shorter than the cycle length of the main rhythm. If this fact is ignored, other beats with abnormal configurations such as escape beats (Chapter 3) and intermittent bundle branch block (Chapter 4) may be misinterpreted as ectopic beats.

The site of origin of an ectopic beat can be determined by careful examination of the ECG. A single rhythm strip may be inadequate. Scrutiny of simultaneous recordings of several ECG leads is often necessary to detect the diagnostic clues (Figures 2.4, 2.5).

Bennett's Cardiac Arrhythmias: Practical Notes on Interpretation and Treatment, Eighth Edition. David H. Bennett.
© 2013 John Wiley & Sons, Ltd. Published 2013 by John Wiley & Sons, Ltd.

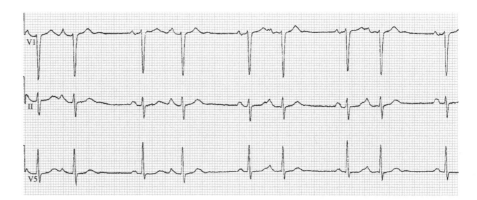

Figure 2.1 The second, fourth, sixth and eighth complexes are atrial ectopic beats. The ectopic P waves are premature and differ in shape from those of sinus origin (the PR intervals of the atrial ectopic beats are prolonged).

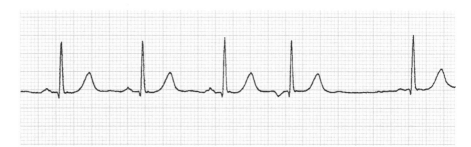

Figure 2.2 The fourth beat is a junctional ectopic beat (lead III). The junctional focus has activated the atria as well as the ventricles, resulting in an inverted P wave which precedes the QRS complex.

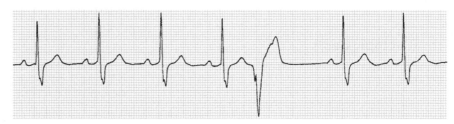

Figure 2.3 The fifth beat is a ventricular ectopic beat.

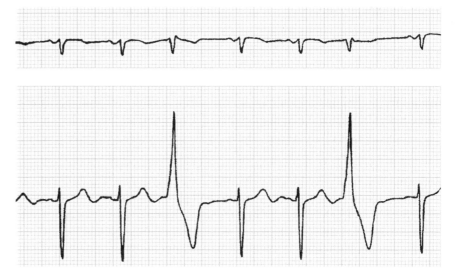

Figure 2.4 Simultaneous recording of leads V1 and V2. The third and sixth beats are unifocal ventricular ectopic beats. Their ventricular origin is not apparent in lead V1 but is obvious in V2.

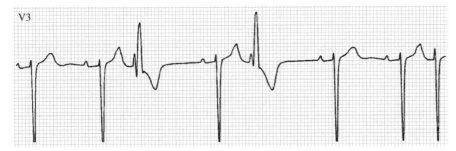

Figure 2.5 Atrial ectopic beats are superimposed on the T waves of the second, fourth and seventh ventricular complexes (lead V3). It can be seen how the T waves of these beats are modified by comparing them with the T wave of the first and sixth ventricular complexes, which are not followed by an atrial ectopic. The first two atrial ectopic beats are conducted with right bundle branch block.

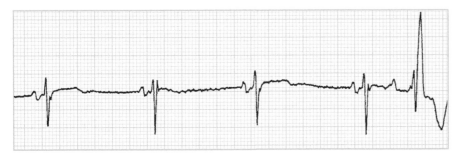

Figure 2.6 The last beat is an atrial ectopic beat conducted with a prolonged PR interval and right bundle branch block.

Atrial ectopic beats

P wave

An atrial ectopic beat results in a P wave that is premature. The site of origin and therefore direction of atrial activation will differ from that during sinus rhythm, so a premature P wave will usually differ in shape to a P wave of sinus node origin (Figure 2.1).

Because atrial ectopic beats are premature, they may be superimposed on and thus deform the T wave of the preceding beat. Careful examination of the ECG is essential to detect ectopic P waves; often, lead V1 is the best lead (Figures 2.5, 2.6).

Atrioventricular and intraventricular conduction

Usually the AV junction and bundle branches will conduct an atrial ectopic beat to the ventricles in the same manner as if the sinus node had activated the atria. Thus the PR interval and QRS complex of the ectopic beat will be identical to those during sinus rhythm (Figure 2.1). If the QRS complex during sinus rhythm is abnormal due to bundle branch block, then so will be the QRS complex of the ectopic beat.

Sometimes, however, atrial ectopic beats, especially those that arise very early in the cardiac cycle, may encounter either an AV junction or a bundle branch which has not yet recovered from conduction of the last atrial impulse and is, therefore, partially or completely refractory to excitation. Partial and complete refractoriness of the AV junction will result in prolongation of the PR interval and blocked atrial ectopic beats, respectively (Figures 2.1, 2.6–2.8). Atrial ectopics that are not conducted to the ventricles have been wrongly taken as an indication for cardiac pacing!

Partial or complete refractoriness of one or other bundle branch (it is usually the right bundle) will correspondingly lead to partial or complete bundle branch block (Figures 2.6, 2.7). This phenomenon of functional bundle branch block is referred to by some as 'phasic aberrant intraventricular conduction'. The resultant QRS

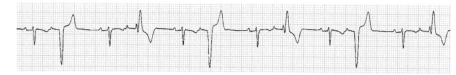

Figure 2.7 Lead V1. Atrial ectopic beats follow each sinus beat. The second, sixth and tenth complexes are atrial ectopic beats conducted with left bundle branch block. The fourth, eighth and twelfth complexes are conducted with right bundle branch block.

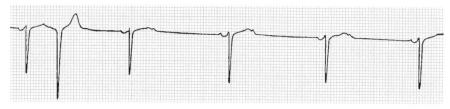

Figure 2.8 Lead V1. Atrial ectopic beats are superimposed on the terminal portion of the T wave of each ventricular complex. The first atrial ectopic is conducted with partial left branch block. The other atrial ectopic beats are not conducted to the ventricles.

complexes are broad and can therefore be confused with ventricular ectopic beats *if the premature P wave preceding the ventricular complex is not detected.*

ECG characteristics of atrial ectopic beats

The P wave of an atrial ectopic beat:
  Is premature
  May be superimposed on and distort the preceding T wave
  Is usually followed by a normal QRS complex
  Is sometimes not conducted to the ventricles, or is conducted with a bundle branch block
    pattern

Significance

Atrial ectopic beats occur in many cardiac disorders but are also commonly found in individuals with normal hearts, particularly the elderly. They are usually benign. However, if they are frequent they may herald atrial fibrillation or atrial tachycardia.

Atrioventricular junctional ectopic beats

AV junctional beats used to be called 'nodal' beats. It is now recognised that at least part of the AV node is not capable of pacemaker activity and that it is not possible to distinguish between beats originating from the AV node and those from the bundle of His. Hence the more general term 'AV junctional' is used. AV junctional ectopic beats are not as common as atrial or ventricular ectopics. Treatment is rarely necessary.

ECG appearance

AV junctional ectopic beats are recognised by a premature QRS complex that is similar in appearance to that occurring in sinus rhythm. The junctional focus may activate the atria as well as the ventricles, leading to a retrograde P wave (i.e. negative in leads II, III and aVF). The retrograde P wave may precede, follow or be buried within the

QRS complex, depending on the relative speeds of conduction of the premature junctional impulse to the ventricles and to the atria (Figure 2.2).

Ventricular ectopic beats

The impulse of a ventricular ectopic beat is not conducted through the ventricles via the His–Purkinje system but through relatively slowly conducting myocardium. The abnormal course and consequent slowing of ventricular activation result in ventricular complexes that are both bizarre in shape and of prolonged duration.

ECG appearance

The complexes are premature, broad (≥ 0.12 s), bizarre in shape and, in contrast to atrial ectopic beats, are obviously not preceded by a premature P wave (Figures 2.3, 2.4).

ECG characteristics of ventricular ectopic beats

The QRS complex of a ventricular ectopic beat is:
   Premature
   Broad (≥ 0.12 s)
   Abnormal in shape
   Not preceded by a premature P wave

Several terms are used to describe the origin, timing and quantity of ventricular ectopic beats:

Focus

Ectopic beats with the same shape and coupling intervals are assumed to arise from the same focus and are termed 'unifocal' (Figure 2.4), whereas differing shapes and coupling intervals suggest more than one focus. These are called 'multifocal' or 'multiform' (Figure 2.9).

Timing

Beats that occur very early in the cardiac cycle will be superimposed on the T wave of the preceding beat and are described as 'R on T' (Figure 2.10). Most episodes of ventricular fibrillation and many episodes of ventricular tachycardia are initiated by 'R on T' ectopics; though by no means do all 'R on T' ectopic beats precipitate these arrhythmias.

A ventricular ectopic beat that occurs only slightly prematurely in the cardiac cycle may fall, by chance, immediately after a P wave initiated by normal sinus node activity: the P wave will not, therefore, in contrast to an atrial ectopic beat, be premature. Such a ventricular ectopic beat is described as 'end-diastolic' (Figures 2.11, 2.12).

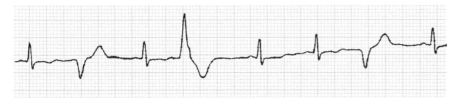

Figure 2.9 Multifocal ventricular ectopic beats. The second ventricular ectopic beat has a different shape and coupling interval from the first and third ectopic beats.

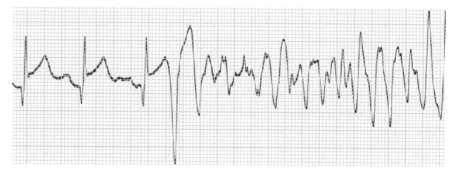

Figure 2.10 An 'R on T' ventricular ectopic beat, which in this case initiates ventricular fibrillation.

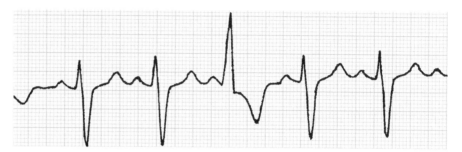

Figure 2.11 The third beat is an end-diastolic ventricular ectopic beat. It is preceded by a normally timed P wave.

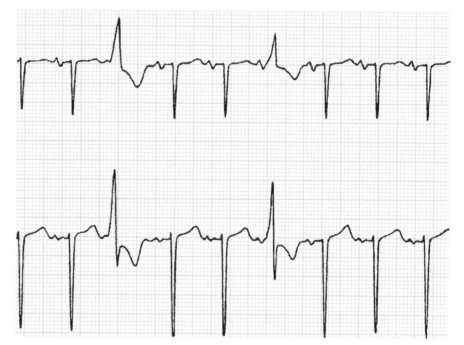

Figure 2.12 Simultaneous recording of leads V1 and V2. Two end-diastolic ventricular ectopic beats. The second mimicking the Wolff–Parkinson–White syndrome.

Usually there is a pause after a ventricular ectopic beat. When there is no such pause and the ectopic beat is thus 'sandwiched' between two normal beats, the ectopic beat is said to be 'interpolated' (Figure 2.13).

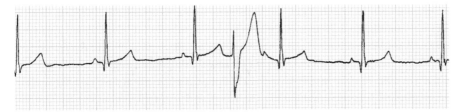

Figure 2.13 Interpolated ventricular beat. The subsequent PR interval is prolonged due to retrograde concealed conduction.

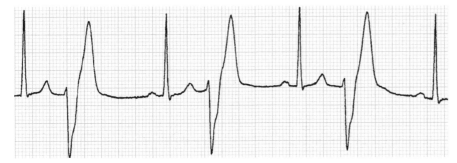

Figure 2.14 Ventricular bigeminy.

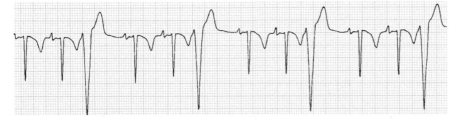

Figure 2.15 Ventricular trigeminy.

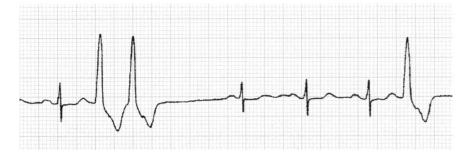

Figure 2.16 The first sinus beat is followed by a couplet of ventricular ectopic beats.

Frequency

When an ectopic beat follows each sinus beat the term 'bigeminy' is applied (Figure 2.14). If an ectopic follows a pair of normal beats there is 'trigeminy' (Figure 2.15). When two ectopics occur in succession (Figure 2.16) they are referred to as a 'couplet'. A 'salvo' refers to more than two ectopic beats in succession.

Atrial activity

The pattern of atrial activity following a ventricular ectopic beat depends on whether the AV junction transmits the ventricular impulse to the atria. If this occurs, the result is an inverted P wave which is often superimposed on and may therefore be concealed

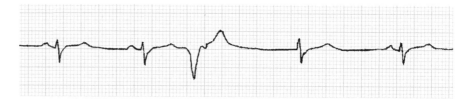

Figure 2.17 The third beat is a ventricular ectopic beat that has been conducted back to the atria, resulting in an inverted P wave (lead aVF). (The ectopic beat is followed by a junctional escape beat.)

by the ventricular ectopic beat (Figure 2.17). When the AV junction does not transmit the ventricular impulse to the atria, atrial activity continues independently of ventricular activity; it is only in these cases that a ventricular impulse is followed by a full compensatory pause (i.e. the lengths of the cycles before and after the ectopic beat will equal twice the sinus cycle length) (Figures 2.3, 2.4).

Sometimes a ventricular impulse only partially penetrates the AV junction. The next impulse arising from the sinus node may therefore encounter an AV junction that is partially refractory and be conducted with a prolonged PR interval (Figure 2.13). This phenomenon of 'retrograde concealed conduction' often occurs following interpolated ventricular extrasystoles.

Causes and significance of ventricular ectopic beats

Ventricular ectopic beats are very common, and their frequency in the general adult population increases with age. Causes of ventricular ectopic beats include acute myocardial infarction; myocardial ischaemia; hypertension; myocardial damage caused by previous infarction, myocarditis or cardiomyopathy; mitral valve prolapse; valvular heart disease and digoxin toxicity; *but frequently, there will be no evidence of heart disease*.

In patients presenting with symptomatic and/or frequent ventricular ectopic beats a cause should be sought by use of non-invasive tests including scrutiny of the 12-lead ECG, echocardiography and, where appropriate, exercise testing.

Occasional ventricular ectopic beats during routine electrocardiography, and even complex ectopic beats (i.e. frequent, multifocal, 'R on T' or those that occur in salvos) during ambulatory electrocardiography, can be found in subjects with otherwise normal hearts and are not necessarily pathological or of prognostic significance. On the other hand, in several surveys of adult, predominantly male, subjects referred for exercise testing, frequent ventricular ectopic beats during and particularly immediately after exercise have been shown to be associated with an increased mortality (approximately × 3) in follow-up periods of 5–15 years.

In patients who have sustained myocardial damage from coronary heart disease, there is a correlation between severity of damage and frequency of ventricular ectopic beats. Recent evidence, however, points to the presence of ectopic beats as an added and independent risk factor, but there is no evidence to show that suppression of ectopic beats by antiarrhythmic therapy improves prognosis. Indeed, several antiarrhythmic drugs have been shown to increase mortality in patients with ventricular ectopic beats after myocardial infarction.

Ectopic beats are usually asymptomatic. Some patients, however, do experience distressing symptoms. They may be upset by the irregularity resulting from the premature beats or by the compensatory pause or 'thump' caused by increased myocardial contractility associated with the post-ectopic beat. They may be anxious that their irregular heart rhythm is a sign of impending heart attack or other major cardiac problem.

There is a group of patients with structurally normal hearts with distressing symptoms caused by ventricular ectopic beats in whom reassurance is inadequate. In these patients, therapy may be necessary for symptomatic purposes. Beta-blockers may help, particularly in patients whose symptoms are related to exertion. Flecainide is useful, provided the patient has a structurally normal heart and there is no evidence of coronary disease. Caffeine avoidance is frequently advised but rarely effective.

The significance of ventricular ectopic beats in acute myocardial infarction is discussed in Chapter 18.

3   Escape Beats

Escape beats may arise from the AV junction or ventricles when there is sinus bradycardia or sinus arrest. In contrast to ectopic beats, the coupling interval of escape beats is greater than the cycle length of the main rhythm. The configuration of junctional escape beats is the same as that of normally conducted beats, whereas ventricular escape beats are of similar appearance to ventricular ectopic complexes. Escape beats themselves require no treatment. If treatment is necessary, it is to accelerate the basic rhythm.

Timing

When there is sinus bradycardia or the sinus node fails to discharge, escape beats may arise from secondary sites in the specialised conducting system. *In contrast to ectopic beats, escape beats are always late*, i.e. the coupling interval is greater than the cycle length of the dominant rhythm (Figure 3.1). Distinction between escape and ectopic

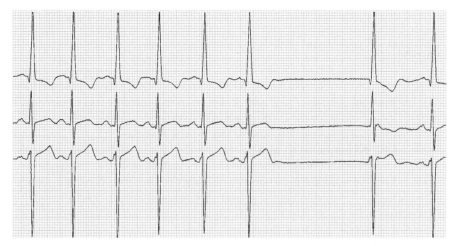

Figure 3.1 Leads I, II and III. After the sixth complex there is a pause in sinus node activity followed by a junctional escape beat.

Bennett's Cardiac Arrhythmias: Practical Notes on Interpretation and Treatment, Eighth Edition. David H. Bennett.
© 2013 John Wiley & Sons, Ltd. Published 2013 by John Wiley & Sons, Ltd.

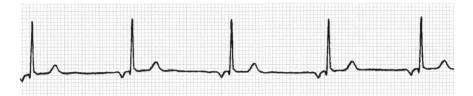

Figure 3.2 Junctional escape rhythm (lead II). The junctional focus has also activated the atria, as indicated by the inverted P wave preceding each QRS complex. (The rhythm has also been termed 'coronary sinus' rhythm.)

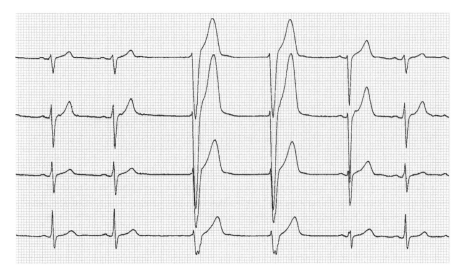

Figure 3.3 Ventricular escape rhythm during sinus bradycardia. After two normally timed sinus beats there are two ventricular escape beats. These are followed by a complex intermediate in appearance between normal sinus and ventricular escape beats which is the result of simultaneous ventricular activation by the sinus node and the ventricular escape focus: a 'fusion beat'.

beats is important, because the former indicate impaired sinus node function. *Escape beats themselves require no treatment*. If treatment is necessary, it is to accelerate the basic rhythm.

Origins

Escape beats usually arise from the AV junction (Figures 3.1, 3.2); less commonly, they originate from the ventricles (Figure 3.3). The ventricular complexes of junctional escape beats are similar to those during normal rhythm because the impulse will be conducted normally via the His bundle and bundle branches. As with junctional ectopic beats, the junctional focus may activate the atria as well as the ventricles, leading to a retrograde P wave, i.e. inverted in leads II, III and aVF. The retrograde P wave may precede, follow or be buried within the QRS complex, depending on the relative speeds of conduction of the premature junctional impulse to the ventricles and to the atria.

Ventricular escape beats have a configuration similar to that of ventricular ectopic beats (Figure 3.3).

Bundle Branch and Fascicular Blocks

Right and left bundle branch block, and block in the left anterior and posterior fascicles of the left bundle branch, are commonly encountered.

Complete bundle branch block prolongs QRS duration to 0.12 s or greater. With right bundle branch block, there will be a secondary R wave in lead V1, resulting in an M-shaped complex. With left bundle branch block, there is no M-shaped complex in V1; there will be a notched complex in left ventricular leads.

Diagnosis of fascicular block requires an understanding of the hexaxial reference system. With left axis deviation, lead I is predominantly positive and both leads II and III are predominantly negative. The criteria for left anterior fascicular block are left axis deviation together with a small initial r wave in leads II and aVF: inferior infarction also leads to left axis deviation but there will be a Q rather than r wave in these leads.

The bundle of His divides into left and right bundle branches. These facilitate very rapid activation of the left and right ventricles. Block in conduction through one or other bundle branch results in delayed and disordered activation of ventricular myocardium, as evidenced on the ECG by a ventricular complex which is prolonged in duration and has an abnormal configuration.

Right bundle branch block

ECG appearance

In right bundle branch block there is delay in activation of the right ventricle, while activation of the interventricular septum and free wall of the left ventricle and hence the initial part of the QRS complex is normal (Figure 4.1). Delayed right ventricular activation results in:

1. an increase in duration of the QRS complex ($\geq$ 0.12 s);
2. a secondary R wave in leads facing the right ventricle (V1 and V2) and hence an M-shaped complex in these leads; and
3. a broad S wave in left ventricular leads and lead I.

Bennett's Cardiac Arrhythmias: Practical Notes on Interpretation and Treatment, Eighth Edition. David H. Bennett.
© 2013 John Wiley & Sons, Ltd. Published 2013 by John Wiley & Sons, Ltd.

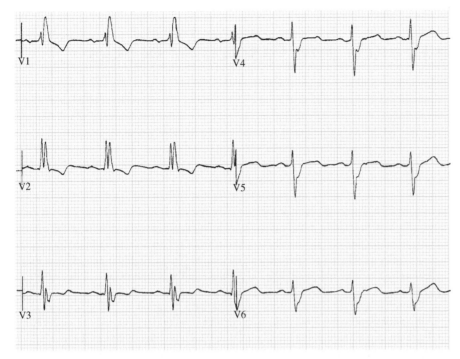

Figure 4.1 Right bundle branch block. There is an M-shaped complex in V1 and a deep slurred S wave in lead V6.

Partial right bundle branch block results in a similar ECG appearance but the QRS duration is 0.10 or 0.11's.

Causes and significance

Right bundle branch block may be an isolated congenital lesion. It often occurs in congenital heart disease, in other causes of right ventricular hypertrophy or strain such as obstructive airways disease, and where there is myocardial damage. Right bundle branch block is common when there is disease of the specialised conducting tissues.

Based on limited data, neither pre-existing nor acquired right bundle branch block are of prognostic significance. However, a recent long-term survey has demonstrated a four-fold increased risk of developing AV block.

Extrasystoles and tachycardias of supraventricular origin may encounter a right bundle branch that is refractory to excitation and be conducted to the ventricles with a right bundle branch block pattern.

Left bundle branch block

ECG appearance

In left bundle branch block, activation of the interventricular septum is in the opposite direction to normal (i.e. from right to left), being initiated by an impulse arising from the right bundle branch. Thus:

1. The initial small, negative q wave normally seen in left ventricular leads (V5, V6, I and aVL) is replaced by a larger, positive R wave.

2. Activation of the left ventricle will be delayed, resulting in a broad and usually notched R wave in left ventricular leads, and prolongation of the duration of the QRS complex (≥ 0.12 s) (Figure 4.2).

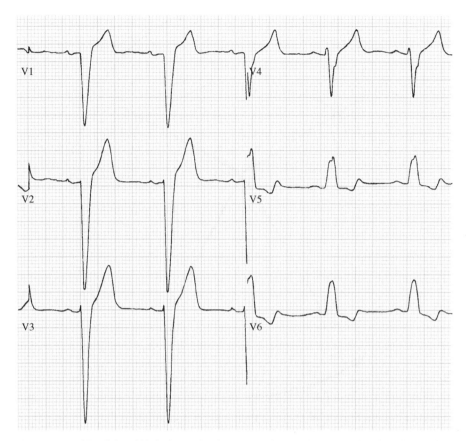

Figure 4.2 Left bundle branch block. There is a broad positive complex in V6. There is no M-shaped complex in lead V1. The QS complex in V1 is also characteristic of left bundle branch block.

Partial left bundle branch block has a similar ECG appearance to complete left bundle branch block, but the QRS duration is 0.10 or 0.11 s.

There is a simple, pragmatic rule to help distinguish right from left bundle branch block. Assuming the absence of Wolff–Parkinson–White syndrome or gross ventricular hypertrophy, if during normal rhythm (or indeed a supraventricular tachycardia) the QRS duration is ≥ 0.12 s then there is bundle branch block. If the ventricular complex in lead V1 is M-shaped there is right bundle branch block, if it is not there is left bundle branch block.

Causes and significance

Causes of left bundle branch block include myocardial damage due to coronary artery disease or cardiomyopathy, and left ventricular hypertrophy. Left bundle branch block can also be caused by disease of the specialised conduction tissues.

Recently acquired left bundle branch block is associated with an increased risk of death: mainly sudden death from coronary disease. In addition, an 18-fold risk of developing AV block in the long term has recently been reported.

Supraventricular extrasystoles and tachycardias may encounter a left bundle branch that is refractory to excitation and be conducted to the ventricles with a left bundle branch block pattern.

Left bundle branch block can be intermittent.

Left anterior and posterior fascicular blocks

The left bundle branch has two main subdivisions, the anterior and posterior fascicles, which conduct impulses to the anterosuperior and posteroinferior regions of the

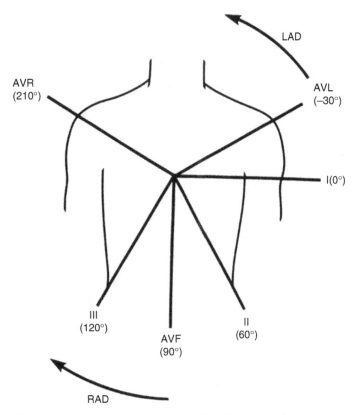

Figure 4.3 Hexaxial reference system. LAD, left axis deviation; RAD, right axis deviation.

left ventricle, respectively. Block can occur in either anterior or posterior fascicle and is known as fascicular block or hemiblock. Left anterior and posterior fascicular block are common in conduction tissue disease, and one or other together with right bundle branch block, i.e. bifascicular block, can herald the onset of high-degree atrioventricular block (Chapter 15).

Diagnosis of the fascicular blocks is based on the hexaxial reference system.

Hexaxial reference system

This is a method of displaying the orientation of the six ECG limb leads to the heart in the frontal plane, i.e. the vertical plane that runs through the centre of the body, dividing it into anterior and posterior regions (Figure 4.3). For example, a superiorly directed impulse will move away from leads II, III and aVF, producing a negative wave in these leads, and towards aVL, producing a positive wave in this lead. The direction of an impulse can be expressed by the number of degrees clockwise (positive) or anticlockwise (negative) of lead I, which is the zero reference point. For example, an impulse towards lead aVL has an axis of −30 degrees and an impulse towards lead III has an axis of +120 degrees (Figure 4.3).

Mean frontal QRS axis

The mean frontal QRS axis describes the dominant or average direction of the various electrical forces that develop during ventricular activation. Normally, the mean frontal QRS axis lies between aVL (i.e. −30 degrees) and aVF (i.e. +90 degrees).

If the axis is to the left of aVL (i.e. less than −30 degrees), it is termed abnormal left axis deviation. If the axis is to the right of aVF (i.e. more than +90 degrees), there is right axis deviation.

Using the hexaxial reference system, the mean frontal QRS axis may be calculated to within a few degrees. However, this degree of precision is unnecessary and most

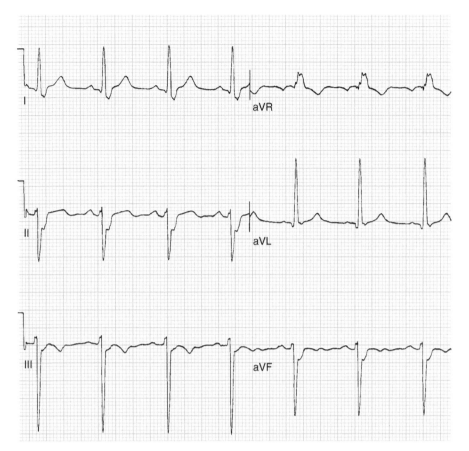

Figure 4.4 Left axis deviation due to left anterior fascicular block.

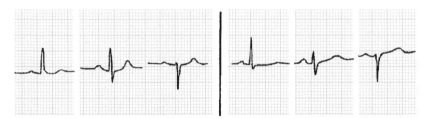

Figure 4.5 Leads I, II and III from two patients. In the first, the mean frontal QRS axis is normal. In the second, lead II is equiphasic and thus there is borderline left axis deviation.

people get the calculation wrong! It is easier to diagnose left and right axis deviation from a simple rule, as follows:

• *In left axis deviation, lead I is mainly positive and **both** leads II and III are mainly negative* (Figure 4.4). Contrary to some older texts, *both* II and III must be mainly negative (i.e. if in lead II the S wave is smaller than the R wave, abnormal left axis deviation is *not* present) (Figure 4.5). If lead II is equiphasic, there is borderline left axis deviation (Figure 4.5).

• *In right axis deviation, lead I is mainly negative and **both** leads II and III are predominantly positive* (Figure 4.6).

Left anterior fascicular block

Block in the anterior fascicle of the left bundle branch causes delay in activation of the anterosuperior portion of the left ventricle. Initial left ventricular activation will be via the posterior fascicle to the posteroinferior region and will therefore be directed

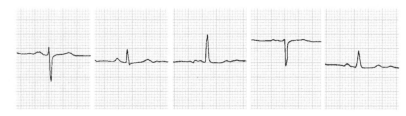

Figure 4.6 Right axis deviation due to left posterior fascicular block (leads I, II, III, aVL and aVF).

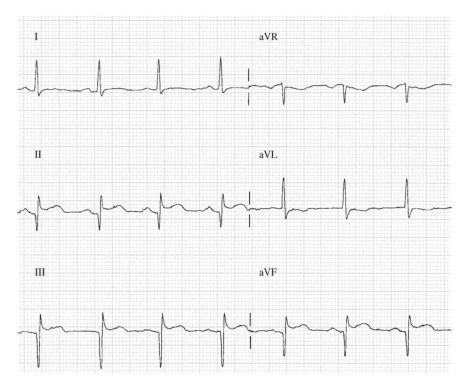

Figure 4.7 Inferior myocardial infarction: the Q waves in the inferior leads have resulted in left axis deviation but there are not the criteria for left anterior fascicular block.

inferiorly and to the right. This results in an initial small positive deflection (i.e. an r wave) in inferiorly orientated leads, i.e. II, III and aVF (Figure 4.4).

The anterosuperior region will be activated by conduction from the posteroinferior region. The resultant wave will therefore be superiorly directed (R wave in I and aVL; S wave in II, III and aVF). Because conduction is through ordinary myocardium rather than the specialised conducting tissues, it will be relatively slow. As a result, activation of the anterosuperior region will be delayed and thus unopposed by activity from the rest of the ventricles. Thus the resultant superiorly directed wave is larger than the initial inferiorly directed wave and the mean frontal QRS axis will also be superiorly directed, i.e. there will be left axis deviation.

Left anterior fascicular block is a common cause of left axis deviation. The other cause is inferior myocardial infarction (Figure 4.7).

To diagnose left anterior fascicular block two criteria must be satisfied:
1. There must be left axis deviation, i.e. lead I must be predominantly positive and both leads II and III predominantly negative.
2. The initial direction of ventricular activation must be inferior and to the right, i.e. there must be an initial r wave in leads II, III and aVF. Inferior myocardial infarction can also cause left axis deviation, but in contrast to left anterior fascicular block the initial part of the ventricular complex in the inferior leads will be a Q wave not an r wave.

Left posterior fascicular block

In left posterior fascicular block, activation of the posteroinferior portion of the left ventricle is delayed. As a result, there will be an initial positive r wave in leads I and aVL and an initial negative q wave in leads II, III and aVF; and there will be right axis deviation, i.e. lead I will be predominantly negative and leads II and III predominantly positive (Figure 4.6).

A diagnosis of left posterior fascicular block can only be made in the absence of other causes of right axis deviation such as right ventricular hypertrophy or strain, lateral myocardial infarction or a young person with a tall, thin build.

QRS complexes

Left axis deviation: lead I predominantly positive, leads II and III both predominantly negative

Right axis deviation: lead I predominantly negative, leads II and III both predominantly positive

Left anterior fascicular block: left axis deviation plus initial r wave in inferior leads

---

Axis deviation and arrhythmias

In the context of arrhythmias, there are several areas where recognition of axis deviation can be significant. As mentioned above, right bundle branch block plus left anterior or left posterior fascicular block can herald complete AV block (Chapter 15). Ventricular tachycardia can arise from left anterior or posterior fascicles and is characterised by ventricular complexes showing left or right axis deviation, respectively (Chapter 12).

Right ventricular apical pacing results in ventricular complexes with left axis deviation, whereas pacing the right ventricular outflow tract can be recognised by right axis deviation (Chapter 22).

5   The Supraventricular Tachycardias

Several tachycardias originate from the atria or atrioventricular (AV) junction and are therefore, by definition, supraventricular in origin: ventricular activation is via the rapidly conducting His–Purkinje system and thus narrow ventricular complexes will usually result. Supraventricular tachycardias are of two main types.

First, there are the AV junctional re-entrant tachycardias. These involve an additional electrical connection between atria and ventricles so an impulse can repeatedly and rapidly circulate between atria and ventricles along a circuit consisting of the AV junction and the additional AV connection. They are usually not associated with any other cardiac pathology.

Secondly, there are the atrial tachyarrhythmias caused by rapid, abnormal activity within the atria, i.e. atrial fibrillation, atrial flutter and atrial tachycardia: the AV node is not an integral part of the tachycardia mechanism but merely transmits some or all of the atrial impulses to the ventricles. They are often associated with other forms of cardiac disease.

Main types

Several tachycardias originate from the atria or atrioventricular (AV) junction and are therefore, by definition, supraventricular in origin. They have one thing in common: because they arise from above the level of the bundle branches, ventricular activation is via the rapidly conducting specialised intraventricular system and thus normal, and therefore narrow, ventricular complexes will usually result. However, it is very important to appreciate that there are significant differences in mechanism, ECG characteristics and treatment. *It is necessary to identify the type of tachycardia and not merely treat all tachycardias with narrow QRS complexes as 'supraventricular tachycardia'.*

Bennett's Cardiac Arrhythmias: Practical Notes on Interpretation and Treatment, Eighth Edition. David H. Bennett.
© 2013 John Wiley & Sons, Ltd. Published 2013 by John Wiley & Sons, Ltd.

Types of supraventricular tachycardia

---

1. Atrioventricular re-entrant tachycardia
2. Atrioventricular nodal re-entrant tachycardia
3. Atrial fibrillation
4. Atrial flutter
5. Atrial tachycardia
6. Sinus tachycardia (Chapter 1)

Atrial origin versus atrioventricular re-entry

Supraventricular tachycardias are of two main types: AV junctional re-entrant tachy-cardias and atrial tachyarrhythmias.

Atrioventricular junctional re-entrant tachycardias

In AV junctional re-entrant tachycardias (Chapter 9) there is an additional electrical connection between atria and ventricles so an impulse can repeatedly and rapidly circulate between atria and ventricles along a circuit consisting of the AV junction and the additional AV connection: the impulse is usually conducted from atria to ventricles via the AV node and then returns from ventricles to atria via the additional connection.

There are two types of additional connection between atria and ventricles:

Accessory pathway

In atrioventricular re-entrant tachycardia (AVRT), the additional connection is an accessory AV pathway which is a strand of myocardium that straddles the groove between atria and ventricles and therefore bypasses the AV node (Figure 5.1). If the accessory AV pathway can also conduct in the direction from atria to ventricles, then the patient will have Wolff–Parkinson–White syndrome (Chapter 10).

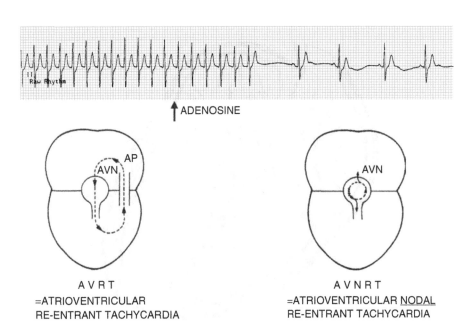

Figure 5.1 The two mechanisms of AV junctional re-entrant tachycardia: AV re-entrant tachycardia (AVRT) due to an accessory AV pathway, and AV nodal re-entrant tachycardia (AVNRT) due to dual AV nodal pathways. Both typically result in a rapid, narrow QRS tachycardia that can be terminated by adenosine. AVN, AV node; AP, accessory pathway.

Dual AV nodal pathways

In atrioventricular nodal re-entrant tachycardia (AVNRT), the AV node and its adjacent atrial tissues are functionally dissociated into fast and slow pathways, i.e. dual AV nodal pathways (Figure 5.1): typically during tachycardia AV conduction is via the slow pathway and ventriculoatrial conduction is via the fast pathway.

Atrial tachyarrhythmias

The second group of supraventricular tachycardias comprises those caused by rapid, abnormal activity *within* the atria, i.e. atrial tachycardia, flutter and fibrillation. The mechanism responsible for the tachycardia is *confined* to the atria. In contrast to the first group, *the AV node is not an integral part of the tachycardia mechanism* but simply transmits some or all of the atrial impulses to the ventricles (Figure 5.2). Arrhythmias in this group are atrial fibrillation (Chapter 6), atrial flutter (Chapter 7) and atrial tachycardia (Chapter 8). These rhythm disturbances are often associated with heart muscle or valve disease or extracardiac pathology, whereas AV junctional re-entrant tachycardias are caused by a specific abnormal electrical connection and no other cardiac condition is likely.

Effects of supraventricular tachycardias

Supraventricular tachycardias may cause major symptoms: syncope or near-syncope, particularly at the onset of the arrhythmia; distressing palpitation; angina, even in the absence of coronary artery disease; dyspnoea; fatigue; and polyuria due to release of atrial natriuretic peptide. Other patients will merely be aware of but not distressed by palpitation or may even be asymptomatic.

Patients may be distressed not only by the symptoms caused by their tachycardia but by the unpredictable nature of the arrhythmia. Some live in dread of their next attack and may be frightened to travel or even to leave their home for fear that a tachycardia might occur.

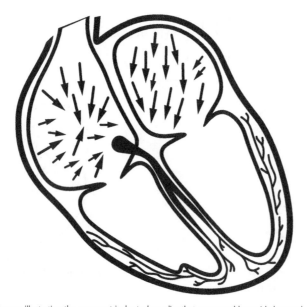

Figure 5.2 Diagram illustrating the supraventricular tachycardias that are caused by rapid abnormal activity originating from within the atria. The AV node is not an integral part of the arrhythmia mechanism but merely conducts some or all of the atrial impulses to the ventricles.

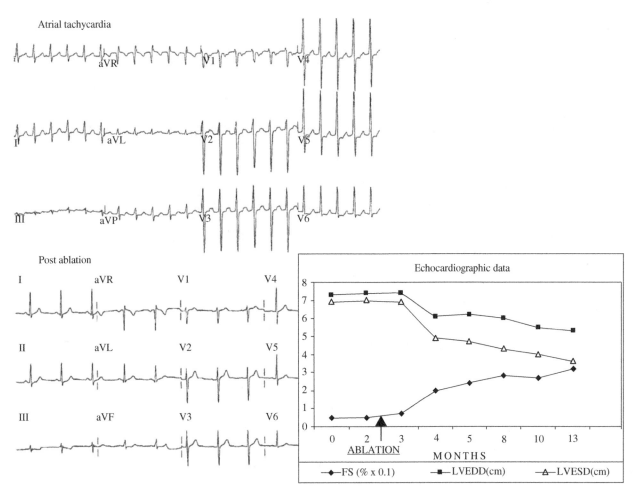

Figure 5.3 ECGs before and after ablation of incessant atrial tachycardia in a patient who presented with severe heart failure. Over the months, left ventricular end-diastolic (LVEDD) and end-systolic (LVESD) dimensions and fractional shortening (FS) returned to normal.

Many patients do not have structural heart disease but they may fear that the arrhythmia is a sign of impending heart attack or other major cardiac catastrophe. They need to be reassured that they have an 'electrical' rather than a 'plumbing' or structural cardiac problem.

If sustained and very rapid, supraventricular arrhythmias can lead to heart failure. The term 'tachycardiomyopathy' is applied. Restoration of normal rhythm will reverse the failure (Figure 5.3).

Occasionally tachycardia can lead to marked ECG changes typical of those caused by myocardial ischaemia in patients without coronary heart disease (Figure 5.4). An elevated troponin level is widely regarded as evidence of acute myocardial infarction. However, small increases are sometimes seen in patients with prolonged tachycardias who have angiographically normal coronary arteries or whose age and coronary risk profile make the possibility of coronary disease most unlikely. *A small troponin rise in a patient presenting with a supraventricular tachycardia should not be assumed to be due to myocardial infarction.*

(a)

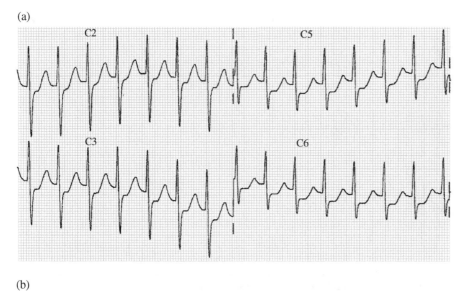

(b)

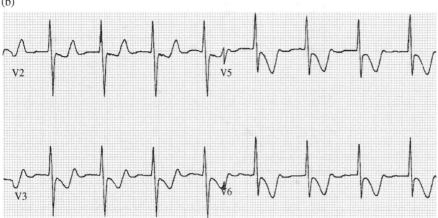

Figure 5.4 Leads V2–V6 during AV re-entrant tachycardia (a), and soon after showing marked ST depression and T wave inversion (b) in a young woman with angiographically normal coronary arteries.

6 Atrial Fibrillation

Atrial fibrillation is characterised by a totally irregular ventricular rhythm and absence of P waves. It may be paroxysmal, persistent or permanent. Causes include hypertension, myocardial infarction, cardiomyopathy, valve disease, hyperthyroidism, sick sinus syndrome and alcohol. Commonly it is idiopathic. Prevalence increases with age: there is a 26% 'lifetime' likelihood of the arrhythmia.

Treatment has to be tailored to the individual according to the cause, clinical effects and associated risks from the arrhythmia. Though cardioversion usually restores sinus rhythm, recurrence is common. Flecainide, amiodarone and sotalol but not digoxin may terminate and/or prevent atrial fibrillation. The ventricular response to atrial fibrillation can be controlled by calcium antagonists or beta-blockers: digoxin may fail to control the rate, particularly during exercise.

Stratification of risk of embolism using the CHA_2DS_2VASc system guides the therapeutic options in non-valvular fibrillation: aspirin, oral anticoagulants (e.g. warfarin or dabigatran), or left atrial occlusion device.

Atrial fibrillation is the most common cardiac arrhythmia. Indeed, as a result of increased life expectancy in the population, and in particular in patients with heart disease, its incidence is increasing.

It is important to be familiar with the arrhythmia's various causes and clinical manifestations, and to appreciate that management of the rhythm disturbance has to be tailored to the individual depending on its aetiology, associated risk and symptoms.

ECG characteristics

During atrial fibrillation, the atria discharge at a rate between 350 and 600 beats/min. The arrhythmia is due to multiple wavelets of electrical activity randomly circulating within the atrial myocardium. The very rapid electrical activity results in loss of effective atrial contraction.

Bennett's Cardiac Arrhythmias: Practical Notes on Interpretation and Treatment, Eighth Edition. David H. Bennett.
© 2013 John Wiley & Sons, Ltd. Published 2013 by John Wiley & Sons, Ltd.

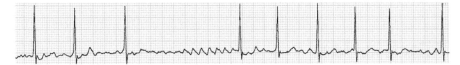

Figure 6.1 Typical f waves and totally irregular ventricular rhythm of atrial fibrillation.

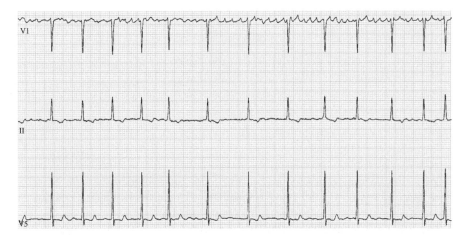

Figure 6.2 Atrial fibrillation: f waves appear coarse in V1, fine in II and are not seen in V5. There is a totally irregular ventricular rhythm.

Atrial activity

The rapid and chaotic atrial activity during atrial fibrillation results in very rapid, small, irregular waves. The amplitude of these f waves varies from patient to patient, and also from ECG lead to lead: in some leads, f waves may not be apparent, whereas in other leads, especially lead V1, the waves may appear so coarse that atrial flutter is suspected, though the atrial activity will be faster than is normally seen in atrial flutter (Figures 6.1, 6.2). Clearly, P waves will be absent.

Atrioventricular conduction

Fortunately, the AV node cannot conduct every atrial impulse to the ventricles: if it could, ventricular fibrillation would result! Some impulses are totally blocked. Others only partially penetrate the AV node. They will not therefore activate the ventricles but may block or delay succeeding impulses. This process of 'concealed conduction' is responsible for the totally irregular ventricular rhythm that is the hallmark of this arrhythmia.

In the absence of P waves, even if f waves are not seen, a totally irregular ventricular rhythm is indicative of atrial fibrillation. Atrial fibrillation with a rapid ventricular rhythm is often misdiagnosed. If the characteristic irregular rhythm is remembered, errors will not be made (Figure 6.3). If, however, there is complete AV block, ventricular activity will, of course, be slow and regular (Figure 6.4).

The ventricular rate during atrial fibrillation is dependent on the conducting ability of the AV node, which is itself influenced by the autonomic nervous system. Atrioventricular conduction will be enhanced by sympathetic activity and depressed by high vagal tone. Typically, ventricular rates are rapid, up to 200 beats/min, when the patient is active, and are slow when the patient is at rest or asleep.

A totally irregular ventricular rhythm is indicative of atrial fibrillation irrespective of whether the ventricular rate is slow or fast.

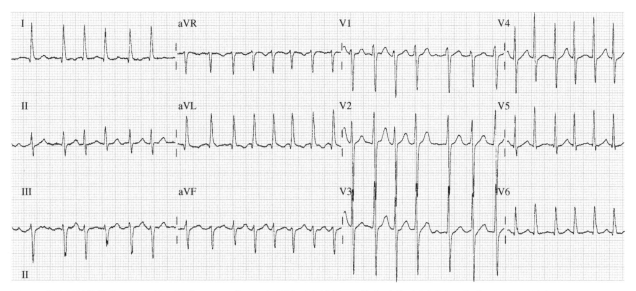

Figure 6.3 Atrial fibrillation with rapid ventricular response (heart rate 180 beats/min). The ventricular rhythm is totally irregular. f waves are not obvious.

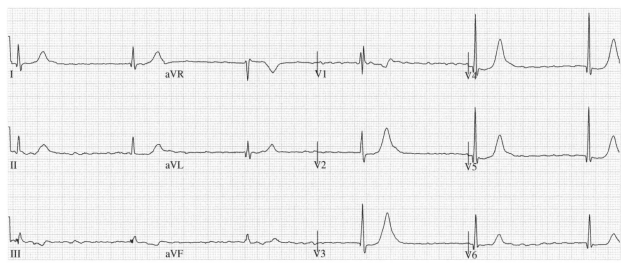

Figure 6.4 Atrial fibrillation with complete AV block. The ventricular rhythm is regular: rate 39 beats/min.

Intraventricular conduction

Ventricular complexes during atrial fibrillation are normal in duration unless there is established bundle branch block (Figure 6.5), Wolff–Parkinson–White syndrome (Chapter 10) or aberrant intraventricular conduction, i.e. rate-related bundle branch block.

Aberrant intraventricular conduction

Aberrant conduction is the result of differing recovery periods of the two bundle branches. An early atrial impulse may reach the ventricles when one bundle branch is still refractory to excitation following the previous cardiac cycle but the other is capable of conduction. The resultant ventricular complex will have a bundle branch block configuration. Because the right bundle usually has the longer refractory period, aberrant conduction commonly leads to right bundle branch block. The duration of the refractory periods of the bundle branches is related to the preceding cycle length. Thus, aberration is likely to occur when a short cycle succeeds a long

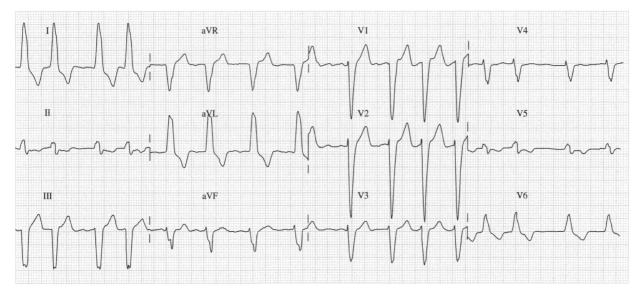

Figure 6.5 Atrial fibrillation with established left bundle branch block. The ventricular rhythm is totally irregular.

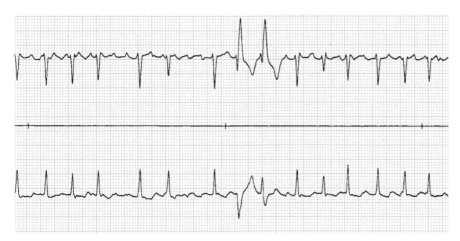

Figure 6.6 Atrial fibrillation. After seven normally conducted ventricular complexes, there are two complexes with right bundle branch block configuration (upper trace is lead V1).

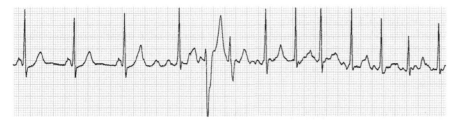

Figure 6.7 An atrial ectopic beat superimposed on the T wave of the third sinus beat initiates atrial fibrillation. Second and third complexes during atrial fibrillation are aberrantly conducted.

cycle (Figures 6.6, 6.7): the 'Ashman phenomenon'. Sometimes a series of aberrantly conducted beats will be misdiagnosed as paroxysmal ventricular tachycardia (see Figure 6.10). However, even though the rate is rapid there will be marked irregularity in the cycle length, and why should there be 'bursts' of a second arrhythmia during atrial fibrillation?

Initiation

Atrial fibrillation is usually initiated by an atrial extrasystole (Figure 6.7). Sometimes atrial flutter or AV re-entrant tachycardia degenerate into atrial fibrillation.

ECG characteristics of atrial fibrillation

Atrial activity:
  P waves absent
  f waves usually seen in at least some leads
Ventricular activity:
  Totally irregular
  QRS duration normal unless persistent or rate-related bundle branch block

---

Causes

The most common causes are damaged or disordered heart muscle caused by myocardial infarction, hypertension or cardiomyopathy; heart valve disease; hyperthyroidism; and sick sinus syndrome. In many cases, atrial fibrillation is idiopathic, i.e. there is no demonstrable cause.

Coronary artery disease, i.e. the presence of a coronary stenosis, does not per se cause atrial fibrillation. However, the arrhythmia often results from myocardial infarction, both acutely and in the long term, and is an indicator of extensive myocardial damage.

Many of the causes can be identified or excluded by clinical examination, electrocardiography and echocardiography. Measurement of serum thyroxine and thyroid-stimulating hormone is necessary to exclude hyperthyroidism. Ambulatory electrocardiography may be required where sick sinus syndrome is a possibility.

Causes of atrial fibrillation

Idiopathic, i.e. no recognised cause (common)
Cardiac
  Acute and past myocardial infarction
  Dilated and hypertrophic cardiomyopathies
  Hypertension
  Myocarditis and pericarditis
  Heart valve disease, especially rheumatic mitral valve disease
  Atrial septal defect
  Cardiac and thoracic surgery
  Constrictive pericarditis
  Sick sinus syndrome
  Atrioventricular junctional re-entrant tachycardias
  Wolff–Parkinson–White syndrome
Non-cardiac
  Hyperthyroidism
  Chronic obstructive airways disease
  Chest infection
  Carcinoma lung
  Pulmonary embolism
  Acute and chronic alcohol abuse
  Obesity
  High-endurance sport training
  Familial, i.e. genetically determined (rare)

Prevalence

Prevalence increases with age. In a survey of male civil servants in the United Kingdom, atrial fibrillation was found in 0.16%, 0.37% and 1.13% of those aged 40–49 years, 50–59 years and 60–64 years, respectively. In a British general practice 3.7% of patients over 65 years were found to have the arrhythmia.

The Framingham study found that 7.8% of men aged between 65 and 74 years had atrial fibrillation. The prevalence increased to 11.7% in men aged 75–84 years. *There is a 26% 'lifetime' likelihood of atrial fibrillation.* Even in people without a history of heart failure or myocardial infarction the risk is in the order of 15%. The arrhythmia is 1.5 times more common in men than in women.

Prognosis

A major determinant of prognosis is the presence or absence of structural heart disease. For example, myocardial infarction, because atrial fibrillation is usually a result of extensive myocardial damage, indicates a poor prognosis. Most studies have shown that idiopathic atrial fibrillation has a good prognosis.

Classification

- **Paroxysmal** – atrial fibrillation terminates spontaneously in less than seven days and usually within 48 hours.
- **Persistent** – atrial fibrillation would continue indefinitely but normal rhythm can be restored by cardioversion.
- **Permanent** – atrial fibrillation has persisted for more than one year, either because restoration of normal rhythm has failed or because it has not been attempted.

Lone atrial fibrillation

Lone, i.e. idiopathic, atrial fibrillation in younger individuals (< 60 years) is very common. While the prognosis is good and the risk of systemic embolism is low (estimated at 1.3% over a 15-year period), lone atrial fibrillation can cause very troublesome symptoms and great anxiety. Like secondary atrial fibrillation, it may be paroxysmal or persistent.

Paroxysmal lone atrial fibrillation

Some patients will experience only a single or a very occasional episode. Others will experience frequent recurrences, perhaps several times in a day. Paroxysms may last for many hours or stop after only a few seconds (Figure 6.8). With time, in some but not all patients, atrial fibrillation will become persistent. Studies have shown that an episode of atrial fibrillation can lead to alterations in the electrical properties of the atria that encourage perpetuation of atrial fibrillation: a process termed 'electrical remodelling'.

Patients often suffer very troublesome symptoms (Chapter 5). Others, including some with frequent episodes and rapid ventricular rates, will be asymptomatic or merely aware of but not distressed by a rapid heart rate.

In a minority of patients there will be an identifiable precipitating event such as exercise, vomiting, alcohol or fatigue. One form of paroxysmal lone atrial fibrillation has been attributed to high vagal activity: the arrhythmia always starts at rest or during sleep (Figure 6.9).

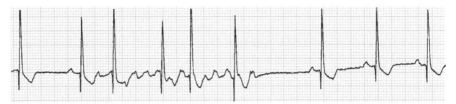

Figure 6.8 A very brief episode of atrial fibrillation.

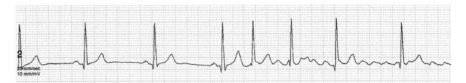

Figure 6.9 Onset of atrial fibrillation at rest during sinus rhythm: rate 50 beats/min.

Management

Management involves ascertaining the cause of the arrhythmia, either restoring normal rhythm or controlling the heart rate during atrial fibrillation, and protecting the patient from systemic embolism.

Management of atrial fibrillation

Ascertain cause
Adopt rate control or rhythm control strategy
Prevent systemic embolism

Systemic embolism

During atrial fibrillation, stasis of blood in the left atrial appendage can occur and lead to thrombus formation and systemic embolism. *Of particular concern is the risk of stroke.* Emboli to the limbs and to the abdominal organs can also occur.

Increased levels of plasma fibrinogen and fibrin D-dimer have been found in atrial fibrillation. Levels return to normal after cardioversion, suggesting that it may be atrial fibrillation itself that causes a 'hypercoagulable' state.

Warfarin, a vitamin K antagonist, has been shown to markedly reduce the risk of embolism, as have the new thrombin inhibitors such as dabigtran, and factor Xa inhibitors such as apixaban and rivaroxaban. Aspirin is far less effective than warfarin (e.g. 19% versus 70% stroke risk reduction): indeed, a recent analysis questioned whether aspirin, which is as likely to cause bleeding as warfarin, had any effect in preventing embolism.

Systemic embolism due to atrial fibrillation can be reduced by:

Vitamin K antagonists, e.g. warfarin
Thrombin inhibitors, e.g. dabigatran
Factor Xa inhibitors, e.g. apixaban
Aspirin (much less effective than the above)

It should be noted that although ischaemic stroke in patients with atrial fibrillation is widely attributed to embolism from the left atrium, up to 25% of strokes in patients with atrial fibrillation may be due to cerebrovascular disease or atheromatous plaque in the carotid arteries or proximal aorta.

Risk

Atrial fibrillation caused by rheumatic mitral valve disease leads to a *very high* (15-fold) risk of stroke. Warfarin is strongly indicated.

'Non-rheumatic' causes of atrial fibrillation, mainly cardiac failure and hypertension, are associated with a moderately high (five-fold) risk of stroke with an incidence of approximately 5% per annum. A history of prior systemic embolism is also associated with high risk. On the other hand, patients with lone atrial fibrillation have a risk of embolism of <1% per annum.

The risk of embolism does not appear to be influenced by whether atrial fibrillation is paroxysmal or persistent.

Two scoring systems, incorporating a number of risk factors, have been devised to assess the risk of stroke in non-valvular atrial fibrillation:

$CHADS_2$ score

C = cardiac failure, H = history of hypertension, A = age ≥ 75 years, D = diabetes, S = history of stroke or transient ischaemic attack (TIA). One point is attributed to each risk factor present except the last, which is assigned 2 points.

Scores of zero, 1, and 2–6 are classified as low, medium and high risk, respectively. Anticoagulation should be considered if the score is ≥ 2. Aspirin or no treatment is recommended if the score is ≤ 1.

However, it has been shown that some patients with a $CHADS_2$ score ≤ 1 may be at a significant risk of stroke. As a result a more complex scoring system has been described to identify those at risk with a $CHADS_2$ score ≤ 1.

CHA_2DS_2VASc score

As above, C = cardiac failure, H = history of hypertension, A = age ≥ 75 years, D = diabetes, S = history of stroke or transient ischaemic attack (TIA). Each of these factors is assigned one point, other than age ≥ 75 years or a history of stroke or TIA, which are given 2 points.

Additional factors are: V = vascular disease (myocardial infarction, complex aortic plaque, peripheral artery disease), A = age 65–74 years, S = sex category (i.e. female). Each of these additional factors is assigned one point.

A score of 0 indicates very low risk and no need for anticoagulation. A score of 1 points to intermediate risk (1.3% per year) and consideration of oral anticoagulants, and ≥ 2 indicates high risk (2.2% per year for a score of 2, rising to approximately 10% per year for scores in excess of 5), in which case oral anticoagulation is strongly indicated.

Oral anticoagulants
Warfarin

Warfarin, a vitamin K antagonist, is well established in clinical practice but has important disadvantages. Regular blood tests are required in order to adjust the dosage to maintain the International Normalised Ratio (INR) at a therapeutic level (between 2 and 3). In a significant proportion of patients, maintenance of anticoagulation in the therapeutic range cannot be achieved. Many drugs interact with warfarin metabolism and can lead to over-anticoagulation, including antibiotics, anticonvulsants, some statins, amiodarone, tamoxifen and alcohol. Concomitant aspirin may increase the risk of haemorrhage. Because of these disadvantages, doctors are sometimes reluctant to prescribe warfarin, and patients sometimes refuse to take it.

Warfarin, prescribed to prevent systemic embolism due to atrial fibrillation, may need to be temporarily stopped prior to surgical procedures. It is common practice to 'bridge' with heparin. However, heparin often leads to bleeding problems and post-operative haematoma. It is in fact rarely necessary to 'bridge': warfarin can be stopped three days before surgery and restarted three days postoperatively.

Newer drugs

Recently, inhibitors of thrombin and factor Xa have become available that can be prescribed in fixed dosages and therefore do not require blood tests for monitoring their effect. They have been shown to be at least as effective as warfarin, to result in less or at least similar bleeding risks (particularly intracranial haemorrhage) and to have few interactions with other drugs. Though clinical trial results are favourable, there is at present limited experience in clinical practice.

Thrombin inhibitors

Dabigatran, 150 mg twice daily, has been shown to be more effective than warfarin in preventing ischaemic stroke, while a dose of 110 mg twice daily has been shown to be non-inferior. In contrast to warfarin, the drug achieves therapeutic levels within two hours of administration and a steady state within two days. Dabigatran is mainly excreted by the kidneys, and it is contraindicated in severe renal impairment or if there is active, significant bleeding. The dose should be reduced to 110 mg twice daily if the patient is over 80 years of age, if the patient is receiving verapamil or if it is felt that the patient is at a higher risk of bleeding. In moderate renal impairment, a twice-daily dose of 75 mg has been suggested.

In the United Kingdom, recent changes to licensing allow the use of new oral anticoagulant drugs such as dabigatran after discussion with the patient about the advantages and disadvantages of these drugs compared with warfarin, but women with a CHA_2DS_2VASc score of 2, aged 65–74 years without other cardiovascular risk factors do not meet current licensed indications.

The main unwanted effects are a moderate incidence of dyspepsia and diarrhoea. Concomitant treatment with systemic ketoconazole, cyclosporine, itraconazole or tacrolimus is contraindicated. Interactions with dronedarone and amiodarone have also been reported.

The drug should be stopped two days before elective surgery; 3–4 days if clearance of the drug is slower due to renal impairment. There is no specific antidote. If converting from warfarin, dabigatran can be started when the INR is less than 2.0.

Factor Xa inhibitors

Rivaroxaban need only be prescribed on a once-daily basis (20 mg). The dosage of apixaban is 5 mg twice daily.

Risk of bleeding

The benefits of anticoagulation have to be weighed against the risk of bleeding. A number of factors associated with an increased risk of bleeding have been incorporated into the 'HAS-BLED' scoring system, which can be used to predict the risk in an individual: **H**ypertension, **A**bnormal renal or liver function, **S**troke, **B**leeding history or predisposition, **L**abile INR, **E**lderly (> 65 years), **D**rugs (e.g. aspirin, non-steroidal anti-inflammatory drugs, steroids, alcohol). More than three factors is regarded as high risk. Diabetes and heart failure have been reported to be additional risk factors.

Several of the risk factors for haemorrhage are the same as those for stroke, i.e. the higher the stroke risk, the higher the risk of bleeding! However, for most patients the risk of stroke is much higher than the risk of haemorrhage. Patients at high risk of bleeding require closer monitoring and, of course, if possible, cessation of drugs which might increase the risk. The small number of patients who have a very low embolic risk but a high bleeding risk should not be anticoagulated.

Anticoagulation following ischaemic stroke

It is recommended that anticoagulation is started on the same day following a transient ischaemic attack, 3–5 days after a mild stroke and 2 weeks following a severe stroke.

Anticoagulant intolerance

Recently, devices for percutaneous occlusion of the left atrial appendage have been developed for use in patients with non-valvular atrial fibrillation thought to be at significant risk of embolism where anticoagulation is contraindicated or cannot be undertaken for other reasons. The devices are deployed via puncture of the interatrial septum. Early experience is encouraging, with high deployment success rates but at the expense of a small incidence of important complications: cardiac tamponade, stroke and device embolisation.

Rhythm management

Choice of treatment depends on whether the purpose is to control the ventricular response to atrial fibrillation or to maintain sinus rhythm. These strategies are termed 'rate control' and 'rhythm control', respectively. In general, *rate control is easier to achieve than rhythm control.*

Atrial fibrillation results in loss of atrial contraction prior to ventricular systole and often an inappropriately fast heart rate. Consequently, cardiac output often falls. One would expect, therefore, that patients would fare better if normal rhythm could be maintained rather than allowing persistent or paroxysmal atrial fibrillation to continue. However, several large studies have shown that a strategy of rhythm control is no better than one of rate control in terms of mortality, hospital admission and quality of life. The patients studied were mainly older, and many had cardiovascular disease. The results cannot necessarily be applied to all patients. For example, younger patients with paroxysmal idiopathic atrial fibrillation are often highly symptomatic and benefit greatly from maintenance of normal rhythm.

Though studies showed that the strategy of trying to maintain normal rhythm was no better than that of rate control, long-term normal rhythm was not achieved in many patients in the rhythm control group. It is very likely that patients in whom normal rhythm is achieved do benefit. This is supported by both recent and old studies that have shown that maintenance of sinus rhythm improves quality of life and exercise capacity. In the event that a safe, relatively cheap therapy can be found that can maintain normal rhythm, rate control will surely be abandoned!

Not all patients with atrial fibrillation are the same. Some experience troublesome symptoms in spite of effective rate control and feel very much better when in normal rhythm. Others, including those who are asymptomatic prior to treatment, do well with a rate control approach. Treatment has to be adapted to the individual patient.

Not infrequently a rhythm control strategy will fail and a rate control approach will have to be accepted, but in highly symptomatic patients an 'aggressive' approach to maintaining normal rhythm is justified.

Rate control

A number of drugs will slow conduction in the AV node (termed a negative dromotropic action) and thereby slow the heart rate during atrial fibrillation.

Calcium channel blockers

Intravenous verapamil quickly and effectively depresses AV conduction and will thereby control a rapid ventricular response to atrial fibrillation within a few minutes. However, it is unlikely to restore sinus rhythm and indeed there is some evidence to suggest that verapamil will encourage the arrhythmia to persist.

Oral verapamil (120–240 mg daily) is usually effective in controlling the ventricular rate during atrial fibrillation, both at rest and on exertion.

Diltiazem (but not the dihydropyridine calcium channel blockers nifedipine and amlodipine) has similar actions to verapamil. In oral form it should be prescribed as a long-acting preparation in a dose of 200 or 300 mg daily.

It is recommended that these drugs should be avoided or used cautiously in patients with cardiac failure.

Beta-blockers

Beta-blocking drugs have similar benefits to the calcium antagonists.

Digoxin

Oral digoxin is widely used to control the ventricular response to atrial fibrillation. It has the advantages that it has long duration of action and may be positively inotropic. However, digoxin not infrequently fails to control the heart rate at rest and is rarely effective at controlling the rate during exertion in spite of appropriate plasma concentrations. Unwanted effects are common (Chapter 19). Increasing age, renal or electrolyte disturbance, or the introduction of other drugs can lead to digoxin toxicity in patients who had been established on an appropriate therapeutic dose.

Intravenous digoxin is often ineffective at promptly reducing the ventricular response to atrial fibrillation. As stated below, digoxin has been shown to be ineffective at terminating or preventing atrial fibrillation. *In view of the many limitations of the drug and the fact that calcium channel blockers or beta-blockers can be used to slow the ventricular response to atrial fibrillation, there is a case for no longer using digoxin.*

Assessing rate control

It is important to remember that though rate control at rest may appear satisfactory, often inappropriately rapid heart rates will occur during exercise. Ideally, ambulatory electrocardiography should be carried out to ensure satisfactory rate control is being achieved. Standard though arbitrarily chosen maxima for satisfactory rate control are heart rates of 60–80 beats/min at rest and 90–115 beats/min during moderate exertion.

Recently, a strategy of 'lenient rate control' with a target of ensuring the ventricular rate was less than 110 beats/min at rest has been compared with standard 'strict rate control'. The former strategy was shown to be 'non-inferior' to the latter strategy. Though 'lenient rate control' may be acceptable in the asymptomatic patient, *good rate control is important in patients with symptoms such as dyspnoea and palpitation and in those with poor ventricular function.*

Fast and slow ventricular rates

Some patients demonstrate both very fast and slow ventricular responses to atrial fibrillation during the daytime (a slow ventricular response to atrial fibrillation during sleep is normal) (Figures 6.10, 6.11). Ventricular pacing may sometimes be required to allow AV nodal blocking drugs to control rapid rates.

Some patients with atrial fibrillation, presumably due to impaired AV nodal conduction (Figure 6.12), are unable to increase their heart rate adequately in response to exercise: 'chronotropic incompetence' (Chapter 16). A rate-responsive pacemaker (Chapter 23) will improve the ability to exercise.

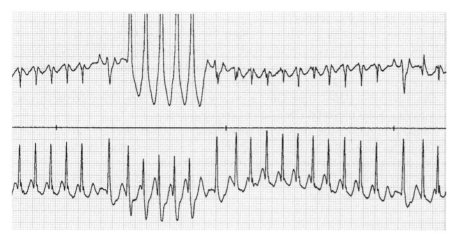

Figure 6.10 Very fast ventricular response to atrial fibrillation. There is aberrant conduction of the seventh to eleventh ventricular complexes.

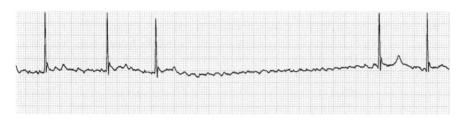

Figure 6.11 Very slow ventricular response during the night in the same patient as in Figure 6.10.

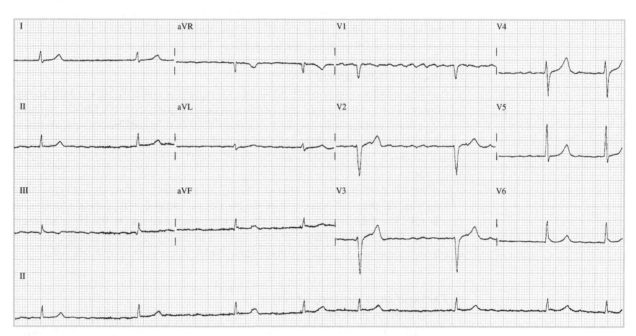

Figure 6.12 Slow ventricular rate (45 beats/min) during atrial fibrillation in spite of absence of AV nodal blocking drugs.

Heart failure

Particular attention should be paid to patients with heart failure and atrial fibrillation. Sustained rapid ventricular rates *may worsen or indeed may be the cause* of heart failure.

As stated above, some patients may have chronotropic incompetence due to impaired AV nodal conduction, whether spontaneous or due to medication such as beta-blockers. It is therefore important to ensure that exertional ability is not being limited by a failure of the heart rate to increase appropriately during exertion.

Rhythm control
Chemical cardioversion
Intravenous therapy

Intravenous flecainide, propafenone, sotalol and amiodarone may restore normal rhythm provided atrial fibrillation is of recent onset, i.e. within seven days. Only amiodarone should be used in patients with heart failure or marked impairment of ventricular function: the other drugs may worsen myocardial function and may cause ventricular arrhythmias. Restoration of normal rhythm can be expected in no more than two-thirds of patients. Amiodarone may take up to 24 hours to work (Chapter 19).

Flecainide and propafenone can sometimes fail to restore normal rhythm but slow the atrial rate and thus convert atrial fibrillation to atrial flutter or atrial tachycardia. Paradoxically, the *lower* atrial rate can lead to a marked *acceleration* of the ventricular rate because the AV node can conduct a greater proportion or all of the atrial impulses (Chapter 19), occasionally necessitating prompt electrical cardioversion.

Dofetilide and ibutilide are newer drugs with a class III antiarrhythmic action (Chapter 19) that have been shown to be moderately effective at terminating atrial fibrillation of recent onset (success rates are higher in atrial flutter). However, there is a significant risk of torsade de pointes ventricular tachycardia (Chapter 13). These drugs are not currently available in the United Kingdom.

Vernakalant is a member of a novel group of drugs that specifically affects the electrophysiology of atrial myocardium. Intravenously, it has been shown to restore normal rhythm within a few minutes in approximately 50% of patients with recent-onset atrial fibrillation.

It should be borne in mind that approximately half of episodes of recent-onset atrial fibrillation will terminate spontaneously within eight hours. Thus, an antiarrhythmic drug may not necessarily get the credit for achieving sinus rhythm in every case!

Ineffective drugs

Digoxin is ineffective at restoring sinus rhythm, and there is evidence that it may actually perpetuate the arrhythmia by shortening the refractory period of atrial myocardium. Beta-blockers and calcium antagonists, though effective in slowing the ventricular response to atrial fibrillation, will not restore normal rhythm.

Oral therapy

Flecainide and propafenone are moderately effective in preventing a recurrence of atrial fibrillation but the same contraindications as for intravenous therapy apply. They should not be used in patients with myocardial dysfunction or with coronary artery disease and ideally should be combined with a beta-blocker or calcium antagonist in case atrial flutter occurs, which might lead to a very fast ventricular rate. The author favours flecainide and would recommend it as a first-line drug provided ventricular function is normal.

Beta-blockers rarely prevent atrial fibrillation but are the drug of choice if the history suggests that fibrillation is induced by exertion or is due to hyperthyroidism. Some, but not all, studies show that sotalol with its class III antiarrhythmic action (Chapter 19) is more effective than other beta-blockers at preventing atrial fibrillation but must be avoided in patients with a prolonged QT interval.

Amiodarone is the most effective drug in preventing atrial fibrillation, but because of the high incidence of unwanted effects it should be reserved for patients with troublesome symptoms who fail to respond to or cannot receive the drugs above. It is a drug of choice in patients with heart failure.

Dronedarone is a derivative of amiodarone which because of reports of a number of cardiac and extracardiac unwanted effects is now only recommended as a second-line drug for adult, clinically stable patients with paroxysmal or persistent atrial fibrillation for the maintenance of sinus rhythm after successful cardioversion.

Quinidine had been used for many years to prevent paroxysmal atrial fibrillation. However, a meta-analysis of studies showed that the drug was associated with a significant increase in mortality, presumably due to a proarrhythmic effect. It is no longer used to prevent atrial fibrillation.

Digoxin shortens the atrial refractory period and may thereby increase the tendency to atrial fibrillation. There is no evidence that it prevents the arrhythmia.

'Upstream therapies'

Angiotensin-converting enzyme (ACE) inhibitors, angiotensin receptor blocking (ARB) drugs, statins, omega-3 fatty acids and eating oily fish have been shown to be associated with a lower incidence of atrial fibrillation. Recently, colchicine given postoperatively has been shown to markedly reduce the incidence of atrial fibrillation following cardiac surgery.

'Pill in the pocket' approach

In order to avoid daily medication, a 'pill in the pocket' approach to paroxysmal atrial fibrillation can be adopted in patients who do not have frequent episodes of atrial fibrillation. A single oral dose of flecainide (200 mg) or propafenone (600 mg) is taken by the patient at the onset of rapid palpitation. If successful, a return to normal rhythm can be expected within 2–3 hours. This strategy may be useful in patients prone to prolonged episodes of atrial fibrillation and may avoid the need for hospital admission. However, some patients with paroxysmal atrial fibrillation experience incapacitating symptoms, and abbreviation of an episode using a 'pill in the pocket' will be inadequate. Furthermore, these drugs should be avoided in patients with coronary artery disease or poor ventricular function, and, because of the significant possibility of them leading to atrial flutter or tachycardia with a very fast ventricular response, should preferably be combined with an AV nodal blocking drug, i.e. a beta-blocker or calcium antagonist.

Electrical cardioversion

Sinus rhythm can be restored by electrical cardioversion in most patients with atrial fibrillation (Chapter 21). However, the arrhythmia frequently returns. Risk factors for recurrence include a long duration of atrial fibrillation, heart failure, marked left atrial enlargement and age. No more than a quarter of patients will be in normal rhythm after one year.

Drugs such as flecainide, sotalol, propafenone and particularly amiodarone reduce the recurrence rate after cardioversion. These drugs may have unwanted effects, and in many patients they should be reserved for repeat cardioversion when restoration of normal rhythm had resulted in major benefit and dictated the need for a further attempt at restoring and maintaining normal rhythm. Digoxin may *increase* the recurrence rate.

While cardioversion only leads to long-term sinus rhythm in a minority of patients, an attempt at restoring sinus rhythm should be considered in those patients with recent atrial fibrillation (less than 12 months) where no cause has been identified or in whom the disorder that has caused the arrhythmia has resolved or is self-limiting. If there is a recurrence, a further attempt at cardioversion, after initiation of antiarrhythmic therapy, should be undertaken in those with troublesome symptoms attributable to the arrhythmia.

There are some reports of restoring and maintaining normal rhythm by cardioversion in up to one-third of patients with atrial fibrillation that has persisted for over

12–24 months. In patients with atrial fibrillation that is difficult to treat, even if long-standing, cardioversion should also be considered, because there is a small chance that normal rhythm will be achieved and maintained.

Transvenous cardioversion is now an established means of restoring normal rhythm (Chapter 21). Higher success rates than for transthoracic cardioversion, especially in very large patients, have been reported.

Most patients undergo cardioversion as an elective procedure, but occasionally urgent cardioversion is required in haemodynamically unstable patients.

Anticoagulation before and after cardioversion

Cardioversion can result in immediate systemic embolism because of dislodgement of pre-existing left atrial thrombus. Also, new thrombus can develop after cardioversion because atrial mechanical activity often does not return for up to three weeks after the procedure and because cardioversion itself can increase blood hypercoagulability. Hence embolism can also occur in the few weeks following cardioversion. It is therefore important that non-urgent cardioversion in patients who have been in atrial fibrillation for more than 24–48 hours is preceded by warfarin to achieve an INR of 2.5 for at least three weeks, and that anticoagulation is continued for at least four weeks after restoration of normal rhythm. Impairment of atrial mechanical function (termed 'stunning') is also recognised to occur following chemical cardioversion.

If urgent cardioversion is required, transesophageal echocardiography can be used to exclude left atrial thrombus or stasis: the signs of atrial stasis are spontaneous echo contrast and reduced atrial appendage flow velocity. If cardioversion has to be carried out urgently it should be preceded by heparin and succeeded by heparin and then warfarin.

Dabigatran has been shown to be as effective as warfarin in stroke prevention associated with cardioversion.

'Refractory' atrial fibrillation
Amiodarone

Amiodarone is a potent drug that will often maintain sinus rhythm or at least control the ventricular response to atrial fibrillation when other drugs have failed. However, in view of its unwanted effects, the drug should be reserved for patients in whom other drugs have failed and for patients in whom the risk of side effects in the long term may not be a major consideration because their prognosis is poor, e.g. the elderly and those with severe myocardial damage.

Catheter ablation

Transvenous catheter ablation involving delivery of radiofrequency energy to sites within the left atrium is being used increasingly widely to prevent paroxysmal atrial fibrillation, and also in some patients with persistent atrial fibrillation. This is discussed in Chapter 25. Occasionally, ablation is carried out surgically – usually with a concomitant surgical procedure.

Radiofrequency ablation of the AV junction is an option in patients with severe symptoms in whom antiarrhythmic drugs are ineffective or cannot be tolerated (Chapter 25). It necessitates pacemaker implantation and continuation of oral anticoagulation, but it is very effective at controlling symptoms and has been demonstrated in several studies to improve patients' quality of life, and it avoids the need for antiarrhythmic therapy.

7 Atrial Flutter

Typical atrial flutter is a common arrhythmia caused by a re-entrant circuit within the right atrium, usually in a counterclockwise direction. It may be paroxysmal or sustained. Atrial activity is registered as F waves at a regular rate in the order of 300 beats/min. Commonly, alternate F waves are conducted to the ventricles with a resultant ventricular rate close to 150 beats/min. In many ECG leads there will be no isoelectric line between atrial deflections, leading to the characteristic sawtooth appearance that is best seen in leads II, III and aVF. However, in lead V1 atrial activity will usually be seen as discrete waves.

Atrial flutter has similar causes to atrial fibrillation. It is often idiopathic. Antiarrhythmic drugs are frequently ineffective and may sometimes cause an increase in ventricular rate. Cardioversion and catheter ablation are both first-line treatments. Embolic risk should be managed as for atrial fibrillation.

Common atrial flutter

The arrhythmia is caused by repeated circulation of an impulse around the right atrium. Usually, the impulse circulates in a superior direction along the interatrial septum and returns in an inferior direction along the lateral border of the right atrium (Figure 7.1). The left atrium is activated by the impulses arising from the right atrium. Atrial flutter may be paroxysmal or sustained.

ECG characteristics

During the typical form of atrial flutter, the atria discharge regularly at a rate of approximately 300 beats/min. In many leads there will be no isoelectric line between atrial deflections, termed F waves, leading to the characteristic sawtooth appearance that is usually best seen in leads II, III and aVF. However, in some leads, especially lead V1, atrial activity will be seen in the form of discrete waves (Figure 7.2).

Commonly, in typical atrial flutter, the atrial impulse circulates counterclockwise within the right atrium, in which case the F waves are predominantly negative in leads II, III and aVF, of very low amplitude in lead I and positive in V1 (Figure 7.2). Uncommonly, the impulse circulates in a clockwise direction when the F waves will be positive in the inferior leads and negative in lead V1 (Figure 7.3).

Bennett's Cardiac Arrhythmias: Practical Notes on Interpretation and Treatment, Eighth Edition. David H. Bennett.
© 2013 John Wiley & Sons, Ltd. Published 2013 by John Wiley & Sons, Ltd.

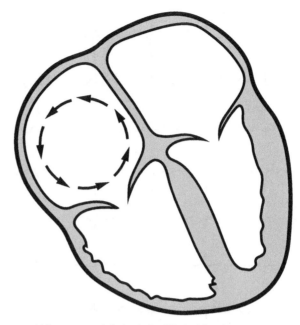

Figure 7.1 Common atrial flutter: counterclockwise circuit within the right atrium.

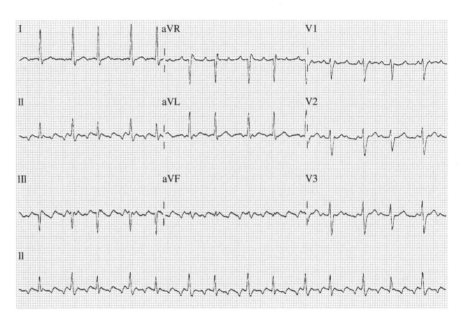

Figure 7.2 Common atrial flutter: negative sawtooth pattern in the inferior leads and positive, discrete F waves in lead V1.

Atypical flutter

In atypical atrial flutter, the atrial rate is faster, ranging from 350 to 450 beats/min. It is not amenable to isthmus ablation (see below) and cannot be terminated by rapid atrial pacing.

Atrioventricular conduction

As with atrial fibrillation, the ventricular response to atrial flutter is determined by the conducting ability of the AV junction. Frequently, alternate F waves are conducted to the ventricles with a resultant ventricular rate close to 150 beats/min (Figure 7.4).

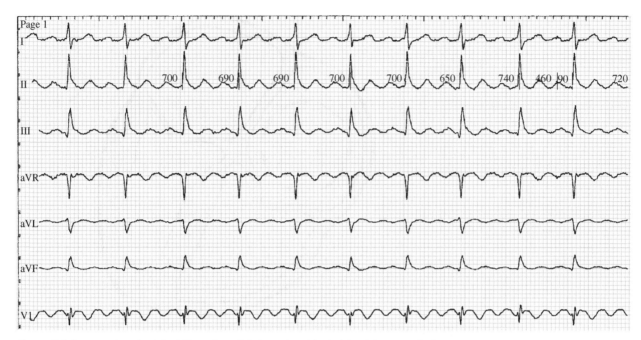

Figure 7.3 Uncommon form of typical atrial flutter due to clockwise rotation within the right atrial re-entrant circuit.

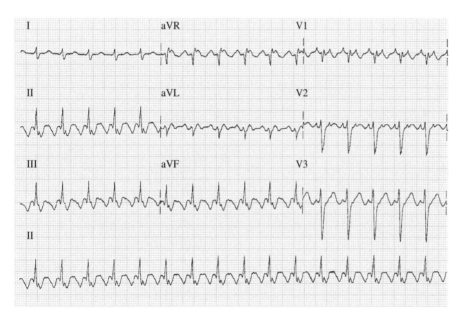

Figure 7.4 Atrial flutter with 2:1 AV block. The limb leads shows a classic sawtooth appearance while V1 shows discrete atrial waves. In V1, each QRS complex is immediately preceded by an F wave and is followed by an F wave which is superimposed on the T wave.

AV nodal blocking drugs, impaired AV nodal function or high vagus nerve tone during the night may lead to a higher degree of AV block (Figure 7.5). High levels of sympathetic nervous system activity, as may occur during exercise, may enhance AV nodal conduction and result in 1:1 conduction and a ventricular rate of approximately 300 beats/min (Figure 7.6).

With high degrees of AV block, atrial activity is clearly discernible and the arrhythmia is easy to diagnose (Figure 7.7). However, during 2:1 atrioventricular conduction,

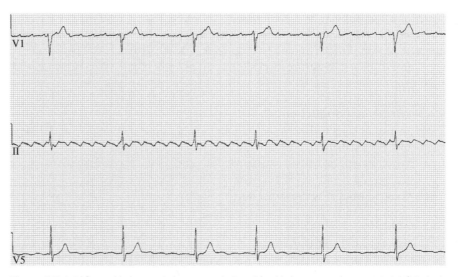

Figure 7.5 Atrial flutter with slow ventricular response. Again, atrial activity has a sawtooth appearance in inferior leads but is seen as discrete F waves in V1.

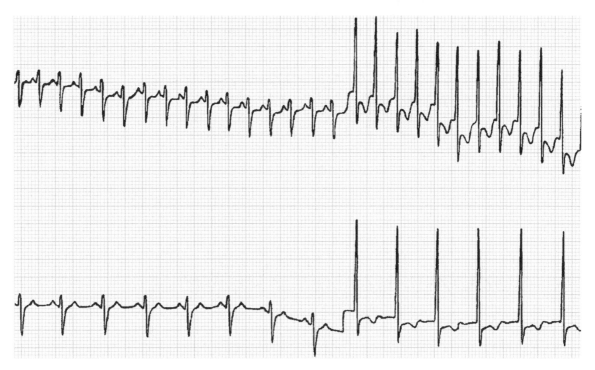

Figure 7.6 Continuous recordings of leads V1 and V4. In the upper trace the ventricular rate is 300 beats/min, suggesting atrial flutter with 1:1 AV conduction. The lower trace shows the effect of carotid massage: the ventricular rate is halved and F waves can be seen in V1 immediately before the QRS complex and superimposed on the T wave.

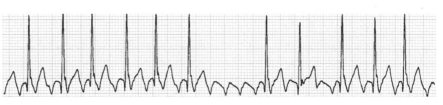

Figure 7.7 Atrial flutter only clearly seen in the sixth cycle during transient increase in AV block.

ventricular T waves may be superimposed on alternate F waves and may obscure the characteristic atrial activity: sinus tachycardia may be mistakenly diagnosed (Figure 7.8). Atrial flutter should be suspected if the heart rate is 150 beats/min at rest. Carotid sinus massage or adenosine can transiently impair AV conduction and aid diagnosis (Figure 7.9).

Intraventricular conduction

Ventricular complexes will be normal in duration unless there is bundle branch block, ventricular pre-excitation or aberrant intraventricular conduction.

ECG characteristics of typical atrial flutter

Atrial activity

F waves at a rate of 300 beats/min
'Sawtooth' appearance in limb leads
Discrete atrial waves in V1

Ventricular activity

Usually, 2:1 or higher degrees of atrioventricular block
Rarely, 1:1 atrioventricular conduction resulting in ventricular rate ≈ 300 beats/min

---

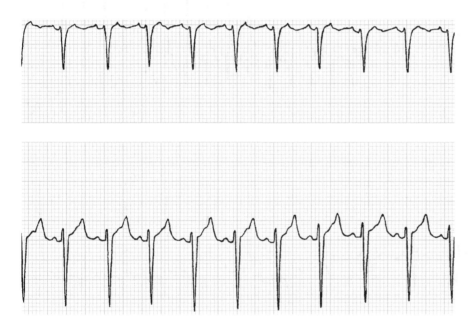

Figure 7.8 Simultaneous recording of leads V1 and V2. Atrial flutter can be diagnosed from V1 (alternate F waves superimposed on the beginning of the ventricular T wave) but V2 looks like sinus tachycardia.

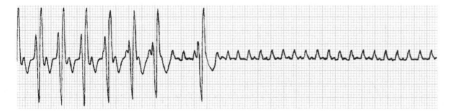

Figure 7.9 Atrial flutter revealed during several seconds of complete AV block induced by adenosine.

Atrial fibrillation

In some patients with atrial flutter there may be separate episodes of atrial fibrillation, and flutter may at times degenerate into atrial fibrillation.

Causes

Atrial flutter has similar causes to atrial fibrillation and may sometimes be caused by antiarrhythmic drugs given to treat atrial fibrillation (Chapter 6). It can also be caused by atrial scarring resulting from cardiac surgery, e.g. atrial septal defect repair.

In recent years it has become clear that atrial flutter may often be idiopathic. An increased incidence of atrial flutter has been reported in those engaging in long-term endurance sports.

Atypical flutter originating from the left atrium is sometimes seen after left atrial ablation procedures for atrial fibrillation.

Prevalence

Atrial flutter is less common than atrial fibrillation. A recent survey reports an annual incidence of 88 per 100 000. As with atrial fibrillation, the arrhythmia is often seen in older patients but does occur in young adults.

Treatment

Attempts to control a rapid ventricular response to atrial flutter by drugs are often unsuccessful. *Where possible, the aim should be to restore and maintain sinus rhythm.*

Catheter ablation

Catheter ablation can be used to interrupt the re-entrant circuit in the right atrium and thereby terminate and prevent typical atrial flutter (Chapter 25). Radiofrequency energy is delivered to the narrowest part of the circuit, i.e. the isthmus, which is between the posterior portion of the tricuspid valve and the inferior vena cava. Success rates are high and compare very favourably with antiarrhythmic therapy and cardioversion: recurrence rates are lower and there is a lesser incidence of hospital readmission. *There is a good case for ablation as first-line treatment for atrial flutter.*

It is usual to initiate anticoagulation before ablation for atrial flutter, and this is very important if the patient has a significant embolic risk as per the $CHADS_2$ score.

Atrial fibrillation sometimes occurs after ablation. On the other hand, some patients with atrial flutter also had episodes of atrial fibrillation, and ablation of flutter can occasionally eliminate fibrillation.

Cardioversion

Sustained atrial flutter can almost always be terminated with a low-energy DC shock (e.g. 50 J). The consensus is that, where possible, cardioversion should be preceded by anticoagulation, as for atrial fibrillation (Chapter 6). The need for anticoagulants is more compelling in patients who have experienced atrial fibrillation in the past.

Atrial flutter will return sooner or later in half of cases, though it is the author's impression that recurrence when the arrhythmia occurs in the early postoperative period after cardiac surgery is less frequent.

Radiofrequency ablation should be considered if atrial flutter does recur after cardioversion. Alternatively, if there has been a long interval before a recurrence, the patient may opt for repeat cardioversion.

Antiarrhythmic drugs

Drugs such as sotalol, flecainide and propafenone may terminate atrial flutter. However, it should be borne in mind that if unsuccessful in restoring sinus rhythm, they may possibly lead to higher ventricular rates because they often slow the atrial rate, facilitating a reduction in the AV conduction ratio and thereby paradoxically leading to an increase in ventricular rate (Figure 7.10).

Ibutilide (only available as an intravenous preparation) and dofetilide can be effective in terminating recent-onset flutter. Both prolong the QT interval and may occasionally cause torsade de pointes tachycardia.

Drugs that may prevent atrial fibrillation (Chapter 6) may be effective in preventing recurrence of atrial flutter.

Amiodarone can be successful in maintaining sinus rhythm when other drugs have failed: even if atrial flutter persists, the drug's actions in both slowing the atrial rate and depressing AV conduction can lead to a substantial slowing of the ventricular rate.

Control of ventricular response

Intravenous verapamil or diltiazem will promptly slow the ventricular rate during atrial flutter. However, not infrequently it is not possible to control the ventricular response with these drugs when they are given orally. Amiodarone may be more effective.

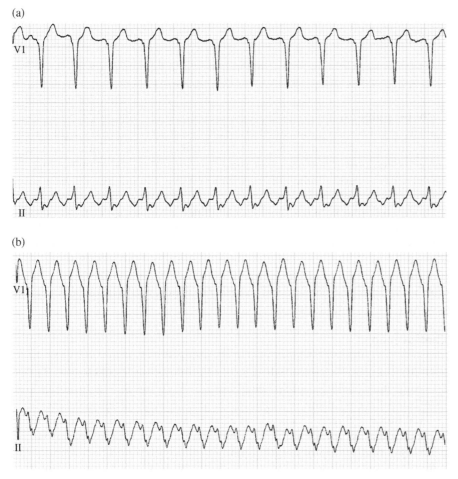

Figure 7.10 (a) Atrial flutter prior to intravenous flecainide; (b) the same patient after intravenous flecainide, which slowed the atrial rate and thereby facilitated a faster ventricular response.

Rapid atrial pacing

Rapid atrial pacing at a rate approximately 25% in excess of the atrial rate for 30 s will often restore sinus rhythm: pacing may have to be repeated several times before atrial flutter is terminated. Atrial fibrillation may sometimes be precipitated, but usually sinus rhythm returns within a few hours and often within a few minutes. It is important to ensure that pacing stimuli do capture the atria: capture is usually reflected by either an increase or decrease in the ventricular rate, depending on the conducting ability of the AV node. It has the advantage that general anaesthesia or hefty conscious sedation is not required.

If flutter develops following cardiac surgery and temporary atrial pacing wires are in place, these can be used to outpace the arrhythmia.

Systemic embolism

As with atrial fibrillation, atrial flutter can cause systemic embolism. The limited available evidence suggests that the risk is lower than for atrial fibrillation, perhaps because there is some preservation of atrial mechanical activity and therefore less likelihood of atrial thrombus, but current recommendations are that patients with atrial flutter should be assessed with a view to anticoagulation using the same stroke risk scoring system as is used in patients with atrial fibrillation (Chapter 6). It is possible that embolism in some cases of atrial flutter is due to these patients also being subject to paroxysmal atrial fibrillation.

Warfarin can be stopped six weeks after successful ablation for atrial flutter provided there is no evidence of paroxysmal atrial fibrillation: it is worthwhile to carry out ambulatory electrocardiography to minimise the possibility of missing this arrhythmia.

8   Atrial Tachycardia

Atrial tachycardia can originate from foci within either the right or left atrium, resulting in abnormally shaped, discrete P waves inscribed at a regular rapid rate, except in multifocal atrial tachycardia, which is characterised by an irregular atrial rate with several P wave morphologies. Causes include myocardial damage, respiratory disease and valvular heart disease. Often, atrial tachycaria is idiopathic.

As with atrial flutter, sometimes the atrioventricular (AV) node can conduct all atrial impulses to the ventricles but frequently there is a degree of AV block. Antiarrhythmic drugs may be effective. Troublesome cases require radiofrequency catheter ablation.

Atrial tachycardia can originate from a focus within either the right or left atrium. It can be sustained or paroxysmal. The practical difference between atrial tachycardia and flutter is that in the former the atrial rate is slower, being between 120 and 240 beats/min. As with atrial flutter, sometimes the atrioventricular (AV) node can conduct all atrial impulses to the ventricles, but often there is a degree of AV block.

ECG characteristics

The atrial rate is slower than in atrial flutter and there is no sawtooth appearance to the baseline (Figures 8.1, 8.2). The ventricular complexes will be narrow unless there is pre-existent bundle branch block, or aberrant intraventricular conduction. Again as for atrial flutter, atrial activity is often best seen in lead V1.

Atrial tachycardia with 1:1 AV conduction may occur (Figure 8.3). Carotid sinus massage is often helpful in the diagnosis (Figure 8.4). Adenosine can also be used to elucidate the diagnosis, but it should be noted that sometimes adenosine will terminate atrial tachycardia without causing transient AV block.

When there is 1:1 AV conduction there can be doubt as to whether the rhythm is atrial or sinus tachycardia. Usually, the PR interval is short during sinus tachycardia because the catecholamines that accelerate sinus node activity also increase the speed of AV nodal conduction. Thus, a longish PR interval points to an atrial rather than sinus tachycardia (Figure 8.3).

Bennett's Cardiac Arrhythmias: Practical Notes on Interpretation and Treatment, Eighth Edition. David H. Bennett.
© 2013 John Wiley & Sons, Ltd. Published 2013 by John Wiley & Sons, Ltd.

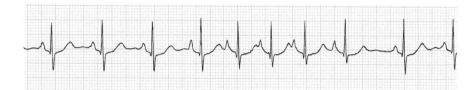

Figure 8.1 After three sinus beats there is a short episode of atrial tachycardia: the atrial rate abruptly increases and there is a change in P wave morphology.

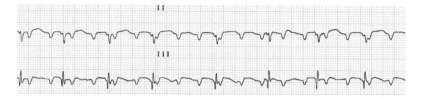

Figure 8.2 Atrial tachycardia with AV block. The atrial rate is 150 beats/min.

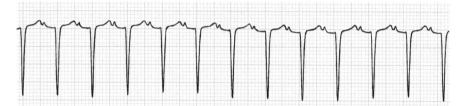

Figure 8.3 Lead V1. Atrial tachycardia with 1:1 AV conduction. The PR interval is longer than is normally seen during sinus tachycardia.

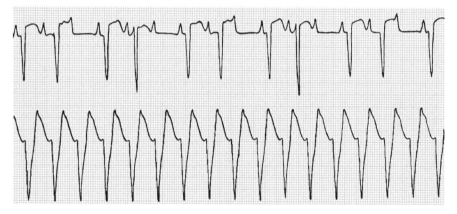

Figure 8.4 Lead V1. Atrial tachycardia before (lower trace) and during carotid sinus massage (upper trace). The atrial rate in the upper trace is identical to the ventricular rate in the lower trace, showing that without carotid massage there is 1:1 AV conduction.

A positive P wave in lead V1 or a negative P wave in leads I or aVL point to a left atrial origin, while a positive P wave in lead aVL points to a right atrial origin (Figure 8.5).

With high grades of AV block, because the ventricular rate is relatively slow, the rhythm may be misdiagnosed as complete heart block and an inappropriate request made for cardiac pacing if it is not appreciated that the atrial rate is rapid!

Atrial tachycardia is often paroxysmal (Figure 8.6). If incessant, however, it may lead to heart failure (Figure 5.3).

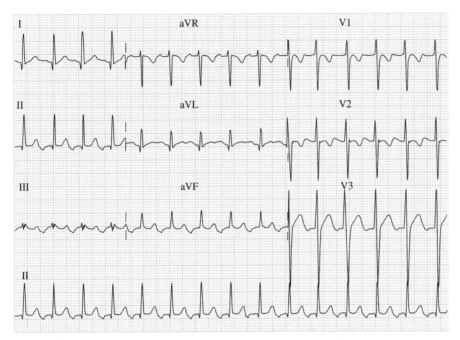

Figure 8.5 Right atrial tachycardia with 1:1 AV conduction. P waves are inverted in inferior leads and positive in aVL.

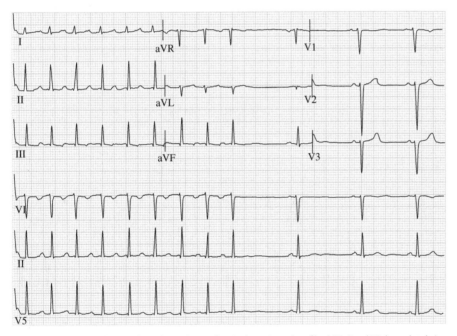

Figure 8.6 Paroxysmal atrial tachycardia terminates after nine beats. Inspection of leads V1, II and V5 shows that during tachycardia there is a P wave superimposed on each T wave.

Causes

Causes of atrial tachycardia include cardiomyopathy, ischaemic left ventricular dysfunction, rheumatic heart disease, surgery for valvular or congenital heart disease, chronic obstructive airways disease and sick sinus syndrome. Not infrequently, it is idiopathic. In left atrial tachycardias, the site of origin is often the junction between

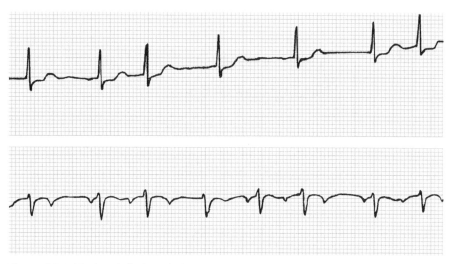

Figure 8.7 Atrial tachycardia (leads II and V1) in a patient with digoxin toxicity. Lead II suggests atrial fibrillation but V1 clearly shows atrial tachycardia with Mobitz I AV block.

atrium and pulmonary vein: these tachycardias have the same mechanism as, and may herald, paroxysmal atrial fibrillation.

The arrhythmia occasionally follows successful slow pathway ablation for atrioventricular nodal re-entrant tachycardia, arising from a site close to where radiofrequency energy had been delivered.

Atrial tachycardia with AV block may be due to digoxin toxicity (Figure 8.7). The arrhythmia has been referred to as 'paroxysmal atrial tachycardia with block'. The term paroxysmal is inappropriate, because the arrhythmia is usually sustained.

Treatment

If a return to sinus rhythm is required, cardioversion or rapid atrial pacing should be performed. Antiarrhythmic drugs such as sotalol, flecainide and amiodarone may be effective in maintaining normal rhythm. AV nodal blocking drugs may control the ventricular rate should atrial tachycardia persist. If the patient is receiving digoxin, toxicity should be suspected and the drug discontinued.

Radiofrequency catheter ablation to the site of origin, which is often in the lateral or low septal wall of the right atrium or near the pulmonary veins in the left atrium, or AV nodal ablation should be considered in refractory cases.

Multifocal atrial tachycardia

Multifocal atrial tachycardia, also termed chaotic atrial rhythm, is characterised by a rapid, irregular atrial rate with several P wave morphologies. It is usually caused by respiratory disease or severe systemic illness such as sepsis.

Atrioventricular Junctional Re-entrant Tachycardias

Atrioventricular junctional re-entrant tachycardias are caused by an additional electrical connection between atria and ventricles, allowing an impulse to repeatedly and rapidly travel around the circuit consisting of the normal atrioventricular (AV) junction and the additional connection.

Atrioventricular re-entrant tachycardia (AVRT) is caused by an accessory pathway: a strand of myocardium, congenital in origin, which straddles the groove between atria and ventricles.

In atrioventricular nodal re-entrant tachycardia (AVNRT), the AV node and its adjacent atrial tissues are functionally dissociated into two pathways: fast and slow. Typically, during AVNRT, AV conduction is via the slow pathway and ventriculoatrial conduction is via the fast pathway.

Both AVRT and AVNRT lead to a regular and usually narrow QRS tachycardia. The tachycardias can be terminated by vagal stimulation or by intravenous adenosine. The best approach to preventing recurrence is radiofrequency catheter ablation.

These supraventricular arrhythmias are caused by an additional electrical connection between atria and ventricles so that an impulse can repeatedly and rapidly travel around a circuit consisting of the normal atrioventricular (AV) junction and the additional AV connection (Figure 9.1). This is in contrast to the atrial arrhythmias discussed in the previous three chapters, where the mechanism responsible for the tachycardia is confined to the atria and the AV node merely transmits some or all of the atrial impulses to the ventricles.

Mechanism

In most cases the heart is structurally normal. If there is valve, myocardial or coronary disease these disorders will be coincidental to but not the cause of the arrhythmia. There are two main types of additional connection between atria and ventricles:

Accessory atrioventricular pathway

In atrioventricular re-entrant tachycardia (AVRT), the additional connection is an accessory AV pathway, which is a strand of myocardium, congenital in origin, which straddles the groove between atria and ventricles and therefore bypasses the AV node.

Bennett's Cardiac Arrhythmias: Practical Notes on Interpretation and Treatment, Eighth Edition. David H. Bennett.
© 2013 John Wiley & Sons, Ltd. Published 2013 by John Wiley & Sons, Ltd.

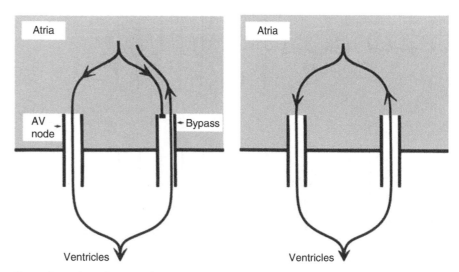

Figure 9.1 Initiation of AV junctional re-entrant tachycardia. An atrial extrasystole arrives at the AV junction while the bypass tract is still refractory to excitation following the last cardiac cycle (left-hand panel). The extrasystole is therefore only conducted to the ventricles via the AV node. By the time the extrasystole has traversed the AV node and reached the ventricles, the bypass tract has recovered and can conduct the impulse back to the atria, thereby initiating the re-entrant mechanism (right-hand panel).

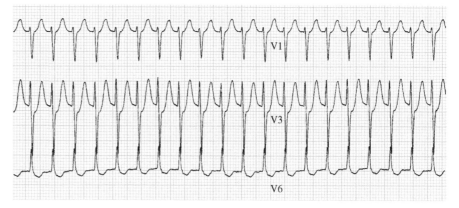

Figure 9.2 AV junctional re-entrant tachycardia. A regular tachycardia with narrow ventricular complexes.

Dual atrioventricular nodal pathways

In atrioventricular *nodal* re-entrant tachycardia (AVNRT), the AV node and its adjacent atrial tissues are functionally dissociated into two pathways: one that can conduct quickly, termed the fast pathway, and another which conducts relatively slowly, termed the slow pathway. The fast pathway has a relatively long recovery or refractory period whereas the slow pathway has a shorter refractory period. Typically during tachycardia, AV conduction is via the slow pathway and ventriculoatrial conduction is via the fast pathway.

ECG characteristics

The tachycardia, whether AVRT or AVNRT, is regular. Usually the QRS complexes are normal and therefore narrow (Figure 9.2) but occasionally pre-existing bundle branch block or bundle branch block resulting from the fast heart rate will lead to broad ventricular complexes (Figures 9.3, 9.4).

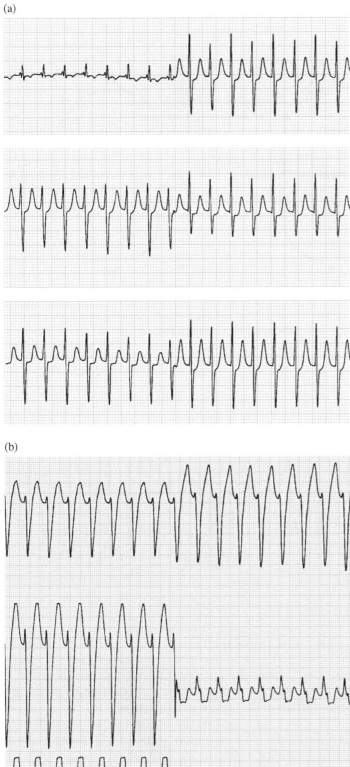

Figure 9.3 AV junctional re-entrant tachycardia, leads V1–V6: (a) with narrow complexes; (b) the same patient a few minutes later, showing broad complexes that have developed due to functional left bundle branch block.

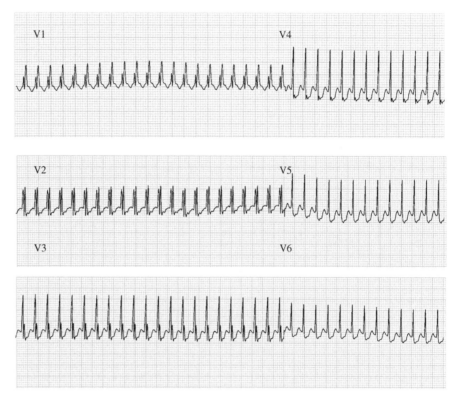

Figure 9.4 AV junctional re-entrant tachycardia with right bundle branch block (leads V1–V6).

The rate during tachycardia can range from 130 to 250 beats/min, and it is influenced by the sympathetic nervous system. For example, sympathetic activity and consequently the speed of AV nodal conduction increase on standing or during exertion so the tachycardia may become faster.

Clearly, normal P waves will not occur during this arrhythmia. Since the circulating impulse re-enters the atria after ventricular activation, each QRS complex will be *followed* by a P wave, though this wave is not always evident (Figures 9.4–9.7). If the atrial rate exceeds the ventricular rate, whether spontaneously or due to a drug or manoeuvre which slows AV node conduction, then the rhythm is not AV re-entrant tachycardia; it is probably atrial tachycardia or flutter. (There is an exception to this important guideline: very rarely, 2:1 AV block can occur during AVNRT.)

ST segment and T wave changes can be caused by the tachycardia and persist for some time after its cessation: they are of no diagnostic significance. The ECG during sinus rhythm is usually normal unless the accessory pathway can *also* conduct from atria to ventricles, in which case the ECG will show the Wolff– Parkinson–White syndrome (Chapter 10).

ECG characteristics of AV junctional re-entrant tachycardias

QRS complexes
  Regular
  Rate 130–250 beats/min
  Usually narrow

P waves
  Inverted, inscribed during or after each QRS complex

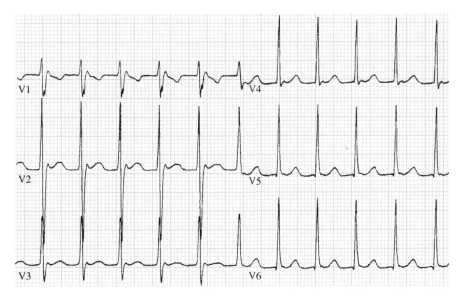

Figure 9.5 AV nodal re-entrant tachycardia. A small P wave can be seen after each QRS. In leads V1 and V2 it could be mistaken for a secondary R wave, but it is clearly also seen in V3–V5.

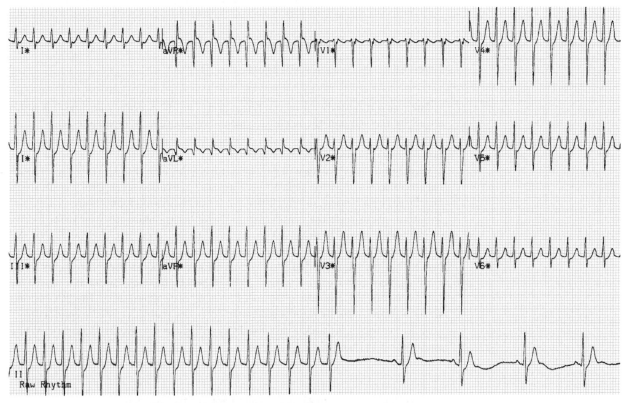

Figure 9.6 AV nodal re-entrant tachycardia. The retrograde P wave can be seen superimposed on the terminal part of lead V1. Sinus rhythm returns during recording of rhythm strip (lead II).

Timing of atrial activity during tachycardia

The timing of atrial activity, if identifiable, will indicate whether the tachycardia is due to an accessory AV pathway, i.e. AVRT, or due to dual AV nodal pathways, i.e. AVNRT. The distinction is important if the patient is being assessed for radiofrequency ablation.

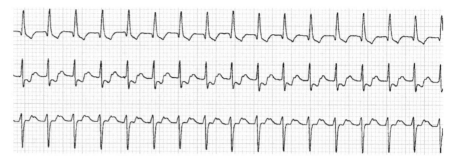

Figure 9.7 AV re-entrant tachycardia. There is a P wave after each QRS complex that is superimposed on the T wave, resulting in its pointed appearance. The inverted P wave in lead I suggests the accessory pathway is left-sided.

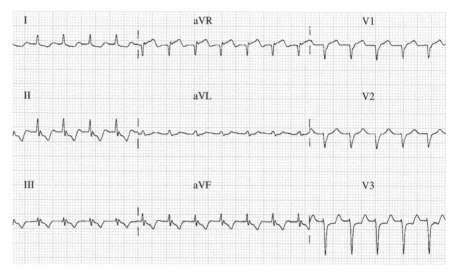

Figure 9.8 AV re-entrant tachycardia (due to left posterior accessory AV pathway).

With typical AVNRT, a P wave immediately follows or is actually superimposed on the QRS complex, because the length of the re-entrant circuit is small (Figures 9.4–9.6). The P wave is often best seen in lead V1. It might be mistaken for the secondary R wave of right bundle branch block, but if this were the case the same wave should be present in lead V1 during sinus rhythm.

The length of the re-entrant circuit is greater in AVRT because the accessory AV pathway is some distance from the AV junction. It therefore takes longer for an impulse to circulate and re-enter the atria. Hence the inverted P wave occurs roughly halfway between QRS complexes, and it will therefore typically be superimposed on the T wave (Figure 9.7). Identification is helped by the fact that superimposition of the P wave on the T wave usually leads to a pointed appearance of the T wave (Figures 9.7–9.9): T waves themselves are rounded, never pointed.

Long RP–short PR tachycardia

Rarely, AVNRT can present in its atypical form in which AV conduction is via the fast pathway and ventriculoatrial conduction is via the slow pathway. This results in a long ventriculoatrial conduction time. As a result, the ECG will show that the interval between the retrograde P wave and the following QRS complex is shorter than the subsequent interval between QRS complex and next retrograde P wave (Figure 9.10). Hence the term 'long RP–short PR tachycardia'. There are, in fact, three causes of a long RP–short PR tachycardia: atypical AVNRT, atrial

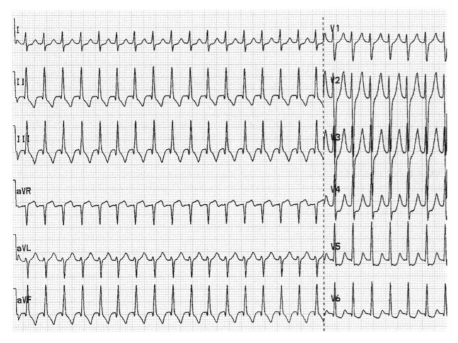

Figure 9.9 AV re-entrant tachycardia. There is a P wave after each QRS complex that is superimposed on the T wave, resulting in its pointed appearance. The inverted P wave in leads II, III and aVF indicates a posteroseptal pathway.

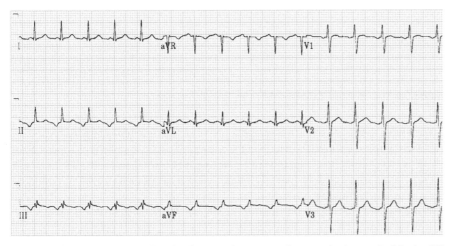

Figure 9.10 Long RP–short PR tachycardia. The retrograde P wave can be seen to be closer to the following QRS complex, rather than occurring just after the preceding ventricular complex.

tachycardia with 1:1 AV conduction (Figure 8.6), and AVRT with a slowly conducting accessory pathway (usually posteroseptal).

Clinical features

These arrhythmias are common. Attacks may start in infancy, childhood or adult life and often recur. Though AVRT is due to a congenitally acquired abnormality the first attack can occur well into adult life. AVNRT can occur at any age but typically starts after the second decade and is more common in females. It is more common than AVRT.

The duration and frequency of attacks varies from patient to patient. They may last for a few minutes or for many hours, and may occur several times per day or be separated by many months. In some patients, attacks are precipitated by exertion. In most, episodes can occur at rest or on exertion, and can be brought on by trivial activities such as bending down. Symptoms will be of sudden onset but their offset may not always be immediate because sinus tachycardia may follow the arrhythmia.

It is usually possible to obtain a full ECG during tachycardia in patients with reasonably frequent and sustained tachycardias. If necessary, diagnosis can often be achieved with ambulatory electrocardiography, but occasionally it is necessary to resort to loop recorder implantation.

Treatment

The patient should be reassured the tachycardia is not dangerous and that it is due to an electrical rather than structural cardiac abnormality: patients often fear the arrhythmia is due to coronary disease and that they are at risk from a heart attack.

Treatment is unnecessary for short episodes of tachycardia that do not cause distress. Several treatments can be used to terminate or to prevent recurrence of the arrhythmia.

Treatments for atrioventricular junctional re-entrant tachycardias

Termination
  Vagal stimulation
  Intravenous drugs, e.g. adenosine, verapamil
  Cardioversion
  Pacing (overdrive or programmed stimulation)
Prevention
  Radiofrequency ablation of additional connection
  Drugs, e.g. sotalol, flecainide

Vagal stimulation

The first approach to termination is vagal stimulation. An increase in vagal tone may temporarily block conduction through the AV node and thereby interrupt the tachycardia circuit.

The Valsalva manoeuvre and carotid sinus massage are the best methods: if possible, they should be carried out with the patient lying down. The former is performed by the patient attempting to forcefully exhale for 10–15 s while sealing the nose and mouth, and then breathing normally. The manoeuvre works because attempted exhalation causes a rise in intrathoracic pressure and resultant hypotension which triggers the autonomic reflex. The patient should be instructed to attempt exhalation until he or she starts to experience dizziness: a sign of hypotension.

Carotid massage is performed by firm digital pressure over either the left or right (but not both!) carotid arteries at the level of the upper border of the thyroid cartilage for 5 s (Figure 9.11a). It should be avoided if there is a carotid bruit or if carotid artery disease is known to be present.

Eyeball pressure is widely quoted as a method for vagal stimulation but is very painful and should *not* be used.

Intravenous drugs

If vagal stimulation fails, the tachycardia can almost certainly be terminated by an intravenous injection of one of several drugs. *Adenosine is the treatment of choice.*

(a)

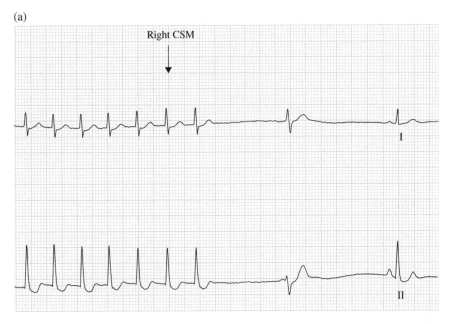

(b)

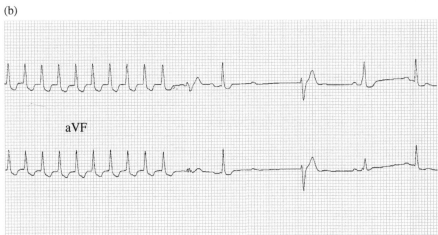

Figure 9.11 Termination of AV junctional re-entrant tachycardia: (a) by carotid sinus massage; (b) by adenosine – there is a short period of AV block after adenosine, as commonly occurs.

Adenosine

Adenosine is a potent blocker of AV nodal conduction that has an extremely short duration of action: < 20 s. It is very effective in terminating AVNRT and AVRT (Figure 9.11b).

It should be given as a rapid (2 s) intravenous bolus, followed by a saline flush. The recommended initial dose in adults and in children is 3 mg and 0.05 mg/kg, respectively. If ineffective, further dosages of 6 mg (0.10 mg/kg) and, if necessary, 12 mg can be given after one-minute intervals up to a recommended maximum of 12 mg (0.20 mg/kg). In adults, however, a dose of 3 mg is rarely effective and there is a good case for starting with 6 mg. Doses as high as 18 mg have been given without significant unwanted effect. If a patient has received adenosine in the past, it would be sensible to start with the dose that was previously shown to be effective.

Many patients will experience chest tightness, dyspnoea and flushing. Though the symptoms last less than 30 s, some patients find the experience very unpleasant. There may be complete AV block for a few seconds following termination of the

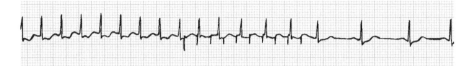

Figure 9.12 Termination of AV junctional re-entrant tachycardia by rapid atrial pacing.

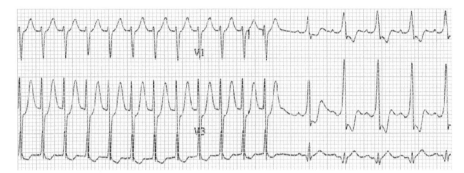

Figure 9.13 Termination of AV re-entrant tachycardia by a couplet of precisely timed atrial premature stimuli, best seen in lead V1, revealing Wolff–Parkinson–White syndrome on return to sinus rhythm.

tachycardia. A few ventricular ectopic beats may also occur. The drug does not have a negative inotropic action.

Adenosine can cause bronchospasm, and avoidance is recommended in asthmatics.

Verapamil

Intravenous verapamil (5–10 mg over 30 s) will usually restore sinus rhythm within a couple of minutes. Verapamil must not be used if the patient has recently received an oral or intravenous beta-blocking drug (Chapter 19) and *must never be given if ventricular tachycardia is possible*: dangerous hypotension can result.

Other drugs

Drugs such as sotalol, disopyramide and flecainide may also be effective (Chapter 19).

Electrical methods
Pacing

Various pacing methods may terminate both AVRTs and AVNRTs. The simplest is pacing the right atrium via a transvenous lead at a rate 10–20% faster than the tachycardia for a few seconds (i.e. overdrive pacing). On abrupt termination of pacing, sinus rhythm will often return; if unsuccessful, pacing should be repeated (Figure 9.12). There is a small risk of precipitating atrial fibrillation, which usually will not last for many minutes before sinus rhythm is restored. However, in patients with the Wolff–Parkinson–White syndrome atrial fibrillation might lead to a very fast ventricular response.

More sophisticated methods require a programmable pacemaker which allows the introduction of precisely timed extra stimuli (Figure 9.13). These methods have been used on a long-term basis by implanting a pacemaker (Figure 9.14), but this approach has now been superseded by radiofrequency catheter ablation.

Cardioversion

If drugs are ineffective or if clinical circumstances necessitate an immediate return to sinus rhythm, cardioversion should be carried out (Chapter 21).

Prevention

There are two main approaches: ablation of part of the re-entry circuit or drug therapy.

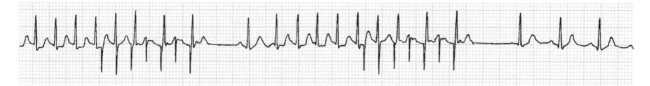

Figure 9.14 Implanted antitachycardia pacemaker. Automatic detection and termination of two episodes of AV re-entrant tachycardia.

Catheter ablation

Radiofrequency energy delivered by a catheter introduced via a vein or artery can be used to ablate an accessory pathway responsible for AVRT, or to modify the slow AV nodal tract involved in AVNRT (Chapter 25). *For most patients, catheter ablation is the treatment of choice, offering a cure and obviating the need for antiarrhythmic drugs.* Success rates well over 90% are being widely achieved and the risks are very low.

Drugs

Selection of a drug which is both effective and well tolerated is often a process of trial and error, and not infrequently it is unsuccessful. The patient should keep a record of the date and duration of any attacks so that the effect of therapy can be assessed. Flecainide (100 mg twice daily) or sotalol (160 mg daily) are first-line drugs.

Amiodarone is likely to be effective where other drugs have failed, but should be reserved for refractory cases where the need for tachycardia control outweighs the drug's possible unwanted effects.

10   Wolff–Parkinson–White Syndrome

> The Wolff–Parkinson–White (WPW) syndrome is caused by an accessory atrioventricular (AV) pathway that bypasses the AV node, thereby pre-exciting ventricular myocardium. It is characterised by a short PR interval and a delta wave. AV re-entrant tachycardia and atrial fibrillation can result.
>
> During AV re-entrant tachycardia there will be no delta waves, unless in its rare antidromic form, and treatment is the same whether or not there is pre-excitation.
>
> During atrial fibrillation, the ventricular rate is often very fast, most complexes will usually have a delta wave configuration and there is a risk of ventricular fibrillation when the minimum interval between delta waves is less than 250 ms. Digoxin and verapamil may be dangerous: a drug which slows conduction in the accessory pathway should be used, e.g. sotalol or flecainide.
>
> Radiofrequency catheter ablation should be considered in all symptomatic patients, and in some circumstances in patients with asymptomatic pre-excitation.

Pre-excitation

Wolff–Parkinson–White (WPW) syndrome is due to an accessory AV pathway: the same pathway that, as discussed in Chapter 9, is the cause of AV re-entrant tachycardia (AVRT). The connection, also referred to as a bundle of Kent, is a strand of normal myocardium that traverses the groove between atria and ventricles. It is congenital in origin.

To facilitate AV re-entrant tachycardia it is only necessary for the accessory pathway to conduct in a retrograde direction, i.e. from ventricles to atria. Many patients with AV re-entrant tachycardia have an accessory AV pathway that is *only* capable of ventriculoatrial conduction. In patients with WPW syndrome the pathway is *also* capable of anterograde conduction, i.e. from atria to ventricles. Unlike the AV node, the accessory connection does not delay conduction between atria and ventricles: consequently the PR interval is very short, and hence the term pre-excitation.

Normally the atria become electrically isolated from the ventricles during fetal development, apart from the AV junction, i.e. AV node plus bundle of His. Incomplete separation leads to an accessory AV pathway. Rarely, WPW syndrome is familial.

Bennett's Cardiac Arrhythmias: Practical Notes on Interpretation and Treatment, Eighth Edition. David H. Bennett.
© 2013 John Wiley & Sons, Ltd. Published 2013 by John Wiley & Sons, Ltd.

The accessory pathway may be situated anywhere across the groove between atria and ventricles. The most common site is the left free wall of the heart. Other locations are posteroseptal, right free wall and rarely anteroseptal. In a minority of patients there is more than one accessory pathway.

Approximately 1.3–3 per 1000 of the population have the electrocardiographic signs of pre-excitation, two-thirds of whom will experience cardiac arrhythmias. One survey reported 4 per 100 000 newly diagnosed cases per annum. The syndrome is more common in young people. With age, fibrosis may sometimes develop in the AV groove and block an accessory pathway.

ECG characteristics

The characteristics of WPW syndrome are a short PR interval, a widened QRS complex due to the presence of a delta wave, *and* paroxysmal tachycardia (Figure 10.1). If tachycardia has not occurred, then, strictly speaking, the patient has ventricular pre-excitation but not WPW syndrome.

During sinus rhythm, an atrial impulse will reach the ventricles via both the accessory pathway and the normal AV node. The AV node conducts relatively slowly. Therefore initial ventricular activation is solely due to accessory pathway conduction, resulting in a short PR interval: ventricular pre-excitation. Because the accessory pathway is not connected to the His–Purkinje system, the rate of early ventricular activation will be slow, leading to slurring of the ventricular complex, i.e. a delta wave, rather than the brisk upstroke that would result from rapid ventricular activation via the specialised conducting tissues. Once the atrial impulse has traversed the AV node, further ventricular activation will proceed rapidly via the His–Purkinje system. During sinus rhythm, therefore, the ventricular complex is a fusion between delta wave and normal QRS complex (Figure 10.1).

Location of the accessory pathway

The syndrome is classified into types A and B, depending on the ventricular complex in lead V1. If predominantly positive, it is type A (Figures 10.2, 10.3), and if negative, type B (Figure 10.4).

Type A is caused by a left-sided accessory pathway. However, type B is not necessarily due to a right-sided pathway, especially if the delta wave is small.

Complex ECG algorithms have been devised for precise location of accessory pathways, but none is reliable. There are a few simple guides. A positive delta wave in lead V1 indicates a left-sided pathway. A negative delta wave in leads III and aVF together with positive waves in leads V2 and V3 indicates a posteroseptal pathway (Figure 10.7b), while a right free wall pathway is usually associated with positive waves in leads II and III and a negative wave in lead V1.

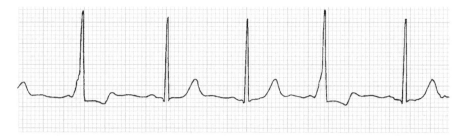

Figure 10.1 Wolff–Parkinson–White syndrome. In this patient, the accessory pathway conducts intermittently. The second, third and fifth complexes are normal whereas the first and fourth complexes show the characteristic short PR interval and delta wave. By comparing pre-excited and normal beats, it can be seen how the delta wave both shortens the PR interval and broadens the ventricular complex.

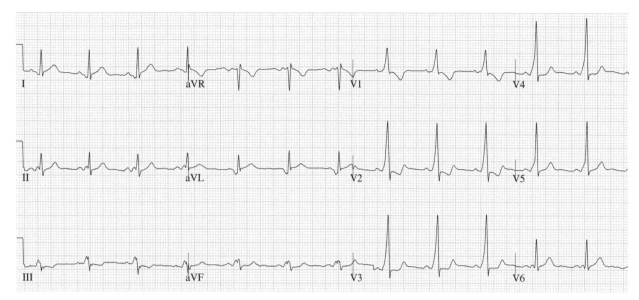

Figure 10.2 Type A Wolff–Parkinson–White syndrome: a positive complex in lead V1.

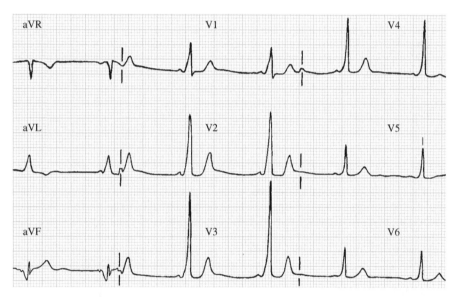

Figure 10.3 Type A Wolff–Parkinson–White syndrome (the negative delta wave in lead aVF could be misinterpreted as a Q wave due to inferior myocardial infarction).

Arrhythmias

Two main arrhythmias can occur in patients with WPW syndrome: atrial fibrillation and, more commonly, AV re-entrant tachycardia (AVRT).

Atrial fibrillation

In patients without pre-excitation the AV node protects the ventricles from the rapid atrial activity during atrial fibrillation (350–600 impulses/min). In WPW syndrome, the accessory pathway provides an additional route of access to the ventricles and can in some patients conduct very frequently. As a result, ventricular rates during atrial fibrillation are often very fast. Usually, most conducted impulses reach the ventricles

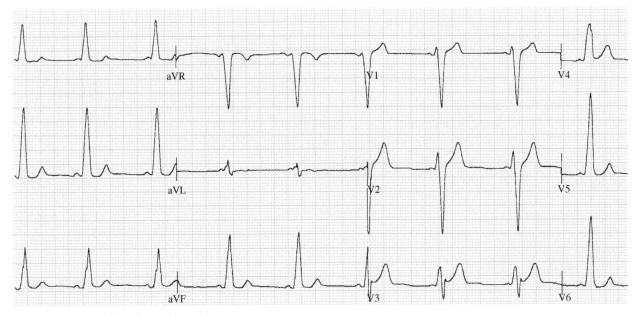

Figure 10.4 Type B Wolff–Parkinson–White syndrome.

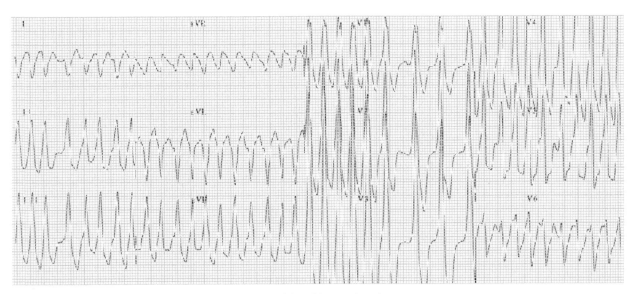

Figure 10.5 Atrial fibrillation: irregular, rapid succession of complexes with large delta waves (type A).

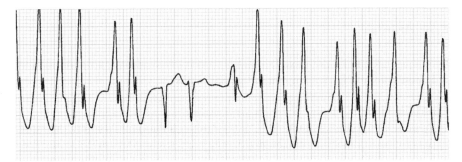

Figure 10.6 Atrial fibrillation: most complexes are delta waves; the seventh and eighth complexes are narrow due to conduction via the AV node.

(a)

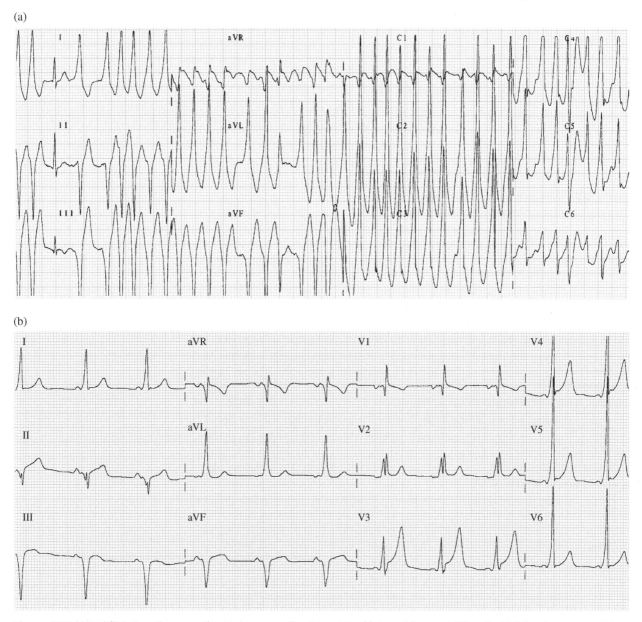

(b)

Figure 10.7 (a) Atrial fibrillation with a very rapid ventricular response. The minimum interval between delta waves is 200 ms. The totally irregular response excludes a diagnosis of ventricular tachycardia. (b) The same patient in sinus rhythm. ECG suggests posteroseptal accessory pathway.

via the accessory pathway and therefore lead to delta waves. The minority of impulses that reach the ventricles via the AV node produce normal QRS complexes. The resultant ECG, which can look very alarming, will show *the totally irregular ventricular response that is characteristic of atrial fibrillation*. Some ventricular complexes will be normal, but usually most will be delta waves (Figures 10.5–10.7).

A very rapid ventricular response to atrial fibrillation may occasionally cause heart failure or shock. If the ventricles are stimulated at a very fast rate there is a risk of ventricular fibrillation: this is the mechanism of sudden death that occasionally occurs in patients with this syndrome. The risk of ventricular fibrillation is small, and it mainly affects those patients where the minimum interval between delta waves during atrial fibrillation is less than 250 ms (Figure 10.7a). The annual risk of sudden

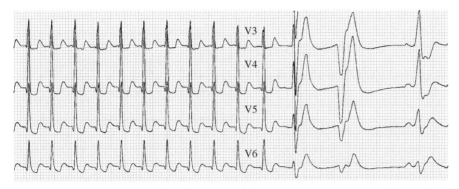

Figure 10.8 AV re-entrant tachycardia terminated by adenosine. After two ventricular ectopic beats there is a sinus beat with short PR interval and delta wave.

death in patients with WPW syndrome is estimated at 0.05%. *Risk is low in those with intermittent accessory pathway conduction, whether demonstrated by resting, ambulatory or exercise ECG* (Figure 10.1), and probably also in asymptomatic patients.

Atrioventricular re-entrant tachycardia

The AV node and accessory pathway differ in the time they take to recover after excitation. Usually, the AV node recovers first. If an atrial ectopic beat arises when the AV node has recovered but the accessory pathway is not yet capable of conduction, the resultant ventricular complex will clearly not have a delta wave and will therefore be narrow. By the time the premature atrial impulse has traversed the AV junction and stimulated the ventricles, the accessory pathway will have recovered and will be able to conduct the impulse back to the atria. When the impulse reaches the atria the AV junction will again be able to conduct and hence the impulse can repeatedly circulate between atria and ventricles, leading to AVRT (Figure 9.1). Similarly, a ventricular ectopic beat during sinus rhythm can be conducted to the atria via the accessory pathway and thereby initiate AVRT.

The ECG during tachycardia will show narrow ventricular complexes (unless there is rate-related bundle branch block) in rapid, regular succession (Figures 10.8, 10.9).

Unlike atrial fibrillation, there will be no delta waves and thus there will be no clue from the ventricular complexes during tachycardia that the patient has WPW syndrome. However, as discussed in Chapter 9, the timing of atrial activity during tachycardia, if identifiable, may point to the tachycardia mechanism. An accessory AV pathway is some distance from the AV junction. Hence the retrograde P wave occurs roughly halfway between QRS complexes (Figure 10.10). If inverted in lead I, the accessory pathway is likely to be left-sided. If inverted in leads II, III and aVF, it is likely the pathway is posteroseptal (Figure 9.9).

Antidromic tachycardia

Antidromic AV re-entrant tachycardia is much less common than the above-mentioned form of AVRT, which is termed orthodromic. The circulating impulse travels in the opposite direction: conduction from atria to ventricles is over the accessory AV pathway and return to the atria is via the AV node. Consequently, ventricular complexes will be in the form of large delta waves (Figure 10.11).

Treatment

Radiofrequency ablation

Radiofrequency ablation of the accessory pathway (Chapter 25) should be considered in all symptomatic patients, particularly if drugs are ineffective or cannot be tolerated, or if there is a fast ventricular response to atrial fibrillation.

(a)

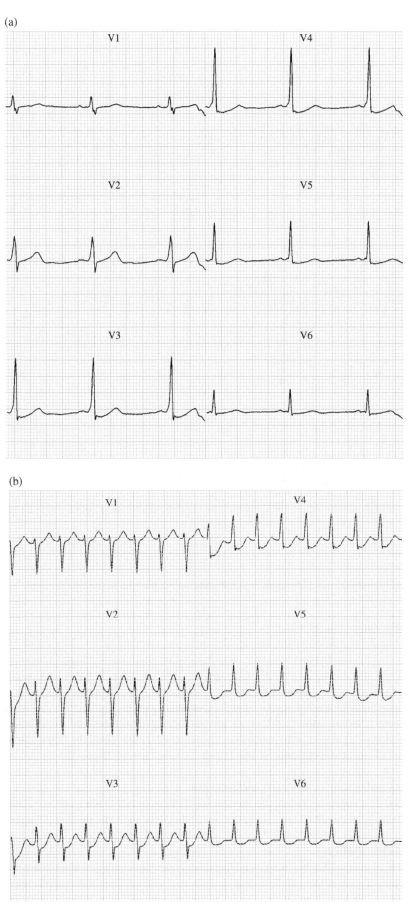

(b)

Figure 10.9 (a) Type A Wolff–Parkinson–White syndrome in sinus rhythm. (b) The same patient in AV re-entrant tachycardia (AVRT).

(c)

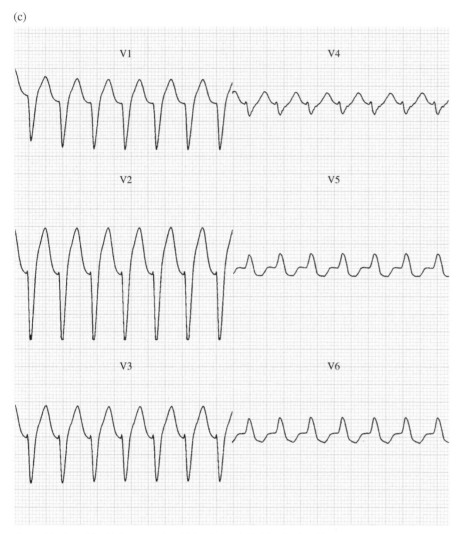

Figure 10.9 (cont'd)   (c) The same patient: left bundle branch block has developed during AVRT.

Asymptomatic patients

Ablation should be considered in asymptomatic patients when the chance finding of ventricular pre-excitation results in employment or insurance difficulties, bearing in mind that some of these patients will experience tachycardias in years to come, or in those who wish to undertake competitive, strenuous sporting activity but in whom investigations have not demonstrated that accessory pathway conduction is intermittent, and who thus do not fall into a low-risk group. The threshold for ablation in asymptomatic patients with pathways close to the AV node should be higher because of the risk of heart block and resultant need for long-term pacing.

Atrioventricular re-entrant tachycardia

Methods for the termination and prevention of AV re-entrant tachycardia are appropriate whether or not the patient has pre-excitation during sinus rhythm (Chapter 9).

Atrial fibrillation

During atrial fibrillation, most atrial impulses reach the ventricles via the accessory AV pathway. Thus AV nodal blocking drugs such as digoxin and verapamil are of little use during atrial fibrillation in WPW syndrome. Indeed, *both digoxin and verapamil*

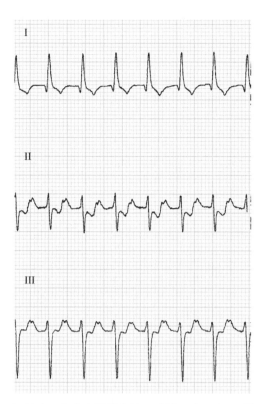

Figure 10.10 AV re-entrant tachycardia due to Wolff–Parkinson–White syndrome. Inverted P waves can be seen halfway between QRS complexes. (The P wave is negative in lead I, suggesting a left-sided pathway.)

can increase the frequency of conduction in the accessory pathway and therefore lead to a faster ventricular rate. These drugs must not be used in those patients who are capable of a rapid ventricular response in case a dangerously fast ventricular rate develops. In patients in whom atrial fibrillation has never occurred, and thus a fast response has not been excluded, the drugs should be avoided.

Intravenous sotalol, flecainide, disopyramide or amiodarone, drugs that slow conduction in the accessory pathway, should be used. These drugs will slow the ventricular response to atrial fibrillation and will often restore sinus rhythm. A simple alternative method of terminating atrial fibrillation is cardioversion, but this is not appropriate if the arrhythmia is frequently recurrent.

For prevention of atrial fibrillation, the drugs listed above that slow conduction in the accessory pathway given orally are often effective, but catheter ablation is the treatment of choice.

T wave memory
During intermittent accessory pathway conduction in patients with WPW syndrome due to a posteroseptal pathway, deep T wave inversion in the inferior leads in non-pre-excited beats can be seen, causing concern that there is myocardial ischaemia. In fact it is due to 'T wave memory': the T wave continues in the same direction as the QRS complex in that lead as occurred in pre-excited beats (Figure 10.12).

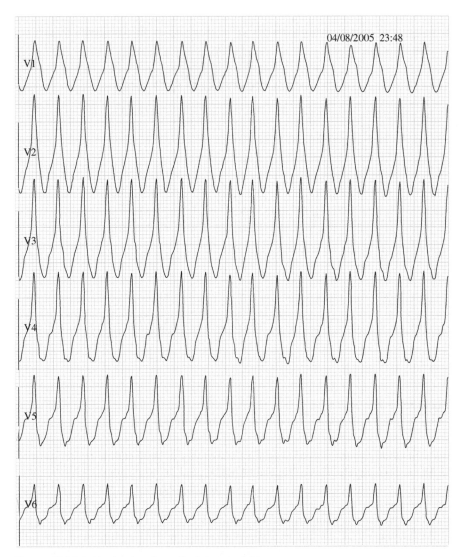

04/08/2005 23:48

Figure 10.11 Antidromic tachycardia resulting in large type A delta waves.

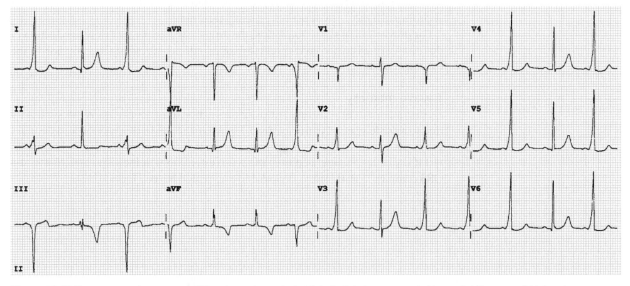

Figure 10.12 T wave memory: deep, symmetrical T inversion can be seen in the inferior leads in the non-pre-excited beats, mimicking myocardial ischaemia.

11 Ventricular Tachyarrhythmias

This chapter is a brief introduction to the following three chapters on monomorphic and polymorphic ventricular tachycardias, torsade de pointes tachycardia, ventricular fibrillation, and the assessment of broad QRS complex tachycardias.

Ventricular tachycardia

Ventricular tachycardia is defined as four or more ventricular ectopic beats in rapid succession (Figure 11.1). Ventricular tachycardias vary in rate, duration and frequency of recurrence. The consequences also vary: severe hypotension or ventricular fibrillation may result, whereas some patients tolerate ventricular tachycardia with few or no symptoms.

Monomorphic and polymorphic

There are two main types of ventricular tachycardia: monomorphic and polymorphic. The latter is also termed 'multiform'.

Monomorphic ventricular tachycardia (Chapter 12) is usually due to heart muscle damage, but there are two specific arrhythmias that occur in patients with a structurally and functionally normal heart: namely, right ventricular outflow tract tachycardia and fascicular tachycardia.

Polymorphic ventricular tachycardia (Chapter 13) is characterised by repeated, progressive changes in the direction and amplitude of ventricular complexes so that they appear to 'twist' about the baseline (Figure 11.2). It can also be caused by heart muscle damage, but often arises in the absence of structural heart disease.

Polymorphic ventricular tachycardia can be associated with a prolonged QT interval preceding the arrhythmia, when it is termed 'torsade de pointes' tachycardia. There may be no structural heart disease. The arrhythmia results from abnormalities in ventricular repolarisation, which can be either acquired or inherited. Treatment is directed to the management of the cause of QT prolongation rather than antiarrhythmic therapy.

Bennett's Cardiac Arrhythmias: Practical Notes on Interpretation and Treatment, Eighth Edition. David H. Bennett.
© 2013 John Wiley & Sons, Ltd. Published 2013 by John Wiley & Sons, Ltd.

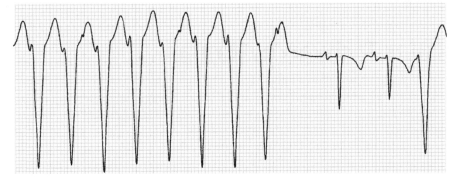

Figure 11.1 Monomorphic ventricular tachycardia: a succession of ventricular ectopic beats, followed by two sinus beats and then a single ventricular ectopic beat.

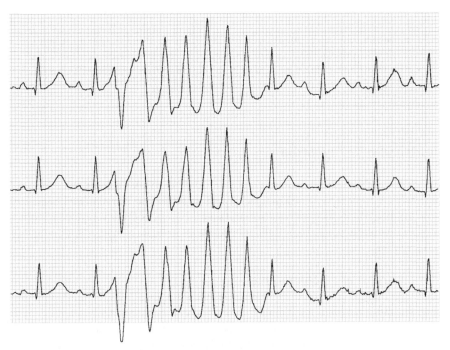

Figure 11.2 Torsade de pointes tachycardia (leads II, V5, III), characterised by repeated, progressive changes in the QRS complex, and prolonged QT interval (QTc = 0.5 s): a brief episode.

Ventricular fibrillation

Ventricular fibrillation (Chapter 13) is usually a consequence of myocardial damage from either coronary disease or cardiomyopathy, but occasionally it is due to a primary electrical disorder such as the Brugada syndrome.

Supraventricular versus ventricular tachycardia

Difficulty is often encountered in distinguishing ventricular from supraventricular tachycardia when the QRS complex during tachycardia is broad. There are a number of pointers that can usually easily help ascertain the origin of a tachycardia (Chapter 14).

12 Monomorphic Ventricular Tachycardia

Monomorphic ventricular tachycardia consists of a rapid, regular succession of ventricular extrasystoles each with the same configuration. QRS duration exceeds 0.12 s and is usually greater than 0.14 s. P waves dissociated from ventricular activity, or fusion or capture beats, indicate independent atrial activity and confirm ventricular tachycardia. Common causes are myocardial infarction and cardiomyopathy: dilated, hypertrophic or arrhythmogenic right ventricular.

Ventricular tachycardia is often a recurrent problem and may lead to sudden death. An implantable defibrillator may be indicated, particularly in patients with poor ventricular function.

Right ventricular outflow tract and fascicular tachycardias arise in structurally normal hearts, have a good prognosis and are ideally amenable to radiofrequency ablation. Accelerated idioventricular rhythm is ventricular tachycardia at a rate less than 120 beats/min: treatment is not required.

Wherever possible, obtain and save a 12-lead ECG during tachycardia for diagnostic purposes.

ECG characteristics

The arrhythmia consists of a rapid succession of ventricular ectopic beats each with the same configuration, hence the term monomorphic (Figure 12.1). As with single ventricular ectopic beats, the complexes will be abnormal in shape, and the duration of each complex will be more than 0.12 s and usually greater than 0.14 s. The rhythm is regular unless there are capture beats (see below) which cause minor irregularities in the rhythm. The rate ranges from 120 to 250 beats/min.

Atrial activity during ventricular tachycardia

With many ventricular tachycardias, the sinus node continues to initiate atrial activity, which is therefore independent of, and slower than, ventricular activity (Figure 12.2). In others, the AV node conducts each ventricular impulse to the atria so a P wave follows the ventricular complex. The P wave is often concealed by the

Bennett's Cardiac Arrhythmias: Practical Notes on Interpretation and Treatment, Eighth Edition. David H. Bennett.
© 2013 John Wiley & Sons, Ltd. Published 2013 by John Wiley & Sons, Ltd.

superimposed terminal portion of the ventricular complex (Figure 12.3). Rarely, second-degree block may occur at the AV junction so only some ventricular impulses are conducted to the atria (Figure 12.15b).

Identification of independent atrial activity during tachycardia excludes an origin at AV node level or above and will thus distinguish ventricular tachycardia from supraventricular tachycardia with broad ventricular complexes. There may be direct or indirect evidence of independent atrial activity.

Direct evidence of independent atrial activity

P waves at a slower rate than and dissociated from ventricular activity are direct evidence of independent atrial activity (Figure 12.2). Inevitably, some P waves will be concealed by superimposed ventricular complexes. Furthermore, not all leads will clearly show atrial activity. A rhythm strip is often inadequate, and scrutiny of a simultaneous recording of several different leads may be necessary. Sometimes there will be doubt whether small waves on the ECG during tachycardia are caused by atrial activity. If they are, they will be separated by similar intervals, or multiples of that interval.

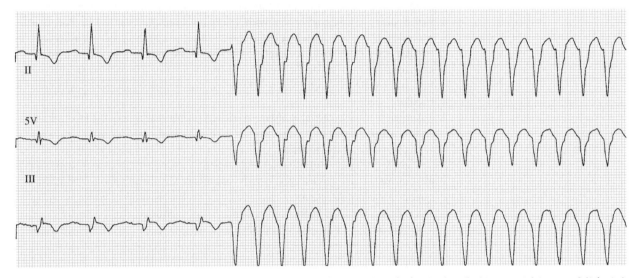

Figure 12.1 Monomorphic ventricular tachycardia. There is a rapid, regular succession of broad complexes after four sinus beats (lead III suggests inferior myocardial infarction).

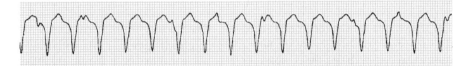

Figure 12.2 Ventricular tachycardia with direct evidence of independent atrial activity. P waves are separated by intervals of 0.75 s, and can clearly be seen after the first, third, sixth, eighth, tenth, thirteenth, fifteenth and seventeenth ventricular complexes.

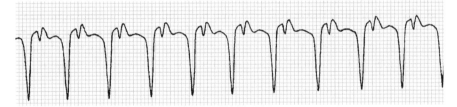

Figure 12.3 Ventricular tachycardia (lead aVF) with retrograde atrial activation. In this case, a P wave can be clearly seen to be superimposed on the T wave of each ventricular complex.

Indirect evidence of independent atrial activity

Capture or fusion beats are indirect evidence of atrial activity. Just one is sufficient to confirm ventricular tachycardia.

Capture beats occur when the timing of an atrial impulse generated by the sinus node during ventricular tachycardia is such that it can be transmitted via the AV junction and activate the ventricles before the next discharge from the ventricular focus. The resultant ventricular complex will be normal in shape and duration and will occur slightly earlier than the next ventricular ectopic beat would have been expected (Figure 12.15a). Fusion beats are caused by a similar process. However, the atrial impulse activates the ventricles slightly later in the cardiac cycle leading to simultaneous activation of the ventricles by the transmitted atrial impulse and the ventricular focus. The result is a ventricular complex with an appearance intermediate between a normal QRS complex and a ventricular ectopic beat (Figure 12.4).

ECG characteristics of monomorphic ventricular tachycardia

Regular rhythm
Broad complexes (≥ 0.12 s and usually > 0.14 s)
Ventricular complexes of uniform appearance
Independent P waves may be present
Capture or fusion beats may be present

Causes

Ventricular tachycardia is most often the result of myocardial infarction or of heart muscle disorders.

Causes of ventricular tachycardia

Acute myocardial infarction or ischaemia
Past myocardial infarction
Dilated cardiomyopathy
Hypertrophic cardiomyopathy
Arrhythmogenic right ventricular cardiomyopathy
Myocarditis
Mitral valve prolapse
Valvular heart disease
Repair of tetralogy of Fallot
Sarcoidosis
Chagas' disease
Digoxin toxicity
Idiopathic

Mechanisms of ventricular tachycardias

Two main mechanisms cause tachycardias: re-entry, which is the commonest mechanism for ventricular tachycardia, and enhanced automaticity, which may be spontaneous or triggered.

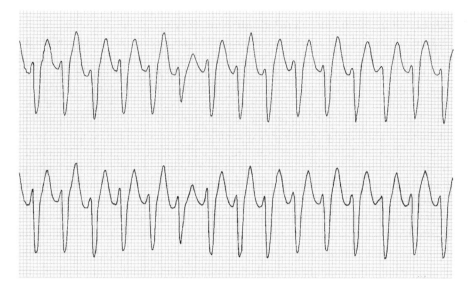

Figure 12.4 Ventricular tachycardia. The sixth complex is a fusion beat.

Re-entry

Two conditions are necessary for a re-entrant tachycardia to occur. The first is the presence of a potential circuit composed of two pathways of tissue with differing electrical characteristics. The second condition is transient or permanent block in one direction in one of the pathways so an impulse arriving at the circuit can be conducted along one pathway and return via the other pathway, thereby re-entering the circuit. The activating impulse is repeatedly conducted around the circuit, exciting the surrounding myocardium at a rapid rate.

Re-entrant ventricular tachycardia

Re-entrant ventricular tachycardia can result from fibrosis or ischaemia that causes delay in activation and hence recovery of an area of myocardium, i.e. one component of the re-entrant circuit. Tachycardia is initiated by a premature beat arriving at the abnormal area to find it is refractory to excitation following the last heartbeat. The impulse is conducted around the damaged area by the adjacent, normally responsive myocardium. By the time the impulse has circumvented the damaged area, the abnormal myocardium has become excitable again and conducts the impulse in the opposite direction, giving rise to a re-entrant circuit. Perpetuation of this process results in ventricular tachycardia.

Ventricular re-entrant tachycardias can be initiated and terminated by precisely timed premature ventricular pacing stimuli.

Enhanced automaticity

Damage or disease can result in a group of myocardial cells acquiring enhanced automaticity, i.e. the cells discharge at a higher rate than the sinus node, taking over control of the heart rhythm. Enhanced automaticity can either be spontaneous or be triggered by after-depolarisations that lead to early reactivation of the myocardium: 'early after-depolarisations' occur at the end of the action potential (phase 3) and 'late after-depolarisations' occur during electrical recovery of myocardial cells (phase 4).

Initiation of tachycardia

A re-entrant circuit or focus of enhanced automaticity provides the substrate for ventricular tachycardia. Initiation of the arrhythmia is usually triggered by an ectopic beat. Ischaemia, increased sympathetic nervous system activity or electrolyte imbalance

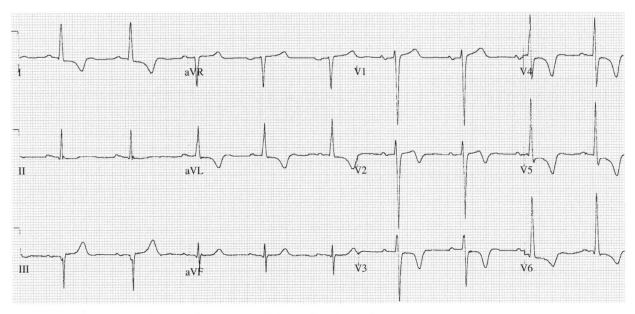

Figure 12.5 ECG shows marked left ventricular hypertrophy caused by hypertrophic cardiomyopathy.

may influence the arrhythmia substrate and may account for a tachycardia occurring at a particular time.

Investigations

The nature and extent of investigations have to be tailored to the individual clinical situation. The aims should be to identify the cause, which may well be of therapeutic and/or prognostic importance, and to assess the role and efficacy of any therapy that may be required.

Twelve-lead ECG

An ECG during sinus rhythm may reveal the cause of tachycardia, e.g. myocardial infarction, or marked left ventricular hypertrophy which in the absence of severe valve disease or hypertension points strongly to hypertrophic cardiomyopathy (Figure 12.5).

Whenever possible, a 12-lead ECG during tachycardia should be recorded. The configuration of the ventricular complexes during tachycardia may indicate its site of origin. A tachycardia with left bundle branch block morphology, i.e. a complex which is positive in V5 and V6 and which is akin to left bundle branch block in its appearance, will usually have a right ventricular origin. A positive complex in lead V1, i.e. with right bundle branch block morphology, points to a left ventricular free wall or septal source. If complexes are negative in V4–V6, a left ventricular apical origin is likely, while Q waves in the inferior leads suggest that the tachycardia is arising from the base of the left ventricle. The ECG appearances of right ventricular outflow tract tachycardia and fascicular tachycardia are diagnostic for those arrhythmias (see below).

Imaging

Echocardiography may help establish the cause of the arrhythmia: for example, by demonstrating dilated or hypertrophic cardiomyopathy, or arrhythmogenic right ventricular cardiomyopathy (ARVC). Magnetic resonance imaging is becoming used more widely. Some regard it as the 'gold standard' for the diagnosis of ARVC. Coronary angiography may be indicated, particularly if myocardial ischaemia might be the cause of the arrhythmia or if surgery is contemplated.

Ambulatory electrocardiography

Ambulatory electrocardiography may be required to assess the frequency and duration of episodes of ventricular tachycardia and the effect of therapy in those patients who have had frequent episodes.

Occasionally, ventricular tachycardia is triggered by bradycardia. This may be revealed if the onset of the arrhythmia is recorded. Prevention of bradycardia in this situation will often prevent ventricular tachycardia.

Exercise testing

Exercise-induced tachycardia is not uncommon. An exercise test can be useful both in its diagnosis and in assessment of response to therapy.

Ventricular stimulation study

Stimulation of the ventricles with up to three precisely timed premature stimuli delivered by a temporary pacing lead introduced via the femoral vein will usually initiate ventricular tachycardia in patients who are prone to this arrhythmia (see Figure 13.15). Stimulation protocols involve progressively aggressive attempts to initiate ventricular tachycardia.

A typical protocol consists of a series of eight paced beats (each termed S1) at a cycle length of 600 ms followed by a single premature stimulus (S2) introduced after 350 ms. This is repeated with progressively shorter S1–S2 intervals until tachycardia is initiated, or S2 fails to activate the ventricles (i.e. the myocardial refractory period has been reached), or an interval of 200 ms has been arrived at. If ventricular tachycardia is not initiated, the process is then repeated with S1–S2 held at 10 ms greater than the refractory period, and a second premature stimulus (S3) is introduced: the S2–S3 interval is progressively reduced until the myocardium is refractory or the cycle length of 200 ms has been reached. If tachycardia has still not been initiated the process is repeated with the addition of a third stimulus (S4) and again S3–S4 is progressively reduced until tachycardia is initiated or the refractory period is reached. If tachycardia has not been induced the whole process is then repeated with the drive-train (S1) shortened to a cycle length of 400 ms. Some only use this faster drive-train.

If monomorphic ventricular tachycardia is induced it can normally be terminated by a burst of rapid pacing, but sometimes cardioversion is required. Non-sustained tachycardia, or ventricular fibrillation initiated by a very aggressive stimulation protocol, is not of diagnostic significance.

The value of a ventricular stimulation study in dilated cardiomyopathy is less than for myocardial damage caused by coronary artery disease.

Signal-averaged electrocardiography

Late potentials are low-voltage, high-frequency signals in the terminal portion of the QRS complex. They indicate an area of delayed myocardial activation and are commonly found in patients subject to ventricular tachycardia caused by a re-entrant mechanism. They are demonstrated by signal-averaged electrocardiography. The ECG is recorded with an orthogonal system, i.e. leads are placed in the fourth intercostal space in both mid-axillary lines, on the front (lead V2 position) and back of the chest, and top and bottom of the sternum. Computerised signal averaging and appropriate filtering of a series of QRS complexes eliminate both electrical noise, which is random, and the main part of the QRS complex, and thereby demonstrate late potentials (Figure 12.6).

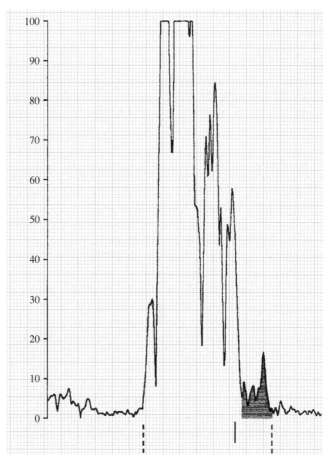

Figure 12.6 Signal-averaged ECG. Shaded area indicates late potential. Filtered QRS = 167 ms; root mean square of terminal 40 ms = 7 μV; duration of high-frequency, low-amplitude signals < 40 μV = 48 ms.

Widely used criteria for presence of late potentials are the presence of two of the following three:

1. Filtered QRS duration > 110 ms
2. Root mean square of last 40 ms of QRS complex < 25 μV
3. Duration of terminal portion of QRS complex which is less than 40 μV > 32 ms

---

Late potentials indicate the presence of the substrate for ventricular tachycardia (i.e. an area of slowed conduction), not that spontaneous ventricular tachycardia will necessarily occur. In patients who present with ventricular tachycardia, late potentials show that the arrhythmia should be inducible at electrophysiological study. Late potentials after myocardial infarction point to a poor prognosis, particularly where there is evidence of extensive myocardial damage.

In practice, the commonest indication for signal-averaged electrocardiography is in the investigation of suspected arrhythmogenic right ventricular cardiomyopathy (see below).

Treatment

Choice of treatment depends on what symptoms or haemodynamic disturbance the arrhythmia causes, whether the arrhythmia is likely to recur, and the prognosis.

Termination of tachycardia
Options include cardioversion, drugs and overdrive pacing.

Cardioversion
If sustained ventricular tachycardia causes cardiac arrest or hypotension, immediate cardioversion is necessary (Chapter 21). Cardioversion should also be undertaken if antiarrhythmic drugs are ineffective, contraindicated or cause haemodynamic deterioration without restoring normal rhythm.

Antiarrhythmic drugs
Lignocaine is a first-line drug to stop ventricular tachycardia, particularly following acute myocardial infarction, because it is unlikely to cause hypotension. Other drugs that are commonly used are sotalol, disopyramide and flecainide. These are negatively inotropic (i.e. they can reduce the force of myocardial contraction) and are best avoided in patients with heart failure or in those known to have extensive myocardial damage. In general, no more than two drugs should be given before considering alternative methods of arrhythmia termination.

Amiodarone is a very useful second-line drug. It does not have a significant negative inotropic action and is extremely effective. However, it seldom works 'at the end of a needle' and can sometimes take up to 24 hours to act. If ventricular tachycardia keeps recurring it may be worth using amiodarone despite its delayed action rather than risking the complications associated with other less effective drugs, even if cardioversion or pacing is required while amiodarone is taking effect.

Though verapamil is effective in controlling supraventricular tachycardia it is, except for fascicular and right ventricular outflow tract tachycardias, useless in ventricular tachycardia and may cause severe hypotension. *It is dangerous practice to use verapamil as a therapeutic test* to ascertain the origin of a tachycardia with broad QRS complexes.

In contrast to most ventricular tachycardias, both fascicular and right ventricular outflow tract tachycardia may be terminated by verapamil, and the latter arrhythmia may also respond to adenosine.

Pacing
Pacing can sometimes be successful in terminating ventricular tachycardia (Figure 12.7). It should be considered when drugs are ineffective, when frequently recurrent tachycardia necessitates multiple cardioversions, or when a temporary pacing wire is already in place for treatment of a bradycardia.

The usual method is overdrive right ventricular pacing. A burst for a couple of seconds at a rate 10–20% in excess of that of the tachycardia will often terminate the arrhythmia. However, there is a significant risk of accelerating the tachycardia or precipitating ventricular fibrillation, in which case immediate cardioversion will be necessary.

Many patients who present with ventricular tachycardia who have poor left ventricular function or a specific form of cardiomyopathy are candidates for an implantable defibrillator (Chapter 24) that provides an automatic antitachycardia pacing facility.

Prevention of recurrence of ventricular tachycardia
Intravenous drugs
Blood levels of most antiarrhythmic drugs fall rapidly after a single bolus. After a bolus has restored sinus rhythm it is usual to give a continuous infusion of the drug. This makes sense if ventricular tachycardia is expected to recur within a short period, e.g. after acute myocardial infarction. However, it is pointless to set up an infusion if either the bolus has failed or the tachycardia is known to occur infrequently.

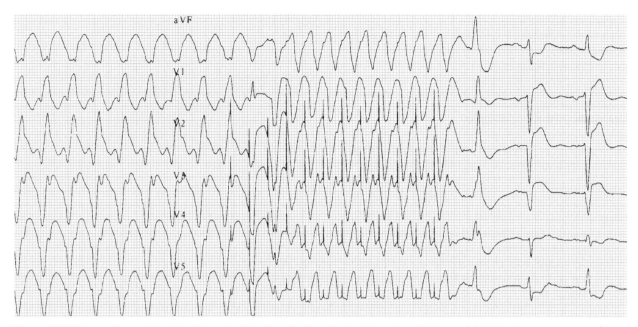

Figure 12.7 Monomorphic ventricular tachycardia terminated by a burst of rapid ventricular pacing: pacing spikes best seen in leads V3 and V4.

Oral drugs

Unless ventricular tachycardia occurs during acute myocardial infarction or other acute event, recurrence is likely and long-term therapy may be required. In patients with poor ventricular function, many antiarrhythmic drugs are negatively inotropic, i.e. they may worsen ventricular function, and they can be 'proarrhythmic', i.e. they may aggravate arrhythmias (Chapter 19). Amiodarone can be given to patients with poor ventricular function and is by far the most effective drug. However, it can cause a number of unwanted effects. In patients who are at high risk from further arrhythmias it is reasonable to use amiodarone and consider alternatives if major side effects occur. Though it may suppress some arrhythmias it has not been shown to improve a patient's prognosis: hence the role of the implantable defibrillator, whose functions and indications are discussed in Chapter 24. Sotalol has been shown to be effective in some patients and in one major study of antiarrhythmic efficacy was more effective than mexiletine, pirmenol, procainamide and propafenone. When ventricular tachycardia has occurred during exertion a beta-blocker is indicated.

Catheter ablation

Delivery of radiofrequency energy via a catheter electrode to the site of origin of tachycardia is very effective in right ventricular outflow tract and fascicular tachycardias.

Only modest rates of success have been achieved in patients with ventricular tachycardia caused by arrhythmogenic right ventricular cardiomyopathy and coronary heart disease.

Surgery

There are several surgical techniques that involve the excision or isolation of the arrhythmia focus. However, potential candidates for surgery often have impaired myocardial function. Cardiopulmonary bypass surgery carries a substantial risk when myocardial function is poor since ventriculotomy may worsen function. Only a few cardiac centres routinely perform surgery for ventricular tachycardia.

There are reports that myocardial revascularisation alone may reduce the incidence of ventricular arrhythmias in some patients with coronary heart disease.

Occasionally, life-threatening, resistant ventricular arrhythmias are an indication for cardiac transplantation.

Coronary heart disease

The commonest cause of ventricular tachycardia, by far, is myocardial damage resulting from infarction. Ventricular tachycardia can occur days, weeks or even years after myocardial infarction. The worse the ventricular function the more susceptible the patient is to this arrhythmia. Usually, ventricular tachycardia occurs in patients whose left ventricular ejection fraction is less than 40% (the normal value is ≥ 60%, not 100%, as is incorrectly assumed by some patients). The lower the ejection fraction below this level the worse is the prognosis.

Acute myocardial infarction can cause ventricular tachycardia. Ventricular tachycardia that occurs within 24–48 hours of acute myocardial infarction is unlikely to recur (Chapter 18.)

Hypertrophic cardiomyopathy

This is a genetically determined disorder of heart muscle that is therefore usually inherited (several dominant gene abnormalities can cause hypertrophic cardiomyopathy) but can arise sporadically as a result of mutation (Figure 12.5). It has been estimated that 1 in 500 of the population is affected. Often the disorder will not cause symptoms or affect prognosis, but heart failure and sudden death can result. Some people can inherit and transmit a genetic abnormality but have no cardiac manifestation of the disorder. It can cause sustained and non-sustained ventricular tachycardia, and sudden death may be the first manifestation of the condition. The annual incidence of sudden death, usually due to ventricular tachycardia or ventricular fibrillation, is reported as 1%. Hypertrophic cardiomyopathy is the commonest cause of sudden death in athletes.

Aborted sudden cardiac death, i.e. successful resuscitation from ventricular tachycardia or fibrillation, and sustained ventricular tachycardia are indications for an implantable defibrillator. Antiarrhythmic therapy, namely amiodarone and beta-blockers, offer little or no improvement in prognosis.

The identification of patients with hypertrophic cardiomyopathy who are at high risk of sudden death and who would therefore benefit from an implantable defibrillator is not a precise science. A number of factors have been identified which are associated with higher risk, as shown in the table.

Hypertrophic cardiomyopathy risk factors

1. Aborted sudden cardiac death
2. Family history of premature sudden cardiac death
3. Left ventricular wall thickness > 30 mm
4. Impaired blood pressure response to exercise testing
5. Unexplained syncope
6. Non-sustained ventricular tachycardia during ambulatory electrocardiography or exercise testing (The literature is inconsistent as to the significance of this rhythm disturbance, particularly if it is brief and infrequent or in older patients)

There is general agreement that the greater the number of clinical risk factors a patient has, the higher the risk of sudden cardiac death. Conversely, *absence of all of the risk factors has a strong negative predictive value, i.e. the patient is at low risk of sudden cardiac death*. Some recommend defibrillator implantation if there is a single risk factor present.

Arrhythmogenic right ventricular cardiomyopathy

Arrhythmogenic right ventricular cardiomyopathy (ARVC) is caused by fatty and/or fibrous infiltration of the right ventricle. Sometimes only localised areas of the ventricle are affected. Impaired function can be demonstrated by magnetic resonance imaging, angiography and sometimes echocardiography. There may be some left ventricular impairment, but it will be less marked than right ventricular dysfunction.

ARVC is the result of inheritance of an autosomal dominant gene. Thus females and males are equally likely to inherit the abnormal gene but males are more commonly affected by its clinical manifestations: ventricular arrhythmias and sometimes heart failure. There is often but not always a family history. Genetic testing is of limited availability, and because a number of mutations can cause ARVC, negative testing does not exclude the condition. Approximately 1 in 2000 of the population is affected.

Typically, during sinus rhythm there is T wave inversion in leads V1–V3 (Figure 12.8a): the QRS duration in these leads is often slightly increased. Because ventricular tachycardia arises from the right ventricle, it has a left bundle branch block morphology (Figure 12.8b,12.9).

An epsilon wave is often present (Figure 12.10). This is a *low-amplitude* wave seen in the terminal portion of the QRS complex in leads V1 and sometimes V2. It represents an area of delayed right ventricular activation and is the surface ECG manifestation of a late potential detected by signal-averaged electrocardiography.

(a)

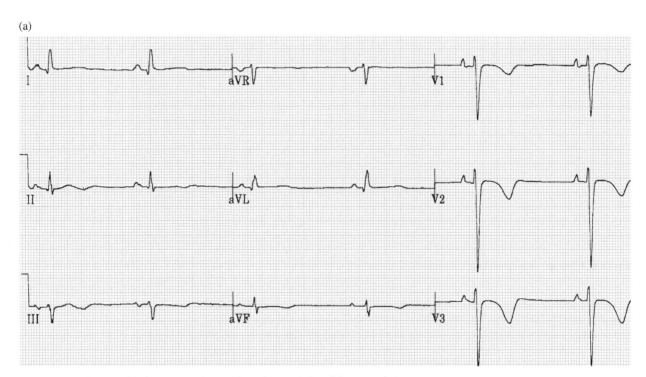

Figure 12.8 (a) Patient with arrhythmogenic right ventricular cardiomyopathy (ARVC) during sinus rhythm.

(b)

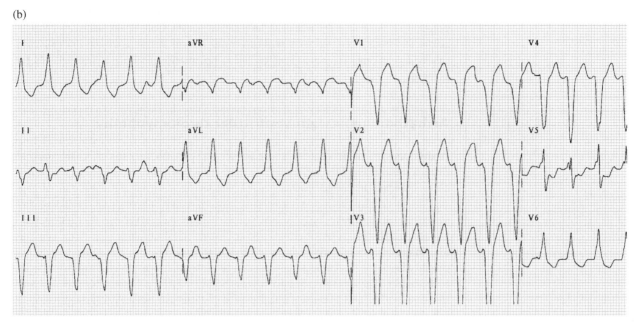

Figure 12.8 (b) Ventricular tachycardia caused by ARVC. The QRS complexes have a left bundle branch block configuration. From the same patient as in Figure 12.8a.

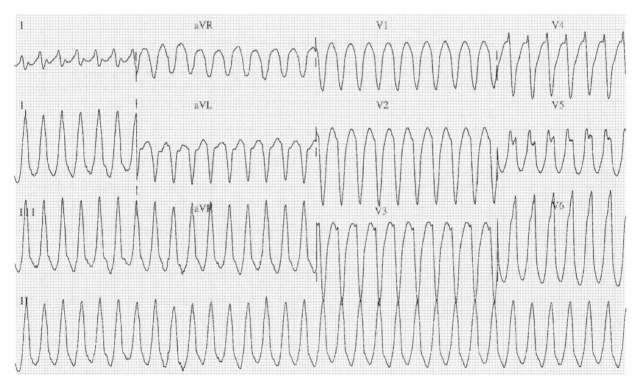

Figure 12.9 Very rapid ventricular tachycardia due to ARVC.

Patients usually present between the ages of 20 and 50 years with palpitation, syncope or near-syncope. Often the arrhythmia is provoked by effort. The disease is progressive and as time goes by lesser degrees of exertion may precipitate ventricular tachycardia. At the time when a patient first presents with ventricular tachycardia, evidence of ventricular dysfunction may not be pronounced. Sudden death can occur and may be the first manifestation of this disorder.

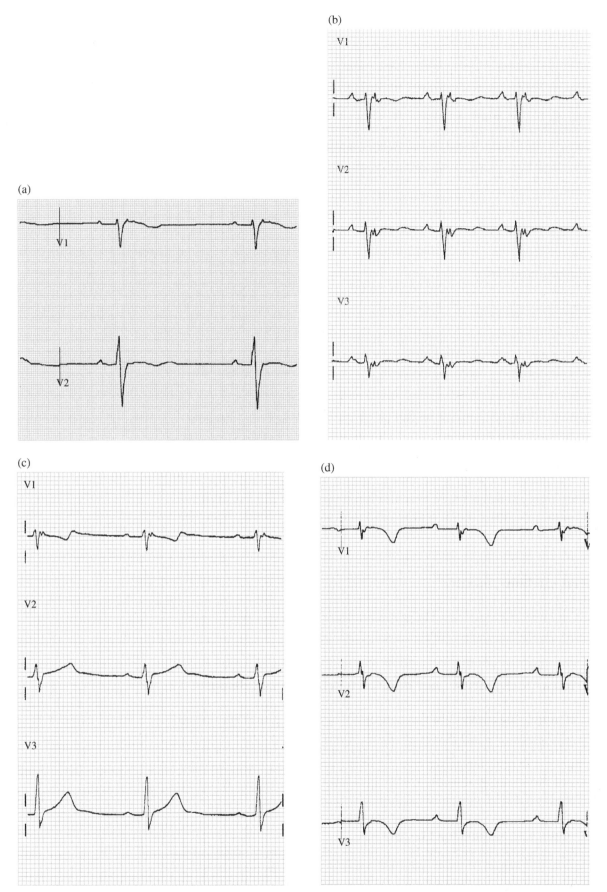

Figure 12.10 (a–d) Patients with ARVC. Epsilon waves, i.e. small deflections in the terminal portion of lead V1, are present. Close inspection of lead V1 is required to identify an epsilon wave.

Recently, a task force has compiled a complex list of major and minor criteria for the diagnosis of ARVC based on imaging, electrocardiography, histology and family history. Major criteria include changes indicating marked right ventricular dysfunction on imaging, T wave inversion in leads V1–V3 (if patient > 14 years old), an epsilon wave, ventricular tachycardia with left bundle branch block morphology and a family history. Minor criteria include minor right ventricular imaging abnormalities, T wave inversion in V1–V2 only, a late potential on signal averaging, and non-sustained ventricular tachycardia or frequent ventricular ectopic beat. The diagnosis is confirmed if there are two major, or one major and two minor, criteria. It should be appreciated that at first clinical presentation it may only be possible to suspect the diagnosis, confirmation coming as the disorder progresses.

Major criteria for ARVC

Marked right ventricular dysfunction on imaging
T wave inversion in leads V1–V3
An epsilon wave
Ventricular tachycardia with left bundle branch block morphology
A family history

Patients should avoid severe exertion and competitive sporting activities. Beta-blockers and/or amiodarone are often effective in preventing ventricular tachycardia. Because of the significant risk and the progressive nature of the disease the implantation of an automatic cardioverter defibrillator should be considered in patients presenting with sustained ventricular tachycardia, syncope, severe right ventricular dilatation or dysfunction or, of course, aborted sudden cardiac death. A family history of sudden cardiac death is not a strong predictor of risk. Exceptionally, cardiac transplantation may be required if ventricular arrhythmias cannot be controlled.

Dilated cardiomyopathy

Dilated cardiomyopathy, which can be genetically determined or acquired, is a common cause of ventricular tachycardia.

Ventricular tachycardias not due to structural heart disease

There are two important ventricular tachycardias that can arise in structurally normal hearts. The more common one arises from the right ventricle, and the other from the left ventricle. Recognition is important because they are associated with a good prognosis, their typical ECG configurations point strongly to the heart being structurally normal, and they are easily amenable to radiofrequency ablation if required for symptomatic purposes (Chapter 25).

Right ventricular outflow tract tachycardia
This tachycardia has a characteristic ECG appearance that reflects its origin in the right ventricular outflow tract, just below the pulmonary valve. Because it arises in the right ventricle the complexes are similar to those seen during left bundle branch block, and because the impulse spreads inferiorly from beneath the pulmonary valve there is an inferior frontal QRS axis, i.e. right axis deviation (Figure 12.11). The origin

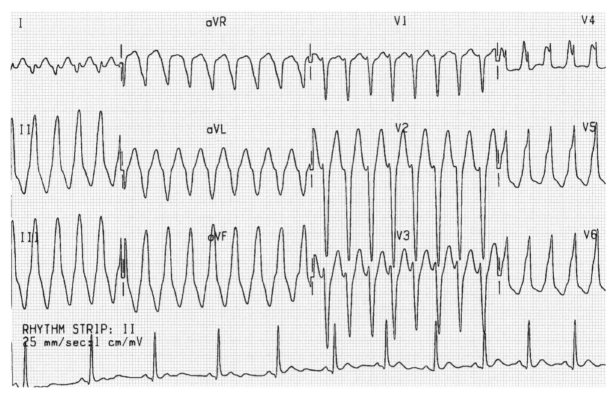

Figure 12.11 Right ventricular outflow tract tachycardia. There is an inferior axis and left bundle branch block configuration. Sinus rhythm returns as the rhythm strip (lead II) is recorded.

of this arrhythmia is fairly close to the AV junction and hence QRS duration is relatively narrow.

There are two types of clinical presentation. Either the tachycardia is paroxysmal and is provoked by effort, or it occurs at rest and is repetitive and non-sustained. In contrast to most ventricular tachycardias, it may be terminated by adenosine and verapamil.

In some patients, frequent ectopic beats rather than tachycardia arise from the right ventricular outflow tract, termed right ventricular outflow tract ectopia (Figure 12.12).

Rarely, a similar tachycardia arises from the left ventricular outflow tract. In contrast to right ventricular outflow tract tachycardia, complexes in leads V1–V3 are usually positive (Figure 12.13).

Some patients have been found to be prone to both right ventricular outflow tract and AV junctional re-entrant tachycardias (Figure 12.14).

Fascicular tachycardia

Fascicular tachycardia is an uncommon arrhythmia which arises from the posterior fascicle or, more rarely, from the anterior fascicle of the left bundle branch.

A posterior fascicular origin results in ventricular complexes during tachycardia with a right bundle branch block and left axis configuration (Figure 12.15), while an anterior fascicular origin leads to right bundle branch block with right axis deviation.

Because the origin is within the specialised conducting system the ventricular complexes are of relatively short duration (0.12 s), and *the arrhythmia is often misdiagnosed as supraventricular tachycardia*. The right bundle branch configuration may be atypical, for example there is a small q wave rather than a primary r wave.

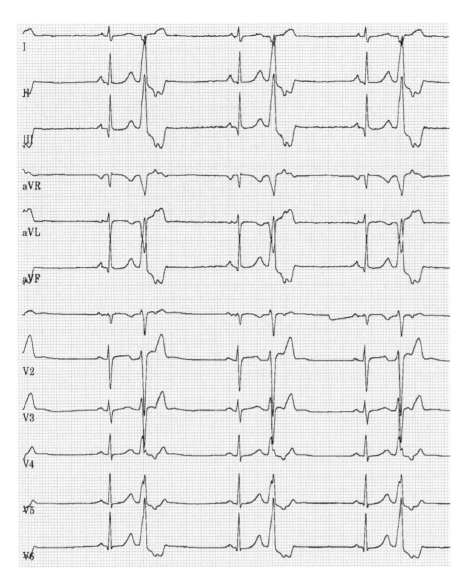

Figure 12.12 Ventricular bigeminy arising from right ventricular outflow tract.

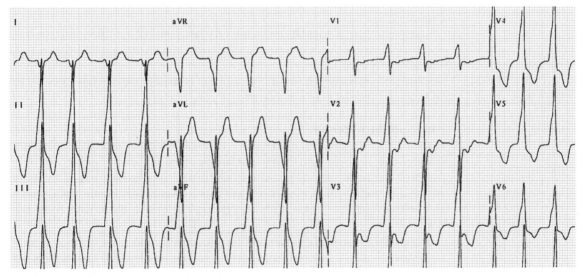

Figure 12.13 Left ventricular outflow tract tachycardia.

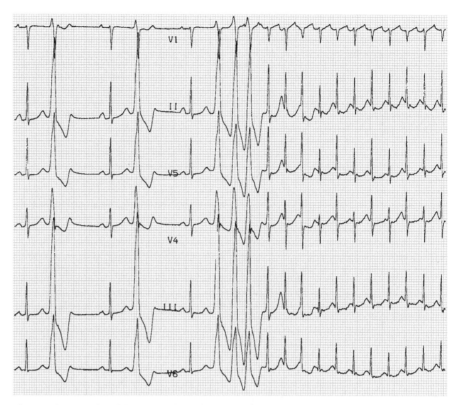

Figure 12.14 Single and then triplet of right ventricular outflow tract ectopic beats, following which AV re-entrant tachycardia is initiated.

(a)

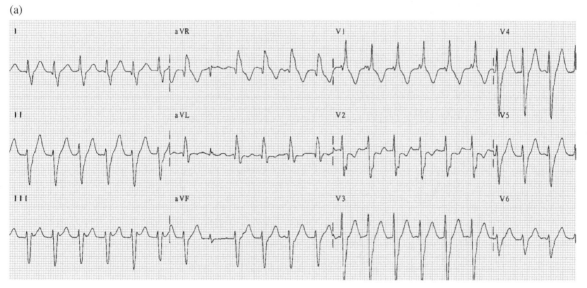

Figure 12.15 (a) Fascicular tachycardia arising from the posterior fascicle. The complexes have a left axis and right bundle branch block configuration. The eighth complex is a capture beat.

(b)

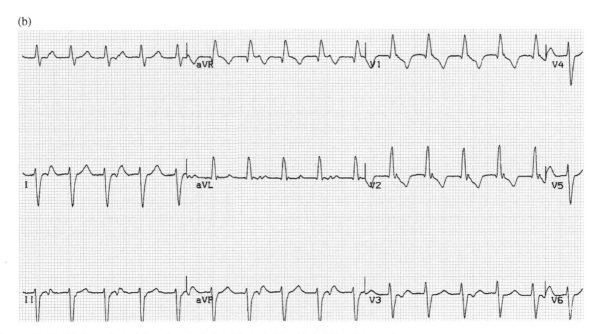

Figure 12.15 (b) Left posterior fascicular tachycardia. In the inferior leads, 2:1 ventriculoatrial condction can be seen.

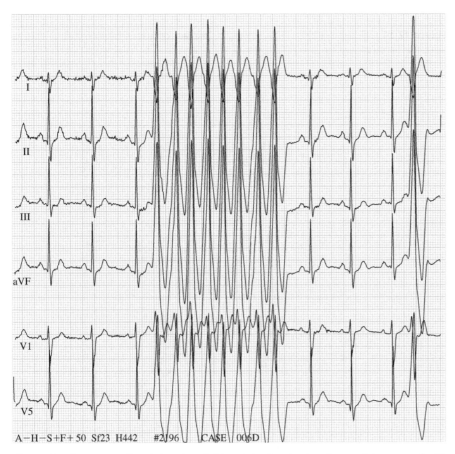

A–H–S+F+ 50 Sf23 H442   #2J96   CASE 006D

Figure 12.16 Non-sustained ventricular tachycardia followed after three sinus beats by a ventricular extrasystole with the same configuration.

Like right ventricular outflow tract tachycardia, it can be terminated by verapamil (but not adenosine).

Non-sustained ventricular tachycardia

Non-sustained ventricular tachycardia is defined as three or more ventricular ectopic beats in succession at a rate in excess of 120 beats/min with return to normal rhythm within 30 s (Figure 12.16).

It rarely causes symptoms but it may be of prognostic significance. Many but not all studies have shown that patients with non-sustained ventricular tachycardia who have suffered a myocardial infarction and who have a left ventricular ejection fraction of less than 40% have a marked increased risk of death either from ventricular arrhythmia or from heart failure. In dilated cardiomyopathy, there is a slight increase in risk of sudden death in those with non-sustained ventricular tachycardia. The arrhythmia is associated with a significant increased risk in symptomatic patients with hypertrophic cardiomyopathy.

Rarely, non-sustained ventricular tachycardia occurs in subjects without structural heart disease and is not indicative of risk.

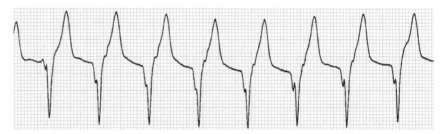

Figure 12.17 Accelerated idioventricular rhythm.

Accelerated idioventricular rhythm

Monomorphic ventricular tachycardia with a rate less than 120 beats/min is termed accelerated idioventricular rhythm or slow ventricular tachycardia (Figure 12.17). Acute myocardial infarction is the most common cause; treatment is unnecessary.

13

Polymorphic Ventricular Tachycardia and Ventricular Fibrillation

Polymorphic ventricular tachycardia is characterised by repeated, progressive changes in the direction and amplitude of ventricular complexes so that they appear to 'twist' about the baseline.

'Torsade de pointes' tachycardia refers to polymorphic tachycardia when there is QT prolongation preceding the arrhythmia: correction of or treatment directed at the cause of QT prolongation is required, rather than antiarrhythmics. Causes of torsade de pointes include bradycardia; drugs (e.g. erythromycin and the antipsychotics) which prolong the QT interval; and the hereditary long QT syndromes. The hereditary long QT syndromes can cause syncope and sudden death: treatment is with beta-blockers and/or an implantable defibrillator.

The Brugada syndrome is a genetic disorder characterised by downsloping ST elevation in the right precordial leads, and it may cause ventricular fibrillation. Catecholaminergic polymorphic ventricular tachycardia (CPVT) is a rare, genetically determined condition, in which polymorphic or bidirectional ventricular tachycardia can be induced by exercise, requiring beta-blockers and/or an implantable defibrillator.

Polymorphic ventricular tachycardia

Whereas monomorphic ventricular tachycardia consists of a rapid succession of ventricular ectopic beats each with the same configuration, polymorphic tachycardia is characterised by repeated progressive changes in the direction and amplitude of ventricular complexes so that they appear to 'twist' about the baseline (Figure 13.1). It may result from myocardial infarction or from cardiomyopathy. In these situations the QT interval during sinus rhythm is normal, and the management of the arrhythmia is the same as for monomorphic ventricular tachycardia.

QT interval
The QT interval is a measure of the duration of the process of ventricular depolarisation and subsequent repolarisation. It is measured from the onset of the QRS complex to the end of the T wave.

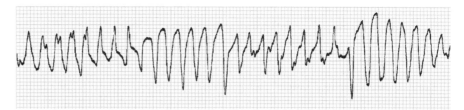

Figure 13.1 Polymorphic ventricular tachycardia.

Normally the QT interval shortens with increasing heart rate, partly due to the increase in rate itself and partly due to the increase in sympathetic nervous system activity which causes sinus tachycardia. When measuring the QT interval it is therefore necessary to correct the measured interval for heart rate. The corrected QT interval (QTc) is calculated by selecting the ECG lead showing the longest QT interval (usually measurements are made from lead II and V5), and then dividing the square root of the cycle length into the measured QT interval (Bazett's formula). For example, a patient with a measured QT interval of 0.38s at a heart rate of 60 beats/min has a cycle length of 1.0s and therefore also has a QTc of 0.38s, whereas with a QT interval of 0.38s at a heart rate of 120 beats/min (cycle length=0.5s), the QTc is prolonged at 0.54s. The normal QTc does not exceed 0.43s in males and 0.45s in females.

Always consider QT prolongation if the end of the T wave approaches the midpoint between QRS complexes.

$$\text{Bazett's formula: QTc(s)} = \text{QT(s)}/\sqrt{\text{R-R interval(s)}}$$

Causes of QT prolongation include the hereditary long QT syndromes, hypocalcaemia, hypothyroidism, a number of drugs, myocardial ischaemia and subarachnoid haemorrhage.

Torsade de pointes tachycardia

'Torsade de pointes' is the term applied to polymorphic ventricular tachycardia *when the QT interval is prolonged preceding the onset of the arrhythmia* (Figures 13.2, 13.3). Recognition is important, because correction of or treatment directed at the QT prolongation is required rather than antiarrhythmic drugs, which may aggravate the

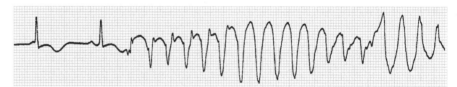

Figure 13.2 Torsade de pointes tachycardia preceded by prolonged QT interval.

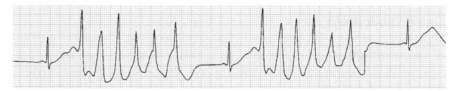

Figure 13.3 Two brief episodes of torsade de pointes tachycardia during sinus bradycardia; there is marked QT prolongation preceding the arrhythmia.

> ## Causes of QT prolongation and torsade de pointes tachycardia
>
> Hereditary prolongation of the QT interval
> Bradycardia due to sinus node dysfunction or atrioventricular block
> Hypocalcaemia, hypomagnesaemia, hypothyroidism
> Antiarrhythmic drugs, e.g. quinidine, disopyramide, procainamide, sotalol, amiodarone, ibutilide, dofetilide, dronedarone
> Antimicrobials, e.g. erythromycin, clarithromycin, ciprofloxacin, fluconazole, ketoconazole, chloroquine, pentamidine
> Psychiatric drugs, e.g. thioridazine, chlorpromazine, pimozide, haloperidol, droperidol, tricyclic antidepressants, methadone, citaloprolam
> Other drugs: prenylamine, bepridil, cisapride, terfenadine, probucol, domperidone, tamoxifen, ondansetron
> Anorexia nervosa

(a)

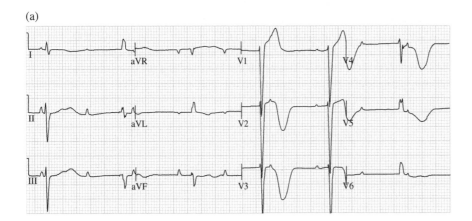

(b)

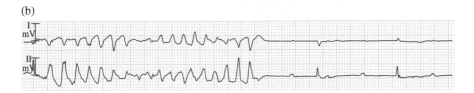

Figure 13.4 Complete AV block leading to (a) a very long QT interval, with (b) episodes of torsade de pointes tachycardia.

tachycardia. Typically the arrhythmia is non-sustained and repetitive, but it can deteriorate to ventricular fibrillation. Onset usually follows a pause in rhythm caused by bradycardia or following an ectopic beat.

Torsade de pointes tachycardia can be caused by disorders that lead to abnormal ventricular repolarisation, by bradycardia (Figure 13.4), or by drugs.

Antipsychotic drugs

Antipsychotic drugs are an important cause of QT prolongation and torsade de pointes tachycardia (Figure 13.5). In a large study, chlorpromazine, haloperidol, pimozide, and thioridazine were shown to increase the risk of sudden cardiac death threefold; female patients and those who had recently started medication were at highest risk. It is recommended that the QT interval be monitored by carrying out a baseline ECG before antipsychotic therapy and repeating it after a few days and

(a)

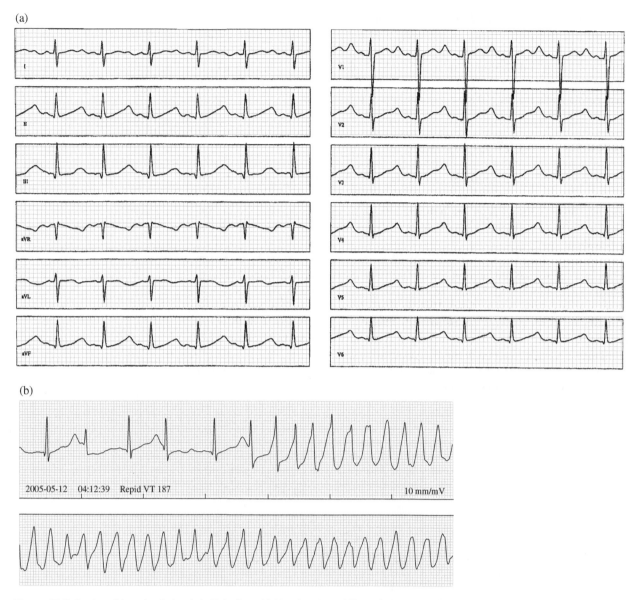

(b)

Figure 13.5 Overdose of the antipsychotic amisulpride leading to (a) QT prolongation and (b) torsade de pointes tachycardia. T wave alternans precedes the arrhythmia.

then every 1–3 months in the early stages of high-dose treatment. Recently, citaloprolam and escitaloprolam have been associated with a dose-dependent QT prolongation: they should be avoided if there is known QT prolongation or hereditary long QT syndrome, or if other drugs that can prolong the QT interval are being prescribed.

Drug interactions

Risk of torsade de pointes may be increased if an interaction between drugs leads to a higher blood level of a potentially proarrhythmic drug. For example, the erythromycins are metabolised by the liver's cytochrome P450 3A enzyme system. Commonly used drugs such as diltiazem and verapamil, as well as a number of antifungal agents, inhibit the enzyme system and have been shown to increase the risk of sudden death when administered together with erythromycin or clarithromycin.

Management of torsade de pointes tachycardia

Treatment consists of reversal of the cause where possible, and cardiac pacing. Intravenous magnesium sulphate may be effective, even when serum magnesium is normal (8 mmol stat; 2.5 mmol/hour infusion). Antiarrhythmic drugs should be stopped: increasing the heart rate to 100 beats/min by pacing will often prevent the tachycardia while the drug(s) are being excreted or metabolised.

Hereditary long QT syndromes

The hereditary long QT syndromes are genetic disorders, with an estimated prevalence of between 1 in 3000 and 1 in 5000, which can cause brief episodes of unconsciousness and sudden death due to torsade de pointes tachycardia or ventricular fibrillation (Figure 13.6). At least 10 types have been described, termed LQT1–10.

LQT1, 2 and 3 are by far the most common forms. They are caused by dominant genes that control the functions of the cardiac cells' potassium (LQT1 and LQT2) or sodium ion channels (LQT3) and are also known as the Romano–Ward syndrome. There is no structural cardiac defect. There is often a family history, but cases can arise by mutation. Some patients can be severely affected and yet others with the same genetic defect can have few or no symptoms and can have a normal ECG (Figure 13.7). Symptoms are most common in childhood and adolescence.

The very rare Jervell and Lange–Nielsen long QT syndrome is due to a recessive gene and is associated with nerve deafness.

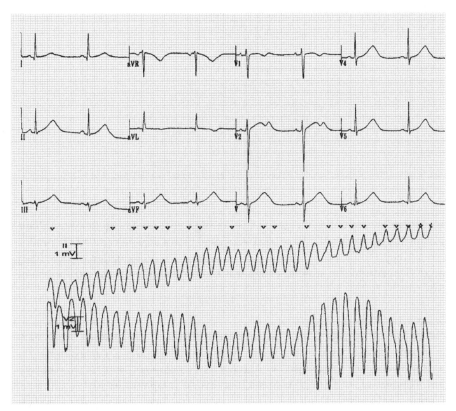

Figure 13.6 Hereditary QT prolongation and resultant torsade de pointes tachycardia. The QT interval is prolonged and the T wave is notched (LQT2 syndrome).

Diagnosis

The clinical diagnosis is based on the ECG: significant prolongation of the QT interval (>450 ms in men, >470 ms in women) and an abnormally shaped T wave. Typically, the T wave is broad in LQT1 syndrome, of low amplitude and notched in LQT2 (Figure 13.6), and has a long isoelectric ST segment in LQT3 syndrome (Figure 13.8). Some patients are prone to marked sinus bradycardia. There may be day-to-day variation in QT duration; it may be normal at times in some patients.

In contrast to normal subjects, the QT interval in patients with long QT syndrome has been shown to lengthen rather than shorten when the sympathetic nervous system is activated by standing or by exercise, and during epinephrine infusion. These

(a)

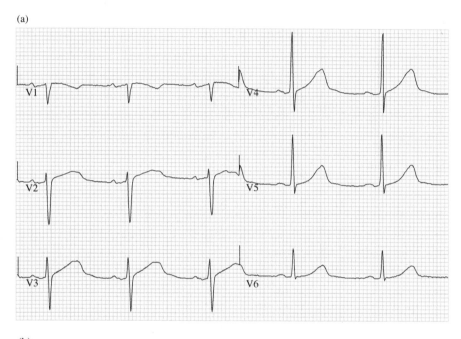

(b)

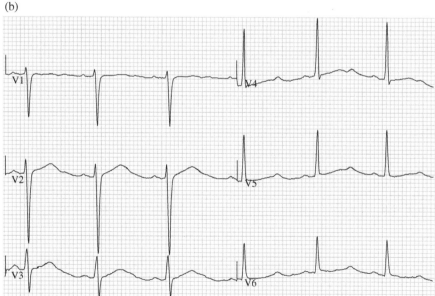

Figure 13.7 Hereditary QT prolongation: ECGs from (a) an asymptomatic father and (b, c) his two highly symptomatic daughters.

(c)

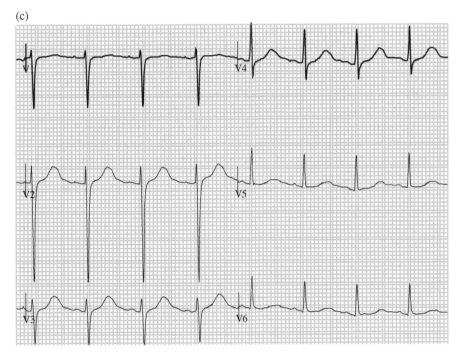

Figure 13.7 (cont'd)

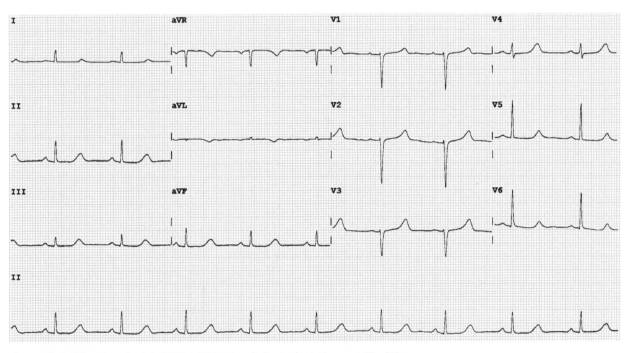

Figure 13.8 LQT3 syndrome. Leads II, AVF, V5 and V6 best show the long isoelectric ST segment. QTc = 510ms.

tests may be useful in confirming the diagnosis in patients with borderline QT prolongation.

Young patients who have experienced collapses due to long QT syndrome are often first referred to a neurologist with a diagnosis of epilepsy: *an ECG is essential in patients presenting with a possible diagnosis of epilepsy.*

First-degree relatives of patients with long QT syndrome should undergo electro-cardiography.

Genetic testing for patients with the long QT syndromes and their relatives is now becoming widely available. Relatives who do carry an abnormal gene but have a normal ECG have been shown to be at an increased risk of sudden cardiac death as compared with relatives who have a normal genetic study.

Arrhythmias

Thirty to forty per cent of patients with hereditary long QT syndrome will experience syncope or cardiac arrest before the age of 40 years, the highest rate being in adolescents. Arrhythmias are usually initiated by exertion (frequently, swimming in LQT1), excitement or fear. Sudden loud auditory stimuli, such as the ringing of a telephone, are also recognised as a common trigger for rhythm disturbances (typically in LQT2 but also in LQT1). In the LQT3 syndrome arrhythmias usually occur during sleep. Males who reach adulthood without an arrhythmia are unlikely to experience one thereafter, whereas females are at risk at least into their fourth decade.

Very marked QT prolongation (QTc ≥ 500 ms), a history of syncope and female gender (LQT1 and LQT2) are associated with a higher risk of death. Arrhythmias are more common at the time of menstruation and in the nine months post partum (particularly LQT2). T wave alternans, i.e. beat-to-beat alteration in T wave direction or amplitude, is also associated with a high risk of arrhythmia (Figure 13.5). It is reported that a family history of sudden cardiac death is not a good guide to a patient's prognosis.

It is likely that patients who develop torsade de pointes tachycardia as a result of a drug or bradycardia have the same genetic abnormalities of cardiac ion channels that cause the congenital long QT syndromes but in a subclinical form. Females are more susceptible.

Treatment

Beta-blockade is effective in 70% of patients. Long-acting drugs should be used: nadolol (80–160 mg daily) has a very long half-life. An implantable defibrillator should be considered in symptomatic patients, especially survivors of cardiac arrest. Asymptomatic patients who are young should receive a beta-blocker. Cardiac pacing in addition to beta-blockers should be considered in those patients with marked bradycardia prior to or because of beta-blockers. Left cervical sympathectomy is occasionally undertaken: it has been shown to reduce but not abolish risk where beta-blockade has failed.

Patients should be advised to avoid highly strenuous activities and, if possible, drugs that may enhance sympathetic nervous system activity, such as decongestants, midodrine, bronchodilators and fenfluramine. *It is very important that they avoid drugs that are recognised to prolong the QT interval*, such as those listed above.

Recently, it has been shown that asymptomatic members of families with long QT syndrome who have a normal QT interval but do have a genetic abnormality are at increased risk of sudden death as compared with the general population. Apparently unaffected family members of patients with a long QT syndrome should, therefore, be advised to follow the same precautions as those with overt long QT syndrome unless genetic testing has been shown no abnormality.

LQT3 is due to a defect in sodium rather than potassium ion transport, and there are reports that flecainide will normalise the ECG and may prevent arrhythmias.

Hereditary short QT syndrome

A rare hereditary short QT syndrome has recently been described. The QTc interval is less than 320 ms. Sudden cardiac death due to ventricular arrhythmias and also atrial

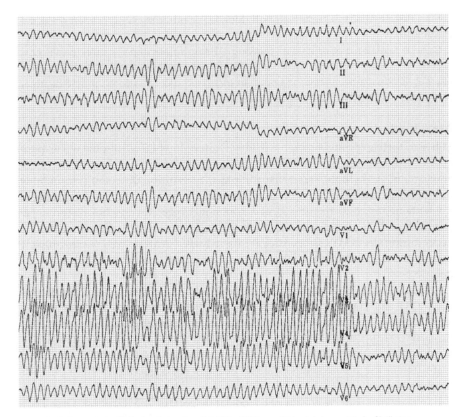

Figure 13.9 Ventricular fibrillation. Unusually, a full 12-lead ECG was obtained during ventricular fibrillation.

fibrillation can occur. It has been suggested that quinidine is effective in prolonging the QT interval and preventing arrhythmias, but implantation of an automatic defibrillator may be necessary.

Ventricular fibrillation

ECG characteristics

Ventricular fibrillation is the very rapid, totally incoordinate contraction of ventricular myocardial fibres. This is reflected in the ECG by irregular, chaotic electrical activity (Figure 13.9). Ventricular fibrillation causes circulatory arrest. Unconsciousness develops within 10–20 s.

Causes

Ninety per cent of deaths caused by acute myocardial infarction are due to ventricular fibrillation. The incidence of fibrillation is highest in the first hour. Ventricular fibrillation can also occur late after infarction and, in patients with severe coronary artery disease, without myocardial infarction. It may be the first clinical manifestation of the disease.

The arrhythmia can result from many other cardiac disorders, such as myocarditis and the cardiomyopathies. It may result from a primary electrical disorder such as the long QT syndromes and the Brugada syndrome (see below).

It is usually initiated by a ventricular ectopic beat but can arise during a pause in cardiac rhythm or result from monomorphic or polymorphic ventricular tachycardia.

Treatment

Very rarely, ventricular fibrillation is a brief event, spontaneously reverting to normal rhythm. Otherwise, without prompt defibrillation, irreversible cerebral and myocardial damage will result.

Recurrent ventricular fibrillation

Acutely, intravenous lignocaine or amiodarone as well as correction of the cause, if possible, may be required. Addition of a beta-blocker can often be effective. Longer-term management is discussed in Chapter 24.

Brugada syndrome

The syndrome is characterised by a typical ECG pattern of downsloping ST elevation in leads V1, V2 and sometimes V3, usually together with partial right bundle branch block, a structurally normal heart and a risk of sudden death due to ventricular fibrillation, or syncope resulting from polymorphic ventricular tachycardia. The estimated prevalence is 1 in 5000.

Diagnosis

The ventricular complex in leads V1 and V2 usually shows the most typical features (classified as type I): the QRS complex ends with a positive component ≥ 2 mm (akin to the J wave seen in hypothermia), followed by a *downsloping ST segment* and negative T wave (Figures 13.10, 13.11). There may be prolongation of the PR interval, and paroxysmal atrial fibrillation is not uncommon (Figure 13.12). Late potentials are often present (Figure 13.13).

In some individuals, the typical ECG abnormalities may be intermittent: at times the ST segment elevation may have a concave or 'saddle-back' morphology (classified as type II or III), appearances which alone are *not* diagnostic of the Brugada syndrome, or may be normal. ECG recording with the chest leads placed one or two intercostal spaces higher then usual can increase the diagnostic yield and should be considered in patients presenting with unexplained syncope or resuscitated from unexplained ventricular fibrillation. Intravenous ajmaline (1 mg/kg over 5 minutes) or, if not available, flecainide (2 mg/kg over 10 minutes) can be used for diagnostic purposes to induce the typical type I pattern in patients suspected of having Brugada syndrome (Figure 13.14. The abnormal ECG pattern can sometimes be induced or accentuated by fever.

Aetiology

The syndrome is a genetically determined abnormality of a cardiac sodium ion channel: several different genetic abnormalities have been linked to the syndrome. Not all patients give a family history of sudden cardiac death; the condition may arise by mutation.

Ventricular fibrillation

Ventricular fibrillation most commonly occurs in middle life. It is rare in the first two decades of life. It usually occurs during sleep or rest. Though Brugada syndrome is due to an autosomal dominant gene, arrhythmias are markedly more prevalent in males.

No antiarrhythmic drugs have been shown to be effective at preventing ventricular fibrillation, but quinidine has been reported to be effective in patients with an 'arrhythmia storm'. The only treatment is implantation of an automatic defibrillator (Chapter 24). Patients who have experienced syncope or have been resuscitated from ventricular fibrillation should receive such a device.

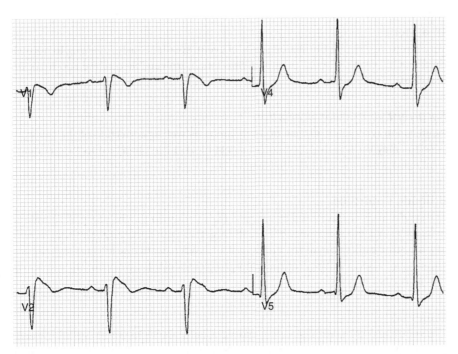

Figure 13.10 Chest leads from a patient with Brugada syndrome resuscitated from ventricular fibrillation that occurred while driving.

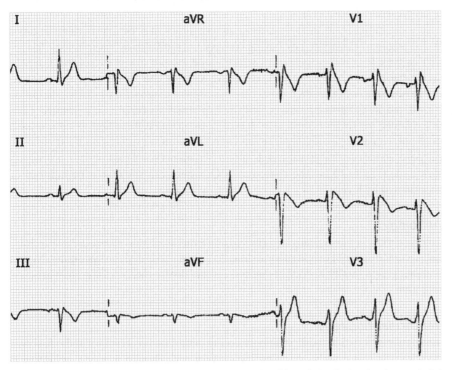

Figure 13.11 Routine ECG showing Brugada syndrome from a member of the medical profession who subsequently died suddenly.

Asymptomatic subjects
Risk factors
Unfortunately reliable criteria are not available to indicate those who are at risk. Studies are limited by relatively small sample size and short follow-up periods, and

marked differences in the incidence of sudden death: some have reported a fairly high incidence of ventricular fibrillation in previously asymptomatic patients, e.g. 8% incidence over a three-year period, whereas others have demonstrated a lower risk, e.g. 2% over five years, 0.5% over 30 months.

A ventricular stimulation study in patients with a type I ECG pattern has been advocated, and implantation of a defibrillator recommended if ventricular fibrillation is initiated (Figure 13.15). However, subsequently a number of studies have not supported the earlier findings.

Late potentials and QRS prolongation have been suggested as possible risk factors, as has augmentation of ST elevation following exercise testing, but a consensus has not been reached. Surprisingly, it seems that a family history of sudden cardiac death is not a risk factor.

(a)

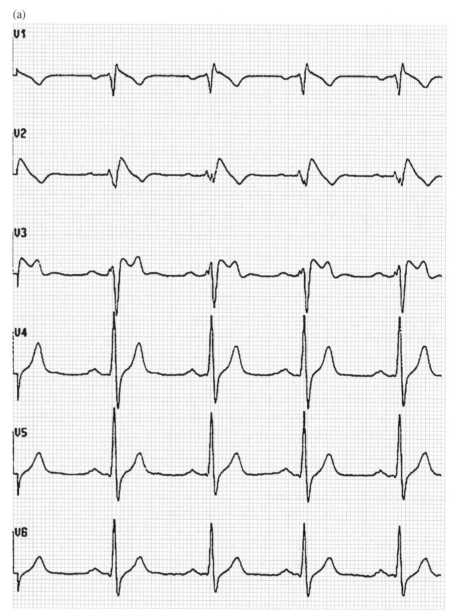

Figure 13.12 Patient with (a) Brugada syndrome who developed (b) atrial fibrillation.

(b)

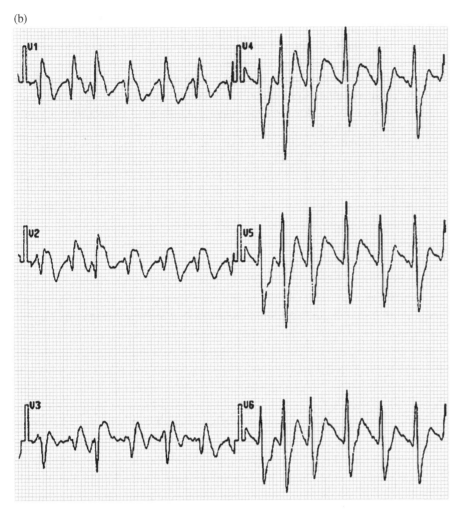

Figure 13.12 (cont'd)

It is generally agreed that patients who do not have a spontaneously abnormal type I ECG are at lower risk.

Management

Routine defibrillator implantation in asymptomatic patients is not warranted in view of the fairly low risk of sudden death and the recognised high complication rate associated with long-term ICD implantation. Recently, it has been suggested that quinidine might be routinely given to asymptomatic patients.

Patients with Brugada syndrome should be advised to avoid class I antiarrhythmic drugs such as flecainide and to seek prompt treatment of any febrile illness.

Early repolarisation syndrome

Early repolarisation, i.e. elevation of the junction between the end of the QRS complex and the beginning of the ST segment (termed the J point) in the inferolateral ECG leads is common, particularly in young men, and has been considered to be innocuous. However, recently J point elevation ≥1 mm, often accompanied by notching on the terminal QRS in the inferolateral ECG leads, has been shown to be associated with a risk of ventricular fibrillation. The absolute risk is low and defibrillator implantation in asymptomatic subjects is not indicated (Figure 13.16).

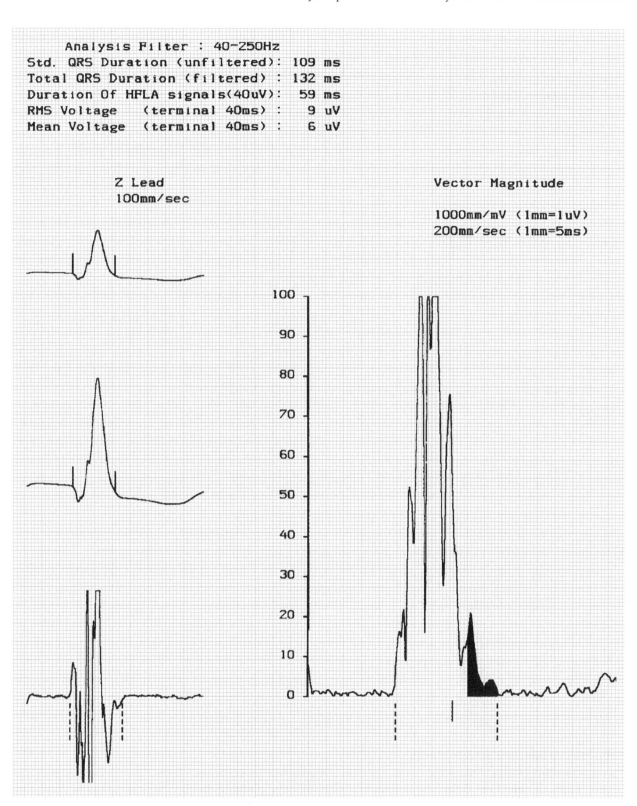

```
Analysis Filter : 40-250Hz
Std. QRS Duration (unfiltered): 109 ms
Total QRS Duration (filtered) : 132 ms
Duration Of HFLA signals(40uV):  59 ms
RMS Voltage   (terminal 40ms) :   9 uV
Mean Voltage  (terminal 40ms) :   6 uV
```

Z Lead
100mm/sec

Vector Magnitude

1000mm/mV (1mm=1uV)
200mm/sec (1mm=5ms)

Figure 13.13 Signal-averaged ECG from patient in Figure 13.10, showing a late potential.

(a)

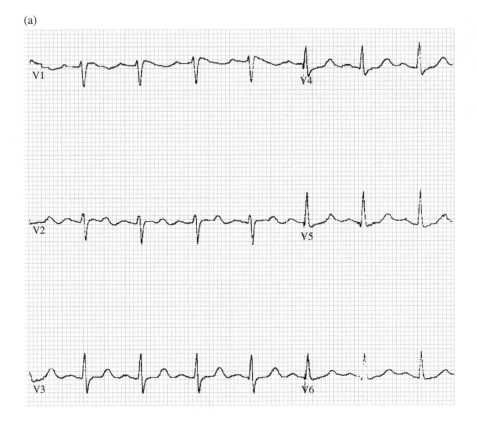

(b)

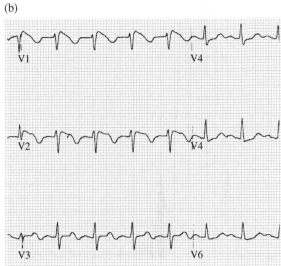

Figure 13.14 (a) Chest leads in a patient with suspected Brugada syndrome. (b) After ajmaline a type I pattern develops.

Bidirectional ventricular tachycardia

This is a rare arrhythmia with two alternating ventricular complex morphologies (Figure 13.17). It cannot be described as either monomorphic or polymorphic! Causes include digoxin toxicity and catecholaminergic polymorphic ventricular tachycardia.

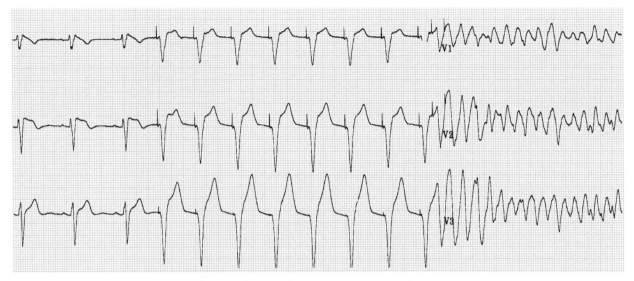

Figure 13.15 Asymptomatic patient with Brugada syndrome (leads V1–V3) who developed ventricular fibrillation during a ventricular stimulation study: after eight paced beats at 120 beats/min a couplet of premature stimuli initiated ventricular fibrillation. (An ICD was implanted and subsequently he received several appropriate shocks.)

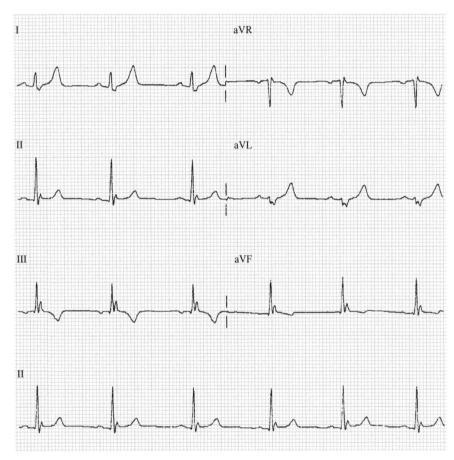

Figure 13.16 ECG (limb leads) showing early repolarisation in inferior leads.

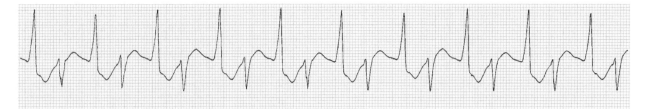

Figure 13.17 Bidirectional ventricular tachycardia.

Catecholaminergic polymorphic ventricular tachycardia (CPVT)

CPVT is a rare, genetically determined condition, affecting cardiac ryanodine receptor calcium release channels, in which polymorphic or bidirectional ventricular tachycardia is induced by exercise or by emotion resulting in syncope or cardiac arrest.

It is due to an autosomal dominant gene. The heart is structurally normal, as is the resting ECG. Ventricular tachycardia can be provoked by exercise testing or by isoprenaline infusion. It is mainly seen in children and young adults. There is a high mortality rate. Beta-blockers are indicated but are not always effective: an implantable defibrillator may be required. Recently, flecainide has been shown to reduce arrhythmias in patients where beta-blockade alone has failed.

14

Tachycardias with Broad Ventricular Complexes

Though bundle branch block can sometimes occur during supraventricular tachycardias and therefore lead to broad ventricular complexes, most broad complex tachycardias are ventricular in origin.

Pointers towards ventricular tachycardia as opposed to supraventricular tachycardia with bundle branch block include the presence of myocardial damage, direct or indirect evidence of independent atrial activity, QRS duration greater than 0.14 s, a concordant pattern in the chest leads, and marked axis deviation. Neither minor irregularities during tachycardia nor the haemodynamic effect of the arrhythmia are useful in ascertaining its origin.

When supraventricular tachycardias are associated with bundle branch block the morphology of the ventricular complexes is usually that of typical left or right bundle branch block. Never use verapamil for a diagnostic test. Wherever possible, record a 12-lead ECG during tachycardia for diagnostic purposes.

Tachycardias of supraventricular origin sometimes result in broad ventricular complexes. Thus they may mimic ventricular tachycardia. Now that this is widely appreciated, the tendency is to misinterpret ventricular tachycardia as supraventricular, rather than the reverse.

Causes of a broad complex tachycardia

Tachycardias with broad ventricular complexes may be due to:
1. ventricular tachycardia;
2. supraventricular tachycardia when bundle branch block has already been present during sinus rhythm;
3. supraventricular tachycardia with rate-related bundle branch block (i.e. bundle branch block develops during tachycardia);
4. Wolff–Parkinson–White syndrome: if atrial impulses during atrial flutter or fibrillation are conducted to the ventricles by the accessory AV pathway, or in the uncommon 'antidromic' form of AV re-entrant tachycardia, when AV conduction is via the accessory pathway.

A number of guides are used to distinguish a supraventricular tachycardia with broad ventricular complexes from ventricular tachycardia.

Useless guidelines

It is often said that whereas ventricular tachycardia leads to major haemodynamic disturbance, supraventricular tachycardia does not. This is wrong. Sometimes ventricular tachycardia causes few or even no symptoms, whereas supraventricular tachycardia, if very fast or in the presence of underlying heart disease, can cause shock or heart failure (Figure 14.1).

Another widely quoted but incorrect rule is that whereas supraventricular tachycardia is regular, ventricular tachycardia is slightly irregular.

Verapamil may terminate supraventricular tachycardia or slow the ventricular response to atrial fibrillation or flutter. It has been used as a 'therapeutic' test of the origin of tachycardia. However, dangerous hypotension may result when the drug is given during ventricular tachycardia. *Never use verapamil to establish the origin of a broad complex tachycardia.*

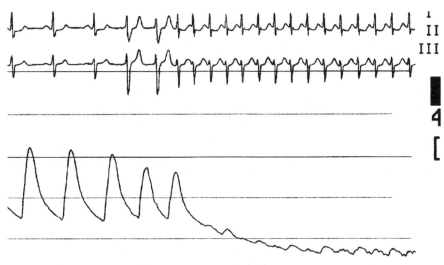

Figure 14.1 Dramatic drop in arterial pressure with onset of AV re-entrant tachycardia.

Useful guidelines

Independent atrial activity

If there is direct or indirect (Figures 12.2, 12.4, 12.10, 14.2, 14.3) evidence of independent atrial activity then supraventricular tachycardia is excluded. As discussed in Chapter 12, scrutiny of several ECG leads may be necessary to identify evidence of atrial activity (Figure 14.4): wherever possible, *a 12-lead ECG during tachycardia should be recorded* (Figure 14.5).

Sometimes, independent atrial activity can only be demonstrated by recording a surface ECG simultaneously with an atrial electrogram acquired via a transvenous lead passed to the right atrium or by an oesophageal electrode positioned behind the left atrium (Figure 14.6). This invasive approach is occasionally required if there is a diagnostic dilemma.

Most implanted pacemakers and defibrillators can facilitate telemetry of the intra-atrial electrogram during a tachycardia.

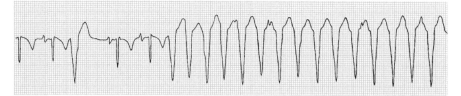

Figure 14.2 The second ventricular ectopic beat initiates ventricular tachycardia. Independent atrial activity can be seen.

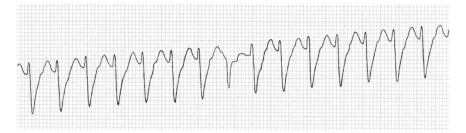

Figure 14.3 Ventricular tachycardia (lead II). The eighth complex is a capture beat.

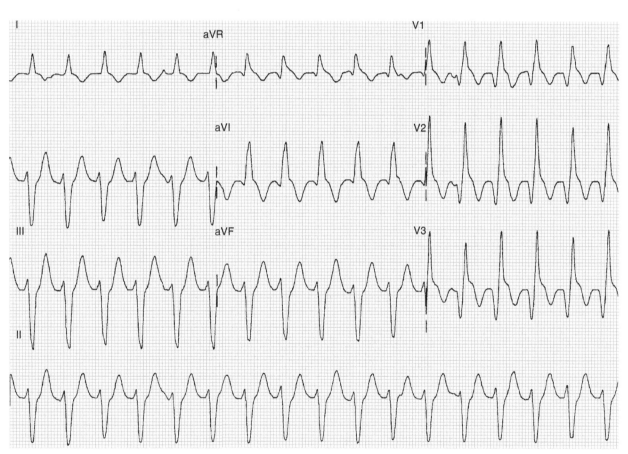

Figure 14.4 Ventricular tachycardia. On close scrutiny, there is evidence of independent atrial activity. In lead I, P waves can be seen on the T wave of the first QRS complex and after the fourth QRS. In lead V1, there is a P wave after the first QRS complex.

Carotid sinus massage

Carotid sinus massage can briefly slow AV node conduction and may thus terminate an AV re-entrant tachycardia, or slow the ventricular rate during atrial flutter or fibrillation, enabling the very rapid atrial activity to be identified.

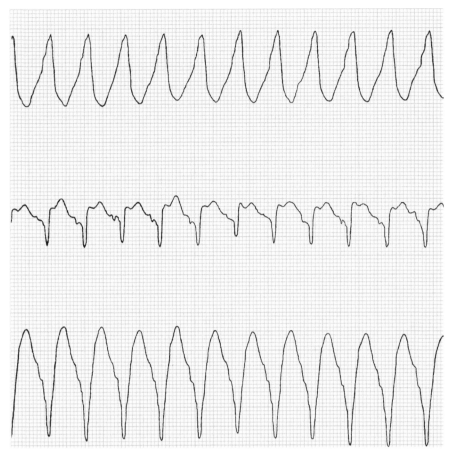

Figure 14.5 Advantage of simultaneous recording of ECG leads (I, II, III). Lead II suggests that there may be a P wave before each QRS complex and thus that the tachycardia is supraventricular rather than ventricular in origin. However, comparison with other leads indicates that the 'P' wave is in fact the initial vector of the ventricular complex.

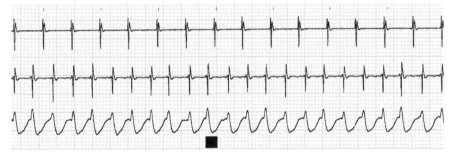

Figure 14.6 Right atrial (upper trace), right ventricular (middle trace) and surface (lower trace) electrograms. Atrial activity is slower than and independent of ventricular activity, confirming ventricular tachycardia.

Carotid sinus massage may not be effective in supraventricular tachycardia, so its failure does not indicate ventricular tachycardia.

Configuration of ventricular complex

The broader the ventricular complex the more likely is a ventricular origin. In ventricular tachycardia, the duration of the ventricular complex is usually 0.14 s or greater.

Marked axis deviation, left or right, also suggests ventricular tachycardia. Another pointer towards this arrhythmia is a 'concordant' pattern in the chest leads, i.e. the complexes are either all positive or all negative (Figures 14.7, 14.8).

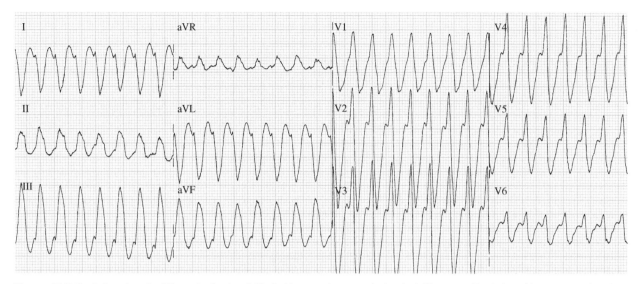

Figure 14.7 Ventricular tachycardia. QRS complex duration = 0.18 s. Positive concordant pattern in chest leads. (The *rare*, antidromic form of AV re-entrant tachycardia in patients with Wolff–Parkinson–White syndrome due to a left-sided accessory pathway can lead to the same positive concordant pattern).

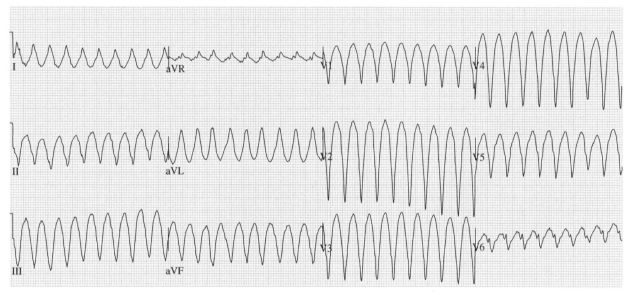

Figure 14.8 QRS complex duration = 0.18 s. Negative concordant pattern in chest leads is diagnostic of ventricular tachycardia.

When supraventricular tachycardias are associated with bundle branch block the morphology of the ventricular complexes is usually that of typical left or right bundle branch block (Figures 14.9, 14.10).

Ectopic beats

If the configuration of the ventricular complex during tachycardia is similar to that of an ectopic beat recorded during normal rhythm, a common origin is probable. It is relatively easy to ascertain the origin of single ectopic beats, especially if a full ECG is available (Figure 14.2).

Adenosine

Adenosine is very effective at terminating supraventricular tachycardia due to an AV junctional re-entrant mechanism, and will transiently slow the ventricular response

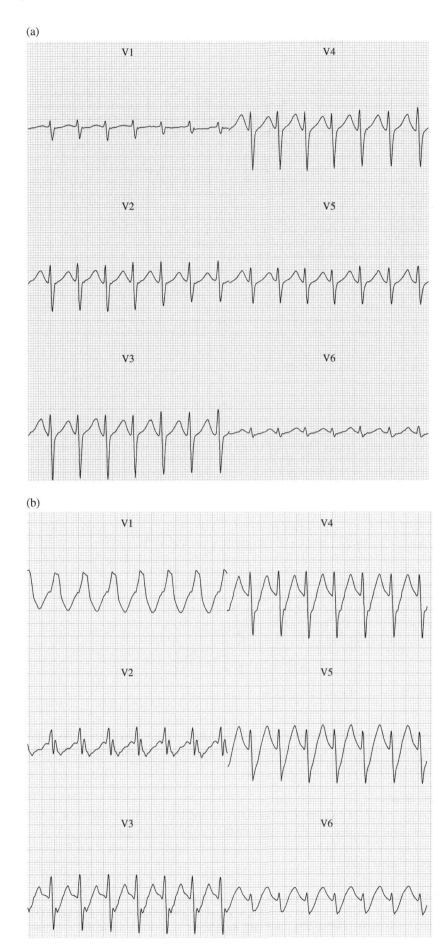

Figure 14.9 AV nodal re-entrant tachycardia recorded during an electrophysiological study. Intraventricular conduction varied from (a) normal to (b) right bundle branch block and (c) left bundle branch block.

(c)

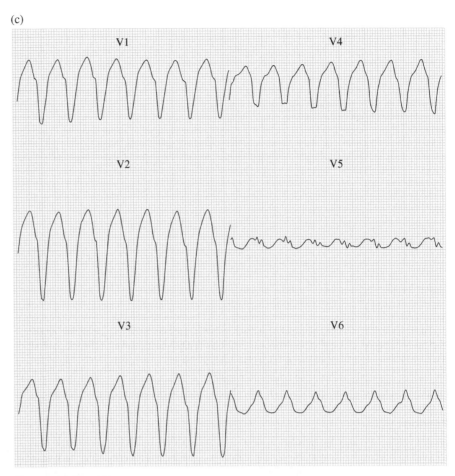

Figure 14.9 (cont'd)

to atrial fibrillation and flutter, making the respective atrial f or F waves easily identifiable for diagnostic purposes. A positive response to adenosine points strongly towards a supraventricular origin to the tachycardia. Because its duration of action is very brief it is a safe drug to give (with the possible exception of patients with asthma).

However, a minority of supraventricular tachycardias will not respond to adenosine, and the drug will terminate right ventricular outflow tract tachycardia. Thus response or lack of response to adenosine is a useful pointer towards the origin of the tachycardia but is not an absolutely reliable guide.

Adenosine is often used in a 'knee-jerk' response to a broad complex tachycardia in patients with known myocardial infarction or cardiomyopathy. Ventricular tachycardia is highly likely, and it is pointless to use adenosine in these situations unless there is a very strong suspicion that the rhythm is atrial flutter or tachycardia with bundle branch block.

Clinical factors

Myocardial damage caused by coronary artery disease, by cardiomyopathy or by other disorders may cause ventricular tachycardia. On the other hand, myocardial damage is not going to create the additional electrical connection between atria and ventricles that is necessary to facilitate an AV junctional re-entrant tachycardia. Thus, *a broad QRS tachycardia in a patient known to have myocardial damage is likely to be ventricular in origin.*

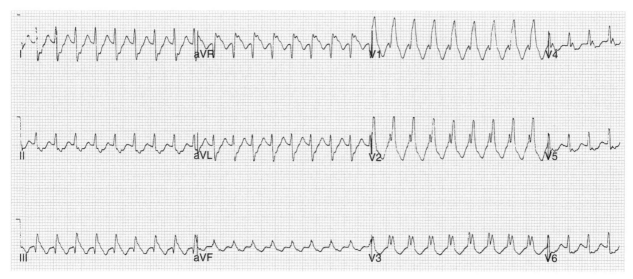

Figure 14.10 Proven AV nodal re-entrant tachycardia at electrophysiological study resulting in right bundle branch block during tachycardia.

Atrial flutter and atrial tachycardia may occur in patients with myocardial damage and may lead to a regular ventricular rhythm with bundle branch block, but they have characteristic features which should lead to their identification (Chapters 7 and 8). *During atrial fibrillation, the ventricular rhythm, whether or not the QRS complexes are broad, is totally irregular, and it should never be confused with ventricular tachycardia.*

Previous ECG

A previous ECG may be helpful. If it shows myocardial infarction, or marked ventricular hypertrophy as may be seen in cardiomyopathy, then ventricular tachycardia is probable. If it shows bundle branch block during sinus rhythm and the same QRS morphology is seen during tachycardia, then a supraventricular origin is very likely.

15

Atrioventricular Block

Atrioventricular (AV) block is classified as first, second or third degree depending on whether conduction of atrial impulses to the ventricles is delayed, intermittently blocked or completely blocked. Second-degree AV block is subdivided into Mobitz I (Wenckebach) and Mobitz II types. With the former, there is progressive lengthening of the PR interval prior to non-conduction of an atrial impulse, whereas the PR interval of conducted atrial impulses is constant in Mobitz II. Bifascicular block may deteriorate intermittently or permanently to complete (i.e. trifascicular) AV block.

Causes of AV block include idiopathic fibrosis of the conduction tissues, myocardial infarction, aortic valve disease, congenital, cardiac surgery and haemochromatosis.

First-degree and Wenckebach block in young people and/or during sleep are usually due to high vagal tone and are benign. High-degree AV block may cause Stokes–Adams attacks (characterised by abrupt, brief losses of consciousness) or may cause sudden death.

Classification

Atrioventricular (AV) block is classified as first, second or third degree depending on whether conduction of atrial impulses to the ventricles is delayed, intermittently blocked or completely blocked.

First-degree atrioventricular block

Delay in conduction of the atrial impulse to the ventricles results in prolongation of the PR interval (Figures 15.1–15.3). The PR interval is measured from the onset of the P wave to the onset of the ventricular complex – whether this is a Q or an R wave – and is prolonged if it is greater than 0.21 s. Since conduction of the atrial impulse is only delayed, the term first-degree AV 'block' is, in fact, a misnomer.

First-degree AV block does not cause symptoms but may sometimes progress to higher degrees of block. In young people it is usually due to high vagal tone and is benign.

Bennett's Cardiac Arrhythmias: Practical Notes on Interpretation and Treatment, Eighth Edition. David H. Bennett.
© 2013 John Wiley & Sons, Ltd. Published 2013 by John Wiley & Sons, Ltd.

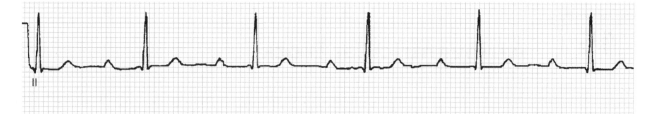

Figure 15.1 First-degree AV block (lead II). PR interval = 0.32 s.

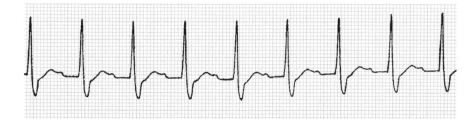

Figure 15.2 First-degree AV block and sinus tachycardia (lead I). PR interval = 0.24 s.

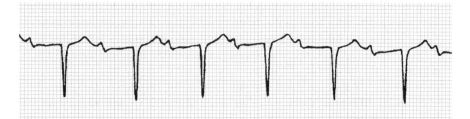

Figure 15.3 First-degree AV block (lead V1). The P wave is superimposed on the terminal portion of the preceding T wave. PR interval = 0.38 s.

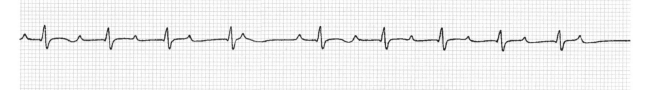

Figure 15.4 Wenckebach AV block.

Second-degree atrioventricular block

In second-degree AV block there is intermittent failure of conduction of atrial impulses to the ventricles. Thus, some P waves are not followed by QRS complexes.

Second-degree block is subdivided into Mobitz type I (also termed Wenckebach) and Mobitz type II block.

Mobitz type I (Wenckebach) atrioventricular block

In this form of second-degree block, delay in AV conduction increases with each successive atrial impulse until an atrial impulse fails to be conducted to the ventricles, i.e. there is progressive increase in PR interval until a P wave is not followed by a QRS complex. After the non-conducted P wave, AV conduction recovers and the sequence starts again (Figures 15.4, 15.5). Typically, the *increments* in PR interval progressively shorten during the sequence, resulting in progressive decrease in the interval between QRS complexes.

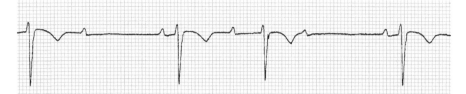

Figure 15.5 Wenckebach AV block. Unlike textbook examples, but as often occurs in practice, the trace does not start with the shortest PR interval.

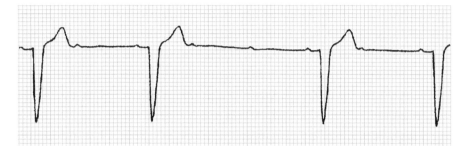

Figure 15.6 Mobitz type II AV block. In this example the ratio between conducted and non-conducted atrial impulses varies.

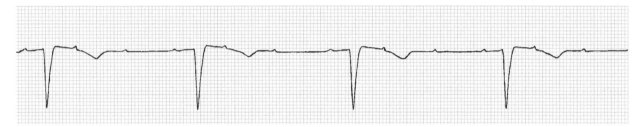

Figure 15.7 Mobitz type II AV block. The QRS complex is broad.

Wenckebach AV block is usually due to impaired conduction in the AV node. However, like first-degree AV block, it can be benign (particularly when it occurs during sleep), being due to high vagal tone. Wenckebach block that cannot be attributed to high vagal tone, e.g. in an older person during waking hours, has a prognosis similar to that of Mobitz type II block.

Unlike textbook examples, often in practice an ECG recording of AV Wenckebach block will not start with the shortest PR interval. *If, at first glance, it is clear that there are non-conducted P waves but it is not obvious what type of AV block is occurring, ask yourself, 'Is this Wenckebach block?' Look for the shortest PR interval and then see if it progressively increases.*

Mobitz type II atrioventricular block

In Mobitz type II block there is intermittent failure of conduction of atrial impulses to the ventricles without preceding progressive lengthening of the PR interval, and thus *the PR interval of conducted beats is constant* (Figure 15.6).

In contrast to first-degree and Wenckebach AV block, Mobitz type II block is usually due to impaired conduction in the bundle branches. Because there is bundle branch disease, the QRS complexes are as a rule broad (Figure 15.7). Block below the AV node is more likely to be associated with Stokes–Adams attacks, slow ventricular rates and sudden death.

The ratio of conducted to non-conducted atrial impulses varies. Commonly 2:1 AV conduction occurs. A similar pattern may be caused by an extreme form of Wenckebach

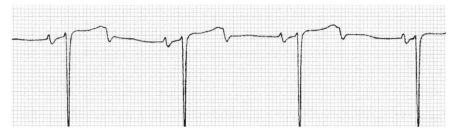

Figure 15.8 2:1 AV block with narrow QRS complexes (lead V1). The non-conducted atrial beats are superimposed on preceding T waves.

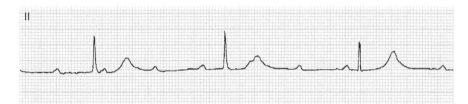

Figure 15.9 Complete AV block with narrow QRS complexes.

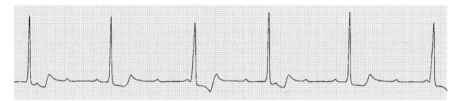

Figure 15.10 Complete AV block with broad QRS complexes.

block, so it is difficult to make prognostic inferences from 2:1 AV block if the QRS complexes are narrow (Figure 15.8).

Third-degree atrioventricular block

Third-degree or complete AV block occurs when there is total interruption of conduction of atrial impulses to the ventricles. Atrial activity will continue to be controlled by the sinus node and will proceed independently of and at a faster rate than the ventricular rhythm.

Third-degree block may be due to interrupted conduction at either AV nodal or infranodal level. When the block is within the AV node, an escape rhythm arises distally from the AV junction, usually discharging reliably at a moderate rate. Unless there is additional bundle branch block, QRS complexes will be narrow (Figure 15.9). In contrast, in infranodal block escape rhythms usually arise in the left or right bundle branches, resulting in broad QRS complexes and slower ventricular rates (Figures 15.10, 15.13). They are less reliable and thus ventricular asystole is more likely.

Complete AV block can occur during atrial fibrillation and flutter (Figures 6.4, 15.11, 15.12).

Occasionally, heart block occurs only during exercise and can be the cause of exertional syncope or weakness.

Supernormal conduction

Rarely, during third-degree AV block, atrial impulses may be conducted to the ventricles. There is a short period immediately after recovery from excitation when AV conduction may transiently improve. This period usually coincides with inscription of the latter portion of the T wave (Figure 15.13). As a result, atrial impulses falling on this part of the T wave will be followed by a premature QRS complex.

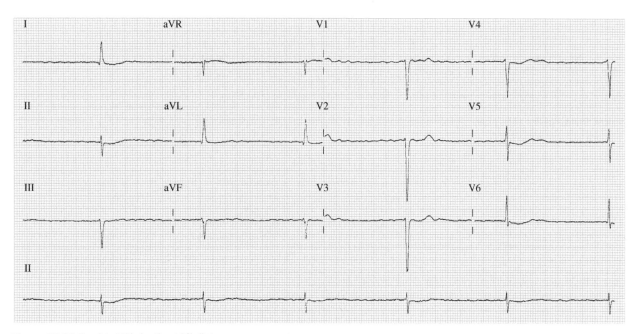

Figure 15.11 Complete AV block with atrial fibrillation.

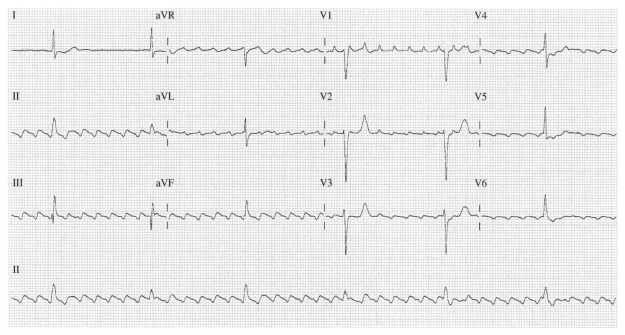

Figure 15.12 Complete AV block with atrial flutter.

Causes of atrioventricular block

Idiopathic fibrosis of the AV junction and/or bundle branches (sometimes referred to as Lenègre–Lev disease) is by far the most common cause. It is a disorder mainly occurring in older patients, but young patients are sometimes affected and familial cases have been documented.

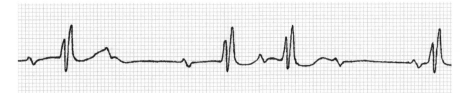

Figure 15.13 Complete AV block. There is supernormal conduction of the atrial impulse that falls on the T wave of the second ventricular complex (lead V1).

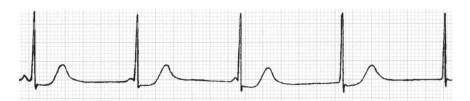

Figure 15.14 AV dissociation. The atrial rate is slower than the ventricular rate: atrial and ventricular rates are 49 and 51 beats/min, respectively. The fourth and fifth P waves are concealed by superimposed QRS complexes.

Causes of atrioventricular block

Idiopathic fibrosis of conduction tissues
Myocardial infarction
Aortic valve disease
Transarterial valve replacement
Congenital isolated lesion
Congenital heart disease (e.g. corrected transposition)
Cardiac surgery
Infiltration (e.g. tumour, sarcoidosis, haemochromatosis, amyloidosis, syphilis)
Inflammation (e.g. endocarditis, ankylosing spondylitis, Reiter's syndrome)
Rheumatic fever
Diphtheria
Dystrophia myotonica
Chagas' disease (South America)
Lyme carditis (tick-borne spirochaetal infection, *Borrelia burgdorferi*, mainly North America)
Rarely, familial

Atrioventricular dissociation

During third-degree AV block, atrial activity is *faster* than and dissociated from ventricular activity. Dissociation between atrial and ventricular activity also occurs when, during sinus bradycardia, an escape rhythm faster than the sinus rate arises from the AV junction (Figure 15.14). The term 'AV dissociation' should be reserved for this latter situation, in which the atrial rate is *slower* than the ventricular rate. If AV dissociation is not distinguished from complete AV block, inappropriate pacemaker insertion may result.

Bilateral bundle branch disease

Infranodal AV block is most often caused by disease in both left and right bundle branches. Although the anatomical situation may be more complex, functionally the bundle of His can be considered to give rise to three divisions: the right bundle branch, and the anterior and posterior fascicles of the left bundle branch (Chapter 4).

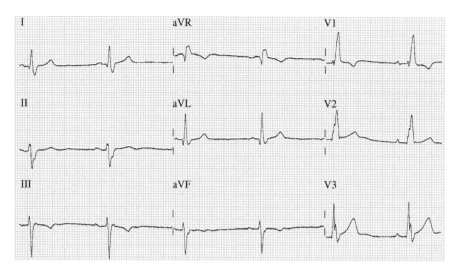

Figure 15.15 Left anterior fascicular and right bundle branch block.

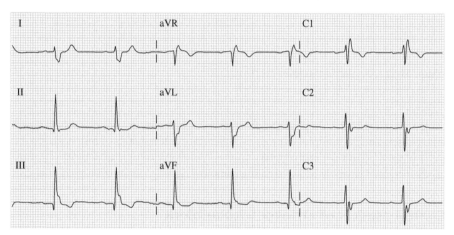

Figure 15.16 Left posterior fascicular and right bundle branch block.

If conduction is blocked in only two of the three fascicles, there is bifascicular block: the functioning fascicle will conduct atrial impulses to the ventricles and maintain AV conduction. Block in the third fascicle will lead to complete AV block.

Bifascicular block

The most common pattern of bifascicular block is right bundle branch plus left anterior fascicular block (Figure 15.15). The posterior fascicle of the left bundle branch is a stouter structure than the anterior fascicle and is therefore less vulnerable. As a result, right bundle branch plus left posterior fascicular block is less common (Figure 15.16).

PR interval prolongation is usually due to impaired AV node conduction, but in the context of bifascicular block it may be due to slow conduction in the functioning fascicle (Figure 15.17). The combination of bifascicular block and a long PR interval is sometimes referred to as 'trifascicular block'. This is incorrect: trifascicular block indicates that there is complete block of AV conduction; 'trifascicular disease' is a better term.

Interrupted conduction in all three fascicles results in complete AV block. In some patients one of the three fascicles is capable of intermittent conduction so that at times there will be sinus rhythm with bifascicular block.

The risk of bifascicular block progressing to trifascicular block is low in patients with right bundle and left anterior fascicular block: it is a few per cent per year. There is little

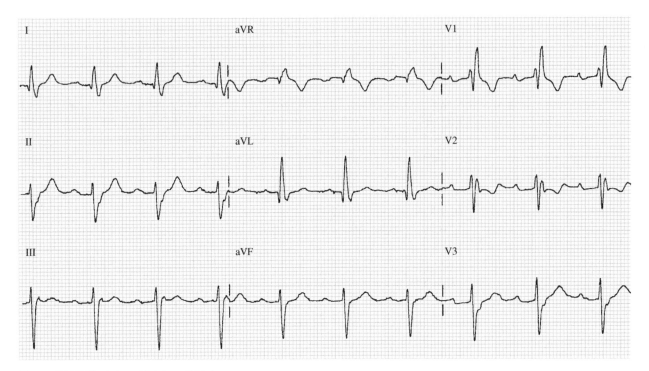

Figure 15.17 Bifascicular and first-degree AV block.

evidence to suggest that prophylactic pacemaker implantation in asymptomatic patients with bifascicular block improves prognosis: the major determinants of prognosis are the states of the myocardium and coronary arteries. The risk of complete AV block is significantly increased when there is alternating complete right and left bundle branch block.

Clinical aspects of atrioventricular block

First-degree and Mobitz type I second-degree AV block do not usually cause symptoms but may progress to higher grades of block. Very rarely, the delay between atrial and ventricular activation can significantly reduce cardiac output and thereby be symptomatic.

In Mobitz type II and complete AV block, a low ventricular rate may cause fatigue, dyspnoea or heart failure. In some patients the focus generating the ventricular escape rhythm may at times discharge very slowly or stop, leading to syncope or, if ventricular activity does not quickly return, sudden death (Figure 15.18). Sometimes, syncope is due to torsade de pointes tachycardia that has resulted from the low ventricular rate during heart block.

Stokes–Adams attacks

Syncope due to transient asystole (or ventricular tachyarrhythmia) – a Stokes–Adams attack – has characteristic features. These are of diagnostic importance because abnormalities of AV conduction and/or sinus node function may be intermittent: it is important to take a detailed history from the patient.

In a Stokes–Adams attack, loss of consciousness is sudden. There is virtually no warning, though the patient will sometimes feel that he or she is going to faint, just before loss of consciousness. The patient collapses, lying motionless, pale and pulseless, and looks as though he or she is dead. Usually, within a minute or two, consciousness returns, and as cardiac action resumes there may be a vivid flush to

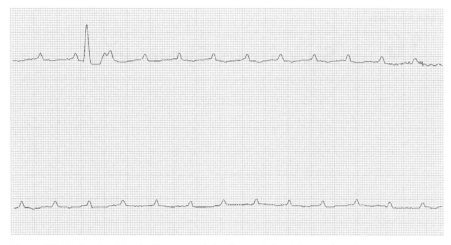

Figure 15.18 Complete AV block with no escape rhythm during ambulatory electrocardiography: just a series of P waves after a single ventricular complex.

the skin. Incontinence does occur occasionally but is not a regular feature as it is in epilepsy. Unlike epilepsy, recovery is quick, and there is no confusion or headache.

Near-syncope

In some patients the rhythm disturbance does not last long enough to cause syncope but the patient feels as though he or she is going to faint and then recovers. The patient may complain of 'dizziness' but on further questioning will admit to light-headedness or faintness not vertigo.

Congenital heart block

In congenital heart block, AV conduction is interrupted at the AV nodal level. Consequently, the subsidiary ventricular pacemaker is situated in the proximal part of the bundle of His, resulting in narrow QRS complexes and a reliable, moderately fast discharge rate (40–80 beats/min), which may accelerate on exercise. Often, there are no symptoms and exercise tolerance is good. However, syncope and sudden death do occur in a minority of patients: symptoms become more common as the patient gets older (Chapter 23).

There is a high incidence of congenital AV block in babies whose mothers have systemic lupus erythematosus.

Acquired heart block

As discussed above, the commonest cause of heart block is idiopathic fibrosis of the AV junction or bundle branches. This mainly affects the elderly but, as with the other causes of AV block, can affect the young and middle-aged as well.

The bradycardia associated with Mobitz type II and third-degree AV block may reduce cardiac output and lead to symptoms such as shortness of breath, tiredness and heart failure. Stokes–Adams attacks will sooner or later occur in about two-thirds of patients with these higher grades of AV block.

Heart block complicating myocardial infarction is discussed in Chapter 18.

Treatment

Cardiac pacing is highly effective at relieving symptoms and improving prognosis. The indications are discussed in Chapter 23.

16 Sick Sinus Syndrome

Sick sinus syndrome is due to impairment of sinus node function or of sinoatrial conduction and may cause sinus bradycardia, sinoatrial block or sinus arrest. A long pause in sinus node activity without an adequate junctional or ventricular escape rhythm will result in near-syncope or syncope necessitating pacemaker implantation. Causes of sick sinus syndrome include idiopathic fibrosis of the sinus node, cardiomyopathy and cardiac surgery.

The bradycardia–tachycardia syndrome is the association of sick sinus syndrome with episodes of atrial fibrillation, flutter or tachycardia, but not AV re-entrant tachycardia. There is a high risk of systemic embolism.

Sick sinus syndrome, also referred to as sinoatrial disease or sinus node dysfunction, is caused by impairment of sinus node automaticity (automaticity is defined as the ability of a cell to initiate an electrical impulse) or of conduction of impulses generated by the sinus node to the surrounding atrial myocardium. It can lead to sinus bradycardia, sinoatrial block or sinus arrest.

In some patients, atrial fibrillation, flutter or tachycardia may also occur. The term 'bradycardia–tachycardia' (often abbreviated to 'brady–tachy') syndrome applies to these patients. AV re-entrant tachycardia is, however, not part of the bradycardia–tachycardia syndrome.

Sick sinus syndrome is a common cause of syncope, dizzy attacks and palpitation. Though found most often in the elderly, it can occur at any age.

Causes

The cause is usually idiopathic fibrosis of the sinus node. Cardiomyopathy, myocarditis, cardiac surgery, antiarrhythmic drugs and lithium toxicity can also cause the syndrome. Rarely, the disorder can be familial.

Bennett's Cardiac Arrhythmias: Practical Notes on Interpretation and Treatment, Eighth Edition. David H. Bennett.
© 2013 John Wiley & Sons, Ltd. Published 2013 by John Wiley & Sons, Ltd.

ECG characteristics

Any one or more of the following can occur. They are often intermittent, normal sinus rhythm being present for most of the time.

Sinus bradycardia
Sinus bradycardia is a common finding (Figure 16.1).

Sinus arrest
Sinus arrest occurs due to failure of the sinus node to activate the atria. The result is absence of normal P waves (Figures 16.2, 16.3).

Sinoatrial block
Sinoatrial block occurs when sinus node impulses fail to traverse the junction between the node and surrounding atrial myocardium. Like atrioventricular block, sinoatrial block can be classified into first, second or third degrees. However, the surface ECG only allows recognition of second-degree sinoatrial block. Third-degree or complete block is indistinguishable from sinus arrest. In second-degree sinoatrial block, intermittent failure of atrial activation results in intervals between P waves that are multiples of (often twice) the cycle length during sinus rhythm (Figure 16.4).

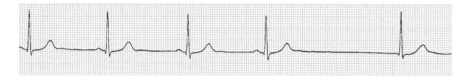

Figure 16.1 Sinus bradycardia. Rate 33 beats/min.

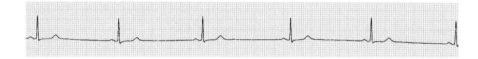

Figure 16.2 Sinus arrest leading to a junctional escape beat.

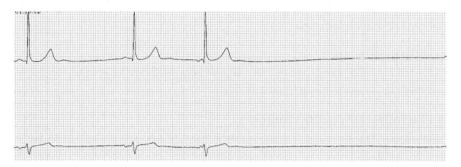

Figure 16.3 Sinus arrest after a junctional beat leading to a prolonged period of ventricular standstill.

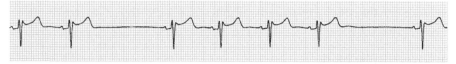

Figure 16.4 Two pauses due to second-degree sinoatrial block during which both the P waves and QRS complexes are dropped for one cycle.

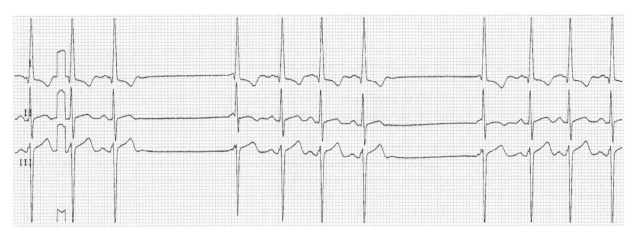

Figure 16.5 Junctional escape beats following sinus arrest.

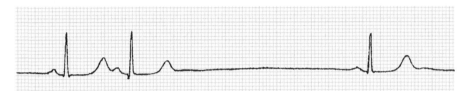

Figure 16.6 Atrial ectopic beat leads to depression of sinus node automaticity.

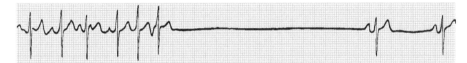

Figure 16.7 Termination of atrial fibrillation followed by sinus arrest.

Escape beats and rhythms

When sinus bradycardia or arrest occurs, subsidiary pacemaker tissue may give rise to an escape beat or rhythm (Figures 16.2, 16.5). A slow junctional rhythm suggests impaired sinus node function.

Atrial ectopic beats

These are common. Long pauses often follow because sinus node automaticity is depressed by the ectopic beat (Figure 16.6).

Bradycardia–tachycardia syndrome

Atrial fibrillation, flutter or tachycardia may occur in patients with the sick sinus syndrome (Figure 16.7). However, AV junctional re-entrant tachycardia is *not* part of this syndrome.

Sinus node automaticity is often depressed by tachycardias, so sinus bradycardia or arrest follows the tachycardia (Figure 16.7). Conversely, tachycardias often arise as an escape rhythm during bradycardia (Figures 16.8, 16.9). Thus, tachycardia often alternates with bradycardia.

Atrioventricular block

AV block sometimes coexists with the sick sinus syndrome. In patients with the sick sinus syndrome who develop atrial fibrillation there is often a slow ventricular

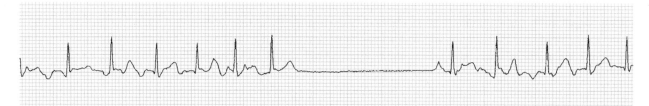

Figure 16.8 Sinus arrest after termination of atrial fibrillation. After a single sinus beat atrial fibrillation recurs.

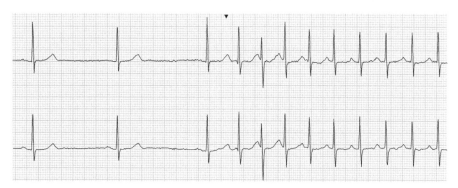

Figure 16.9 Bradycardia–tachycardia syndrome. Atrial tachycardia arises during sinus bradycardia.

response without AV nodal blocking drugs, suggesting coexistent impaired AV nodal function.

Clinical features

Sinus arrest without an adequate escape rhythm may cause syncope or near-syncope, depending on its duration. Tachycardias often produce palpitation, and subsequent sinus node depression may lead to syncope or near-syncope as palpitation ceases.

Some patients will experience symptoms several times each day, whereas in others symptoms will be infrequent.

Systemic embolism is common in the bradycardia–tachycardia syndrome.

Chronotropic incompetence

Impaired sinus node function may result in an inadequate increase in heart rate during exertion, resulting in an impaired ability to exercise. Chronotropic incompetence is defined as the inability to achieve a heart rate of 100 beats/min in response to maximal exertion.

Diagnosis

Suspect sick sinus syndrome when there is syncope, near-syncope or palpitation in the presence of sinus bradycardia or a slow junctional rhythm. Prolonged sinus arrest or sinoatrial block confirms the diagnosis.

Sometimes the standard ECG will provide diagnostic information, but often ambulatory electrocardiography, or with infrequent symptoms an implantable ECG loop recorder, will be necessary.

It should be noted that *sinus bradycardia and short pauses during sleep are normal* and are not evidence of the sick sinus syndrome. Furthermore, pauses in sinus node activity of up to 2.0 s during the daytime due to high vagal tone may be found in fit, young people. Ambulatory electrocardiography in a normal subject will inevitably show sinus bradycardia during sleep and sinus tachycardia during exercise. Sometimes these are wrongly taken as evidence of the bradycardia–tachycardia syndrome!

Treatment

Atrial or dual-chamber pacing is necessary to control symptoms (Chapter 23). Antiarrhythmic drugs often worsen sinus node function. A pacemaker is usually necessary if drugs are needed to control tachycardias. Tachyarrhythmias often arise during sinus bradycardia or pauses. Atrial pacing may prevent these arrhythmias.

The risk of systemic embolism in the bradycardia–tachycardia syndrome is high. Anticoagulation is indicated.

Vasovagal and carotid sinus syndromes are due to abnormal autonomic nervous system reflexes that can cause syncope due to bradycardia and/or hypotension. The malignant vasovagal syndrome, also termed neurocardiogenic syncope, is characterised by recurrent, abrupt syncope when sitting or standing, and a positive tilt-table test that can be used to demonstrate the cardioinhibitory and/or vasodepressor elements of the syndrome. Pacing may prevent syncope when caused by the former element but will not influence symptoms if due to the latter. A generous intake of both water and salt can be effective in preventing symptoms.

The diagnosis of carotid sinus syndrome is made in patients who suffer from near-syncope or syncope in whom carotid sinus massage causes sinus arrest or complete AV block for 3 s or more.

'Situational faints' are triggered by a variety of factors such as sight of blood, venepuncture, pain, emotion or oppressive environment.

Syncope is defined as transient loss of consciousness due to global cerebral hypoperfusion of abrupt onset and short duration, and spontaneous complete recovery.

The term neurally mediated syncope refers to the vasovagal syndrome, carotid sinus syndrome and less common syndromes such as micturition syncope, in which triggering of an autonomic nervous system reflex results in syncope due to inappropriate bradycardia, and/or hypotension caused by vasodilatation.

Neurally mediated syncope should be considered in patients with unexplained syncope when there is no electrocardiographic evidence of the sick sinus syndrome or atrioventricular (AV) block.

Malignant vasovagal syndrome

The malignant vasovagal syndrome, also termed neurocardiogenic syncope, is characterised by recurrent, abrupt syncope when standing or sitting (including car driving), and a positive tilt-table test. Tests for sick sinus syndrome and atrioventricular block are negative. The term 'malignant' is used to indicate that episodes occur

Bennett's Cardiac Arrhythmias: Practical Notes on Interpretation and Treatment, Eighth Edition. David H. Bennett.
© 2013 John Wiley & Sons, Ltd. Published 2013 by John Wiley & Sons, Ltd.

without obvious prodromal symptoms or an apparent triggering stimulus such as occurs in situational faints.

Syncope is thought to result from pooling of blood in the lower extremities during standing or sitting. Reduced venous return leads to hypotension which is detected by baroreceptors in the aortic arch and carotid arteries and leads to reflex-enhanced sympathetic nervous system activity and thus increased force of myocardial contraction. Because of reduced venous return, the left ventricle in diastole is relatively empty. Systole results in *excessive* stimulation of ventricular mechanoreceptors, which in patients with the vasovagal syndrome trigger *inappropriate* reflex vasodilatation and bradycardia. Reflex control of venous tone has also been shown to be abnormal. In some patients 'cardioinhibition' (i.e. bradycardia, either sinus arrest or AV block) predominates, while in others it is the 'vasodepressor' element (i.e. vasodilatation) that is the main problem.

Even though a period of asystole may occur, the syndrome is not a cause of sudden death. Frequency of recurrence of attacks is variable and unpredictable; episodes may occur in clusters. It occurs in both young and elderly people. In contrast to syncope caused by the sick sinus syndrome or AV block, loss of consciousness may be prolonged due to persistent hypotension, and fitting and incontinence can sometimes occur.

Tilt-table test

The patient is gently secured on a tilt table and rapidly tilted from the supine position to a 60-degree angle, and then stays in this position, standing on a footplate, for up to 45 minutes. The ECG and blood pressure are continuously monitored. The test is positive if the patient's *typical spontaneous symptoms* result from profound bradycardia (often asystole) and/or hypotension (Figures 17.1–17.3). Blood pressure and heart rate are rapidly restored on returning to a horizontal position (Figure 17.4).

Isoprenaline or glyceryl trinitrate are sometimes used to increase the sensitivity of the test (i.e. more positive results are obtained), but these drugs also reduce the test's specitivity (i.e. a positive test may occur in a person who has not experienced spontaneous reflex syncope). If these drugs are used and lead to a positive test, it is even more important to ensure that the patient's typical symptoms were experienced before making a diagnosis of vasovagal syndrome.

It should be appreciated that sometimes a predominantly vasodepressor response will be observed during tilt-table testing and yet a cardioinhibitory response is responsible for spontaneous symptoms.

Treatment of vasovagal syndrome
Prevention

Patients should undertake measures to prevent venous pooling: they should avoid standing or sitting for prolonged periods and should regularly tense and contract the

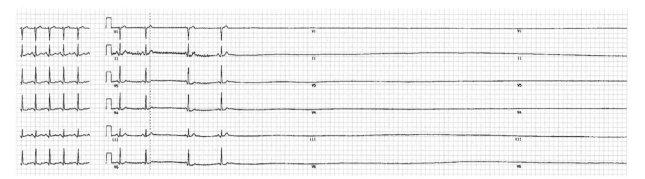

Figure 17.1 Vasovagal syndrome. Asystole and then fitting developed after three minutes on a tilt table.

muscles in their legs to aid venous return. Dehydration should be avoided: a high intake of water should be encouraged. A generous salt intake should also be encouraged: not infrequently, patients presenting with this syndrome completely avoid salt during cooking and at the table.

One study has shown that a programme of progressively prolonged periods of 'enforced upright posture' or 'tilt-training' can be effective. For example, the patient

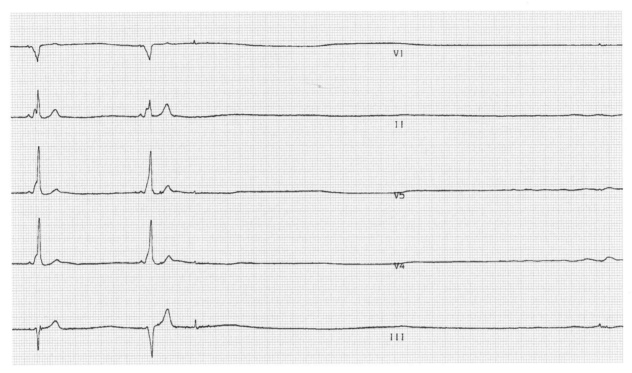

Figure 17.2 Positive tilt-table test in a patient with the Wolff–Parkinson–White syndrome whose syncope was thought to be due to paroxysmal tachycardia.

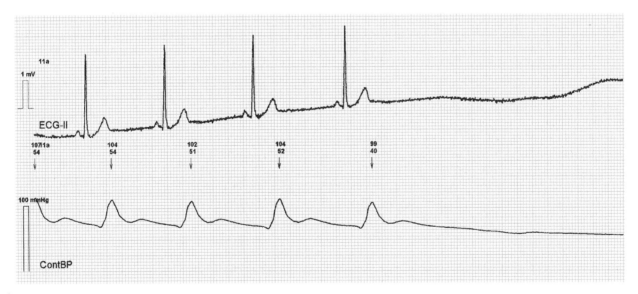

Figure 17.3 Predominantly cardioinhibitory response to tilt-table test.

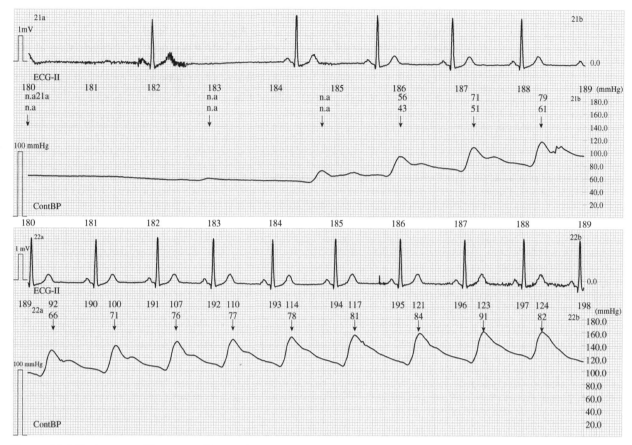

Figure 17.4 Blood pressure and heart rate rapidly restored to normal on returning to a horizontal position after profound bradycardia and hypotension during tilt-table testing.

should, each day, stand against a wall with his or her feet 15 cm from the wall for periods of up to 40 minutes.

Treatment

Isometric arm muscle contraction at the first signs of an impending vasovagal attack has been shown to elevate blood pressure and to avoid syncope: the patient should extend both arms and then very forcefully push one hand against the other. Another effective measure is squatting. If feasible, assuming a horizontal position should quickly terminate an episode.

Dual-chamber cardiac pacing should be considered to treat the cardioinhibitory element of the syndrome in patients who have experienced frequent blackouts. Because pacing will not prevent the vasodepressor element of the syndrome, some symptoms may continue. It should be noted that a few clinical trials have failed to demonstrate a benefit from pacing, but the results may be a reflection of the nature of patients enrolled into the studies. In the author's experience, patients with frequent cardioinhibitory syncope not responding to preventive measures do benefit greatly from pacing. A rate-drop algorithm is probably the best method of pacing: a sudden reduction in heart rate, e.g. to 40 beats/min, will trigger pacing at a high rate, 90–130 beats/min; the high rate may compensate for the vasodepressor effect.

Treatment of the vasodepressor component is difficult. A number of drugs have been tried: beta-blockers, disopyramide, scopolamine skin patches, paroxetine, midodrine and fludrocortisone. None has been shown to be very effective.

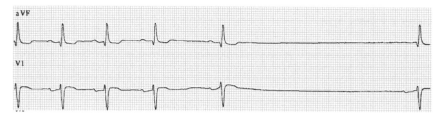

Figure 17.5 Carotid sinus syndrome. Carotid sinus massage causes 3 s sinus arrest.

Simple faint

Syncope due to the vasovagal syndrome must be distinguished from the 'simple faint' that is particularly common in young people. This is triggered by a variety of 'situational factors' such as unpleasant sights, e.g. blood or needles, pain, extreme emotion or stuffy rooms. Common places for fainting are churches, hospitals and restaurants. In contrast to the malignant vasovagal syndrome, where syncope is of abrupt onset, there is a history of preceding dizziness, sweating and nausea prior to loss of consciousness. Witnesses often report marked pallor. Weakness and nausea usually occur during recovery.

Acute diarrhoea or sudden major blood loss can also cause syncope.

Carotid sinus syndrome

The diagnosis of carotid sinus syndrome is made in patients who suffer from near-syncope or syncope in whom *unilateral* carotid sinus massage for 5 s causes sinus arrest or complete AV block for 3 s or more (Figure 17.5). There is a very small risk of stroke resulting from carotid massage and there are occasional reports of ventricular fibrillation, so some would only perform carotid massage with resuscitation facilities available. Carotid sinus massage should not be performed in patients with a history of stroke, known carotid artery disease or carotid bruit. If right-sided carotid massage is negative, the test should be repeated on the left carotid artery. Sensitivity of the test can be increased by performing carotid massage in the head-up tilt position. In some patients, severe hypotension due to vasodilatation occurs as well as bradycardia.

Cardiac pacing (Chapter 23) may improve or abolish symptoms when they are caused by bradycardia; however, in some patients, the vasodepressor element continues to cause symptoms.

Some *asymptomatic* subjects, particularly among the elderly, may develop a marked bradycardia on carotid massage. Carotid sinus syndrome should only be diagnosed in patients with typical spontaneous symptoms.

Postural orthostatic tachycardia syndrome

This syndrome (often abbreviated to POTS) is characterised by an intolerance to standing due to symptoms such as palpitation, light-headedness, near-syncope and fatigue, together with a rise in heart rate by 30 beats/min or to a rate in excess of 120 beats/min without significant hypotension. It is commoner in females and typically affects people 20–40 years of age. It can be demonstrated by tilt-table testing.

A number of treatments may help: small doses of a beta-blocker, high salt and fluid intake, and an exercise training program initially concentrating on activities such as swimming and rowing which avoid standing.

Causes of syncope

When a patient presents with syncope it is important to bear in mind the many possible causes, as listed in the table.

Causes of syncope

Cardiac arrhythmias

  Sinus node disease
  Atrioventricular block
  Paroxysmal supraventricular tachycardia
  Paroxysmal monomorphic ventricular tachycardia
  Paroxysmal polymorphic ventricular tachycardia

Neurally mediated syncope

  Simple, common faint
  Carotid sinus syndrome
  Vasovagal syndrome

Structural heart disease

  Aortic stenosis
  Hypertrophic cardiomyopathy
  Atrial myxoma
  Acute myocardial ischaemia
  Pulmonary embolism

Orthostasis

  Disorders of autonomic nervous syndrome: primary, and caused by diabetes, amyloidosis
  Haemorrhage
  Diarrhoea
  Addison's disease
  Postural orthostatic tachycardia syndrome

18 Arrhythmias Due to Myocardial Infarction

Ventricular fibrillation occurs during the first hour of acute myocardial infarction in more than 10% of patients, necessitating immediate defibrillation. Frequent and 'R on T' ventricular ectopic beats, and other 'warning arrhythmias' are common in acute infarction and are not in fact predictive of ventricular fibrillation. Ventricular fibrillation or tachycardia during the first 24 hours of infarction is unlikely to recur. Atrial fibrillation and ventricular arrhythmias arising 24 hours or more after acute infarction are usually associated with extensive myocardial damage.

Sinus and junctional bradycardia, and complete atrioventricular (AV) block due to inferior infarction, do not require treatment unless causing symptoms or marked hypotension. AV block due to acute inferior infarction will resolve and is not an indication for permanent pacemaker implantation. Bilateral bundle branch damage or high-degree AV block caused by anterior infarction imply extensive myocardial damage and a poor prognosis.

Acute myocardial infarction causes a wide variety of arrhythmias, some of which require immediate action, whereas for others no treatment is necessary. Arrhythmias are most frequent in the early hours after infarction.

The main sustained arrhythmias are ventricular fibrillation, atrial fibrillation and ventricular tachycardia. In recent years, serious cardiac arrhythmias due to acute myocardial infarction seem less prevalent: presumably due to the reduction in infarct size resulting from the widespread use of thrombolytic therapy and primary angioplasty. Arrhythmias are more common in myocardial infarction with ST elevation (STEMI).

Incidence of arrhythmias in a series of patients within four hours of myocardial infarction

Ventricular fibrillation	16%
Ventricular tachycardia	4%
Ventricular ectopic beats	93%
Supraventricular arrhythmias	6%
Sinus or junctional bradycardia	34%
Second- or third-degree atrioventricular block	7%

Bennett's Cardiac Arrhythmias: Practical Notes on Interpretation and Treatment, Eighth Edition. David H. Bennett.
© 2013 John Wiley & Sons, Ltd. Published 2013 by John Wiley & Sons, Ltd.

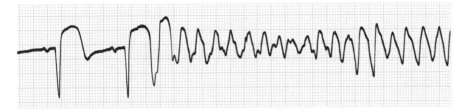

Figure 18.1 Ventricular ectopic beat initiating ventricular fibrillation.

Ventricular fibrillation

Ninety per cent of deaths caused by acute infarction are due to ventricular fibrillation. The incidence of fibrillation is highest in the first hour after the onset of chest pain and decreases progressively thereafter. Forty per cent of deaths occur within the first hour. Thus, many patients die before they can receive medical aid.

In those patients who reach hospital, however, ventricular fibrillation and other arrhythmias are sufficiently common to necessitate continuous ECG monitoring for 24–48 hours in an area where facilities for resuscitation are immediately available, i.e. a coronary care unit. Between 3% and 10% of patients with acute myocardial infarction develop ventricular fibrillation while in a coronary care unit. The shorter the delay before admission, the greater will be the incidence of ventricular fibrillation.

Ventricular fibrillation is most often initiated by an 'R on T' ventricular ectopic beat (Figure 18.1).

Treatment

On a coronary care unit, a defibrillator ought to be immediately available so little or no time need be spent on cardiopulmonary resuscitation. A 150–200 J biphasic shock will successfully defibrillate 90% of cases. If unsuccessful, further shocks at the same energy level may be effective. Sequential shocks, delivered by means of two defibrillators with separate pairs of electrodes, should be considered in any patient who is not defibrillated with repeated shocks.

In the past, following restoration of normal rhythm, an infusion of lignocaine has been given to prevent further ventricular fibrillation, but there is little evidence to show that lignocaine or other antiarrhythmic drugs are effective in this situation. Lignocaine is best reserved for the few patients with recurrent fibrillation. If lignocaine fails, alternative drugs including beta-blockers and amiodarone may be effective.

If ventricular fibrillation develops in a heart that was functioning satisfactorily during normal rhythm it is termed 'primary' fibrillation, whereas if it occurs in the context of cardiac failure or cardiogenic shock it is termed 'secondary'. Successful defibrillation is less likely in secondary ventricular fibrillation.

Ventricular flutter

Ventricular flutter is a very rapid ventricular rhythm in which there are continuous changes in waveform, distinction between QRS complexes and T waves being impossible (Figure 18.2). For practical purposes, it is the same as ventricular fibrillation.

Prevention of ventricular fibrillation in acute infarction

Conventional teaching used to be that ventricular ectopic beats that were frequent, multifocal, 'R on T' or repetitive – the 'warning arrhythmias' – heralded ventricular fibrillation or tachycardia (Figures 18.3–18.6). It was common practice to suppress these ectopic beats with antiarrhythmic agents.

However, analysis of continuous ECG recordings has shown that ventricular ectopic beats occur in almost all cases of acute infarction, and warning arrhythmias

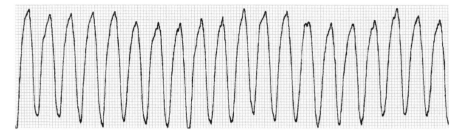

Figure 18.2 Ventricular flutter.

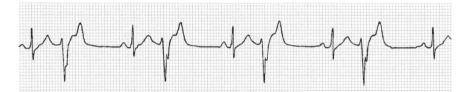

Figure 18.3 Frequent unifocal ventricular ectopic beats.

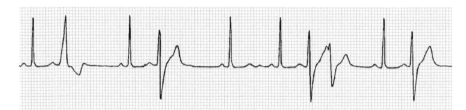

Figure 18.4 Frequent multifocal ventricular ectopic beats. The first ectopic beat arises from a different focus from that of subsequent ectopic beats. There is a couplet of ectopic beats after the fourth sinus beat.

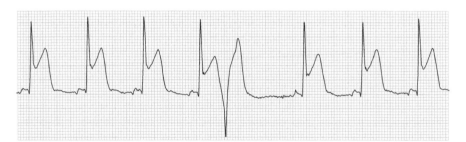

Figure 18.5 'R on T' ventricular ectopic beat.

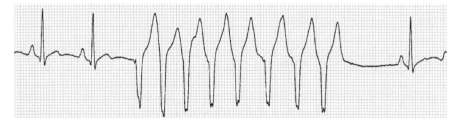

Figure 18.6 Salvo of ventricular ectopic beats.

are as common in patients who do not develop ventricular fibrillation as in those who do. Furthermore, warning arrhythmias may not precede ventricular fibrillation, and when they do occur, staff in even the best coronary care units often fail to detect them.

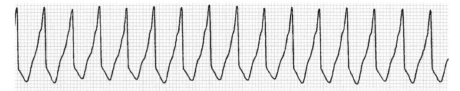

Figure 18.7 Monomorphic ventricular tachycardia.

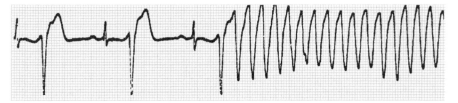

Figure 18.8 The third ventricular 'R on T' ectopic beat initiates ventricular tachycardia.

Since 'warning arrhythmias' do not in fact warn, it has been advocated that all patients should receive lignocaine. Several recent studies in the 'thrombolytic era' showed that lignocaine does reduce the incidence of ventricular fibrillation but mortality from acute infarction is not reduced: in fact, a trend to increased mortality has been shown. The consensus is that prophylactic lignocaine is not advisable. Oral mexiletine, a class IB drug like lignocaine, has been shown to increase mortality in acute infarction.

Ventricular tachycardia

Ventricular tachycardia may be self-terminating (Figure 18.6) or sustained (Figure 18.7). Ventricular tachycardia may be initiated by either 'R on T' or later ventricular ectopic beats (Figure 18.8). It may be monomorphic or polymorphic.

Sometimes ventricular tachycardia will result in shock or circulatory arrest. On the other hand, ventricular tachycardia may cause few or no symptoms. In myocardial infarction a regular tachycardia with broad ventricular complexes is usually *ventricular* in origin, even in the absence of haemodynamic deterioration.

Non-sustained ventricular tachycardia is very common in the first 24 hours following acute infarction. Only sustained ventricular tachycardia requires treatment. If cardiac arrest or shock occurs, immediate synchronised cardioversion (Chapter 21) is necessary. Otherwise intravenous lignocaine should be given. If lignocaine fails, second-line drugs include sotalol and amiodarone. Cardioversion may be necessary if a second-line drug fails. Overdrive ventricular pacing may be effective in terminating recurrent ventricular tachycardia.

Reperfusion arrhythmias

Reperfusion of an occluded coronary artery by thrombolysis or by balloon angioplasty can lead to a reperfusion arrhythmia: ventricular fibrillation, accelerated idioventricular rhythm (see below) or ventricular tachycardia.

Arrhythmias subsequent to recent myocardial infarction

A study using implantable loop recorders in patients following recent myocardial infarction with marked myocardial damage (ejection fraction < 40%) demonstrated

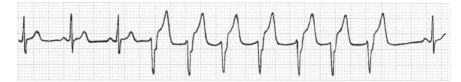

Figure 18.9 Accelerated idioventricular rhythm.

episodes of atrial fibrillation (28%), second- or third-degree AV block (10%), non-sustained ventricular tachycardia (13%), sustained ventricular tachycardia (3%), and ventricular fibrillation (3%).

Long-term significance of ventricular arrhythmias

Ventricular tachycardia and fibrillation within the first 24 hours after myocardial infarction are unlikely to recur after that period. While most studies suggest that early ventricular arrhythmias are not related to the degree of myocardial damage and are not of long-term prognostic significance, there are some that suggest that early primary ventricular fibrillation is associated with an impaired prognosis and may be a mark of extensive infarction.

Relation of ventricular tachycardia/fibrillation to infarct size and long-term treatment		
	Related to infarct size	Long-term treatment
Early	Probably not	Not indicated
Late	Yes	Indicated

In contrast to early arrhythmias, ventricular tachycardia or fibrillation occurring more than 24–48 hours after infarction is likely to recur days, weeks or even months later. Long-term antiarrhythmic therapy such as sotalol or amiodarone should be prescribed. A study in which defibrillators were implanted within six weeks after myocardial infarction which had resulted in an ejection fraction ≤ 35% showed no reduction in mortality. Defibrillator implantation should be considered beyond that period. Most patients with late arrhythmias will have poor ventricular function and should therefore benefit from an angiotensin-converting enzyme inhibitor and beta-blockade.

The more extensive the myocardial damage the worse the prognosis. The incidence of late ventricular arrhythmias is related to the size of the infarct. However, ventricular arrhythmias are also an independent predictor of prognosis. That is, a patient with both extensive myocardial damage and late ventricular arrhythmias has a poorer prognosis than a patient with the same degree of myocardial damage but no arrhythmia.

Frequent ventricular ectopic beats at the time of hospital discharge have been shown to indicate extensive myocardial damage and hence a poor prognosis but not an increased risk of arrhythmic death. There is no evidence that suppression of ventricular ectopic beats or non-sustained ventricular tachycardia improves prognosis. Studies have shown that class I antiarrhythmic drugs actually worsen prognosis.

Accelerated idioventricular rhythm

This is also referred to as 'slow' ventricular tachycardia: the rate will be less than 100 beats/min. It is benign and treatment is not necessary (Figure 18.9).

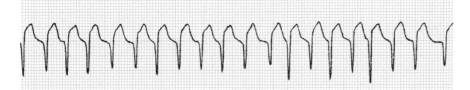

Figure 18.10 Atrial fibrillation with rapid ventricular rate in anterior infarction (lead V3).

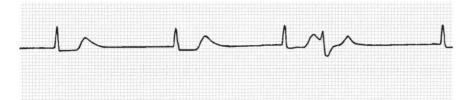

Figure 18.11 Junctional bradycardia. The fourth beat is an 'R on T' ventricular ectopic.

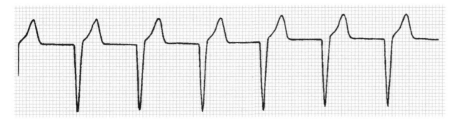

Figure 18.12 Junctional escape rhythm as a result of sinus bradycardia in anterior infarction (lead V4).

Supraventricular tachycardias

When supraventricular tachycardia is diagnosed in a patient with acute infarction, the diagnosis is usually atrial fibrillation or flutter, or erroneously ventricular tachycardia. AV junctional re-entrant tachycardia can only occur if there is an additional AV connection (Chapter 5): thus, it is highly unlikely to present for the first time during acute myocardial infarction.

Atrial fibrillation

In atrial fibrillation, which occurs in approximately 10% of patients in the first few days after myocardial infarction, the resultant rapid ventricular rate and reduction in cardiac output from loss of atrial systole can sometimes cause severe hypotension (Figure 18.10) and may necessitate immediate cardioversion. Otherwise, a rapid ventricular rate can be lowered by an intravenous beta-blocker, or verapamil or diltiazem (provided the patient is not already receiving an oral beta-blocker or is in left ventricular failure), or amiodarone. Spontaneous reversion to sinus rhythm is not uncommon.

Atrial fibrillation is usually associated with extensive myocardial damage or older patients and hence a poor prognosis. Frequent atrial ectopic beats often herald atrial fibrillation.

Sinus and junctional bradycardias

Sinus and junctional bradycardias are common, particularly in inferior infarction (Figures 18.11, 18.12). If uncomplicated, no treatment is required. Bradycardia may be

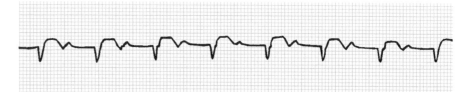

Figure 18.13 First-degree AV block (lead aVF).

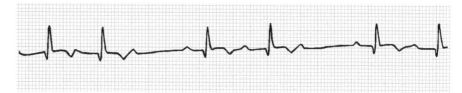

Figure 18.14 Wenckebach AV block in inferior infarction (lead aVF).

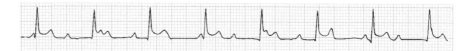

Figure 18.15 Inferior infarction complicated by complete AV block (lead II).

beneficial in acute infarction in that myocardial oxygen consumption is related to heart rate, and low oxygen consumption might limit infarct size.

However, if bradycardia causes hypotension (systolic blood pressure less than 90 mmHg), mental confusion, oliguria, cold peripheries or ventricular arrhythmias, intravenous atropine (initially 0.5 mg) should be given. Temporary cardiac pacing is occasionally necessary and is preferable to frequent doses of atropine. If hypotension persists after rate correction, consider right ventricular infarction (the ECG typically shows ST elevation in lead V1), in which case intravenous fluids may be necessary.

Atrioventricular block

The management and prognosis of AV block in inferior and anterior infarction differ markedly.

Inferior infarction

In inferior infarction, AV block is common and is often due to ischaemia of the AV node. Permanent AV node damage is exceptional. The prognosis for inferior infarction is widely accepted as good, but some studies do indicate increased in-hospital mortality.

First-degree and Mobitz type I second-degree (Wenckebach) AV block require no action other than stopping drugs that may worsen AV nodal conduction (e.g. verapamil, diltiazem, beta-blockers) (Figures 18.13, 18.14).

If complete AV block develops, subsidiary pacemakers in the bundle of His will control the ventricular rate (Figure 18.15). These pacemakers usually discharge at an adequate rate. However, sometimes the ventricular rate does fall very low (less than 40 beats/min), when hypotension, oliguria or ventricular arrhythmia may occur. In these circumstances, temporary pacing is necessary. There is no place for steroids or catecholamines, although in the first six hours atropine may be effective.

AV block will almost always resolve within three weeks of infarction, and it is highly unlikely that long-term cardiac pacing will be necessary.

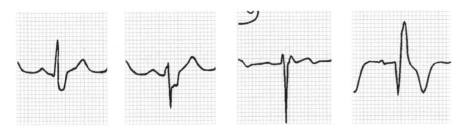

Figure 18.16 Left anterior fascicular and right bundle branch block in anterior infarction (leads I, II, III and V1).

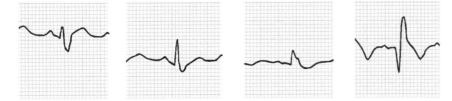

Figure 18.17 Left posterior fascicular and right bundle branch block in anterior infarction (leads I, II, III and V1).

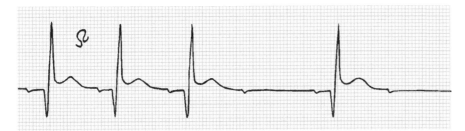

Figure 18.18 Intermittent Mobitz type II AV block in a patient with bifascicular block due to anterior infarction (lead V2).

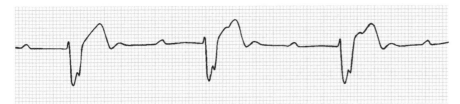

Figure 18.19 Complete AV block in anterior infarction.

Anterior infarction

In anterior infarction, it is the bundle branches rather than the AV node which are usually the site of ischaemic damage. AV block is more serious than in inferior infarction for two reasons. First, subsidiary pacemakers that arise below the level of the block in the distal specialised conducting system tend to be slower and less reliable. Thus hypotension due to a low ventricular rate is common and asystole often occurs. Second, an extensive area of infarction is necessary to affect both bundle branches. Prognosis after myocardial infarction is related to the extent of infarction. Hence it is poor in patients with anterior infarction complicated by AV block.

Evidence of bilateral bundle branch damage (alternating right and left bundle branch block, or right bundle branch block with left anterior or posterior hemiblock) often precedes the onset of second-degree (Mobitz type II) or complete AV block (Figures 18.16–18.19). The chance of bilateral bundle branch damage progressing to second-degree or complete heart block is approximately 30%. The first manifestation of these higher degrees of block may be ventricular standstill (Figure 18.20). Temporary transvenous pacing should be considered if there is evidence of bilateral

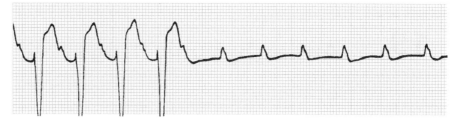

Figure 18.20 Ventricular asystole due to complete AV block in a patient with bifascicular block due to anterior infarction.

bundle branch damage, provided an experienced operator is available, otherwise the risks of temporary pacing will outweigh the advantages of pacing.

Second- and third-degree AV block due to anterior infarction are always indications for temporary pacing. Sinus rhythm often returns after a few days, but in some patients AV block will persist and may necessitate long-term pacing.

Mortality is high in the first three weeks after anterior infarction complicated by AV block, and long-term pacing should not be undertaken until the patient has survived this period.

If sinus rhythm does return, bifascicular block often persists. Complete AV block may recur in the weeks and months after acute infarction, but there is no conclusive evidence to show that implantation of a pacemaker will improve prognosis. This is because the extensive myocardial damage associated with this situation will often lead to ventricular fibrillation or heart failure.

Atrioventricular dissociation

In contrast to complete AV block, in AV dissociation the atrial rate is *slower* than the ventricular rate: no treatment is necessary (Figure 15.14).

Antiarrhythmic Drugs

Antiarrhythmic drugs are of limited efficacy and often cause unwanted effects. They are better at terminating arrhythmias than at preventing their recurrence. Drugs can be proarrhythmic, particularly if ventricular function is impaired.

Flecainide is effective at preventing atrial fibrillation but is contraindicated in patients with poor ventricular function or coronary disease. Adenosine is the treatment of choice for termination of atrioventricular junctional re-entrant tachycardias. Intravenous verapamil will quickly control the ventricular response to atrial fibrillation and flutter. Sotalol may be effective in treating supraventricular and ventricular arrhythmias but caution is required because it prolongs the QT interval. Digoxin toxicity is common, and alternative antiarrhythmic drugs can be used in most situations. Amiodarone is the most effective agent currently available but because of its unwanted effects its use should be confined to patients with arrhythmias that are dangerous or are refractory to other forms of treatment.

Limitations

Drugs are widely used in the treatment of arrhythmias, but their limitations should be appreciated. Antiarrhythmic drugs are of limited effectiveness: in other words, a drug prescribed in the correct dose for an appropriate indication may fail to work. With many drugs it is difficult to maintain consistent therapeutic drug levels. Considerable insight into the mode of action of antiarrhythmic drugs has been gained, but selection for an individual patient of a drug that is both effective and well tolerated is often a process of trial and error. Unwanted effects often occur: the most common are hypotension, heart failure, impairment of the specialised cardiac conducting tissues and symptoms from the gastrointestinal and central nervous systems.

Proarrhythmic effect

Many antiarrhythmic drugs, particularly those in class IA and IC (see below), can sometimes worsen or cause arrhythmias, sometimes with fatal consequences. Patients with poor ventricular function are at greatest risk, while the risk is low in those with structurally normal hearts.

Bennett's Cardiac Arrhythmias: Practical Notes on Interpretation and Treatment, Eighth Edition. David H. Bennett.
© 2013 John Wiley & Sons, Ltd. Published 2013 by John Wiley & Sons, Ltd.

> **Limitations of antiarrhythmic drugs**
>
> Limited efficacy
> Difficulty in maintaining therapeutic drug levels
> Selection of an effective drug is often based on trial and error
> Unwanted effects are common
> Proarrhythmic

Choice of treatment

Drugs are only one form of treatment, and in some situations other approaches – i.e. catheter ablation, cardioversion, artificial pacing or surgery – may be better.

A number of factors influence the choice of treatment: the type of arrhythmia, the urgency of the situation, the need for short- or long-term therapy and the presence of impaired myocardial performance, sick sinus syndrome or abnormal AV conduction.

It is important to consider whether an antiarrhythmic drug is being given to terminate an arrhythmia, to prevent its recurrence or to slow the heart rate during the arrhythmia. In some situations drugs are given to control symptoms, whereas in others the purpose may be to prevent dangerous arrhythmias.

Modes of action

The modes of action of antiarrhythmic drugs can be classified according to their effects in the intact heart (clinical classification) or according to their effects at cellular level as established by *in vitro* studies (action potential classification). The latter classification is widely referred to, although it is of limited practical value.

Clinical classification

In this classification, drugs are divided into three groups according to their main site or sites of action in the intact heart.

> **Classification of antiarrhythmic drugs according to principal site(s) of action in intact heart**
>
> | Site of action | Examples |
> | --- | --- |
> | AV node | Verapamil, diltiazem, adenosine, digoxin, beta-blockers |
> | Ventricles | Lignocaine, mexiletine |
> | Atria, ventricles, accessory AV pathways | Quinidine, disopyramide, amiodarone, flecainide, procainamide, sotalol, propafenone |

The first group consists of drugs whose chief action is to slow conduction in the atrioventricular (AV) node. These drugs may therefore be useful in the treatment of arrhythmias of supraventricular origin. In the second group are drugs that work mainly in ventricular arrhythmias. The third group comprises drugs that act on the atria, ventricles and, in cases of Wolff–Parkinson–White syndrome or AV re-entrant tachycardia, accessory AV pathways. Thus, they may be effective in both supraventricular and ventricular arrhythmias.

Action potential classification

In this classification, drugs are divided into four main classes depending upon their electrophysiological effects at cellular level.

Classification of antiarrhythmic drugs according to electrophysiological effects

	I	II	III	IV
A	Quinidine Procainamide Disopyramide	Beta-blockers	Amiodarone Sotalol Dofetilide Dronedarone	Verapamil Diltiazem
B	Lignocaine Mexiletine			
C	Flecainide Propafenone			

Class I

Class I drugs impede the transport of sodium across the cell membrane during the initiation of cellular activation and thereby reduce the rate of rise of the action potential (phase 0). They are subdivided into classes A, B and C according to their effect on the duration of the action potential (which is reflected in the surface ECG by the QT interval). IA drugs increase the duration of the action potential, IB drugs shorten it and IC drugs have little effect. The antiarrhythmic action of IB drugs is confined to the ventricles, whereas IA and IC drugs affect both atria and ventricles. IA and particularly IC drugs slow intraventricular conduction, and IA drugs can significantly prolong the QT interval.

Class II drugs

Class II drugs interfere with the effects of the sympathetic nervous system on the heart. They do not affect the action potential of most myocardial cells but do reduce the slope of spontaneous depolarisation (phase 4) of cells with pacemaker activity and thus the rate of pacemaker discharge.

Class III drugs

Class III drugs block potassium ion transport across the cell membrane. They prolong the duration of the action potential and hence the length of the refractory period and the QT interval, but do not slow phase 0.

Class IV drugs

Class IV drugs antagonise the transport of calcium across the cell membrane which follows the inward flux of sodium during cellular activation. Cells in the AV and sinus nodes are particularly susceptible. It should be noted that the dihydropyridine calcium channel blockers, nifedipine and amlodipine, do not have an antiarrhythmic action.

Limitations of action potential classification

The majority of drugs are in class I, and drugs within this class differ significantly in their clinical effects. Some drugs have more than one class of action: amiodarone has class I, II and IV actions as well as its main class III effect! Furthermore, some drugs (e.g. digoxin and adenosine) cannot be classified.

Notes on individual drugs

Flecainide

Flecainide is a potent drug which can be given both orally and intravenously. Its indications include paroxysmal atrial fibrillation, pre-excitation syndromes and ventricular arrhythmias. It is very effective at suppressing ventricular ectopic beats but less so in the treatment of ventricular tachycardia.

It has a long half-life of approximately 16 hours, which facilitates twice-daily oral administration. The usual oral dosage is 100 mg twice daily. If side effects occur then reduction of the daily dosage by as little as 50 mg can help. Rarely, a twice-daily dose of 50 mg is effective, and occasionally 300 mg daily is required. There is a once-daily, slow-release preparation available, the dose being 200 mg daily.

The intravenous dose is 1–2 mg/kg body weight over 10 minutes; it should be given more slowly in patients with impaired ventricular function. Flecainide is both metabolised by the liver and excreted by the kidney.

The drug has a narrow therapeutic range, i.e. it can be difficult to achieve a therapeutic action without unwanted effects. High levels can cause visual disturbance, particularly on rotating the head, light-headedness and nausea. Marked QRS prolongation (>25%) during treatment indicates that the blood level may be too high. The drug has been shown to increase the threshold of pacemaker stimuli.

The drug does have an important negative inotropic action and should be avoided in patients in heart failure or with extensive myocardial damage. It can be proarrhythmic, particularly in patients with a history of sustained ventricular tachycardia and/or poor ventricular function. In a major study of patients with ventricular extrasystoles following myocardial infarction, flecainide was found to increase mortality. It is now generally agreed that *the drug should not be given to patients known to have coronary artery disease*.

Flecainide causes slight prolongation of the QRS complex and hence the QT interval: it does not prolong the JT component of the QT interval, as do quinidine and disopyramide.

Flecainide is effective and safe when used to prevent atrial fibrillation and AV re-entrant tachycardias in patients with structurally normal hearts. It is also indicated in patients with highly symptomatic idiopathic ventricular extrasystoles.

Occasionally, like other class I drugs, flecainide can worsen atrial arrhythmias: either converting atrial fibrillation to flutter or increasing the ventricular rate during atrial flutter (Figure 19.1).

The drug must not be given to patients with the Brugada syndrome.

Propafenone

This drug has both IC and mild beta-blocking properties and has been shown to be effective in both supraventricular and ventricular arrhythmias. It can be proarrhythmic and should not be given to patients with impaired ventricular function or with the Brugada syndrome. In the author's experience, non-cardiac unwanted effects are common.

Amiodarone

Amiodarone has several advantages over other drugs. It is highly effective in both supraventricular and ventricular rhythm disorders: even in arrhythmias refractory to other drugs there is a 70% success rate. It has a remarkably long half-life (20–100 days), so that the drug need only be given once daily or even less frequently. It does not significantly impair ventricular performance and can be given to patients in heart failure. However, amiodarone has important unwanted effects, dictating that its long-term use is confined to patients with arrhythmias that are dangerous or resistant to other drugs, or where the risk of side effects is not a major consideration because the patient's prognosis is poor, e.g. in the elderly and those with severe myocardial damage.

Though it is effective in the treatment of ventricular arrhythmias, recent studies have shown that it has no role in 'primary prevention' in patients with poor ventricular function, i.e. it does not reduce the incidence of fatal ventricular arrhythmias in these patients. Nevertheless, many patients with implantable defibrillators require amiodarone to reduce ventricular arrhythmias in order to prevent frequent shock delivery.

(a)

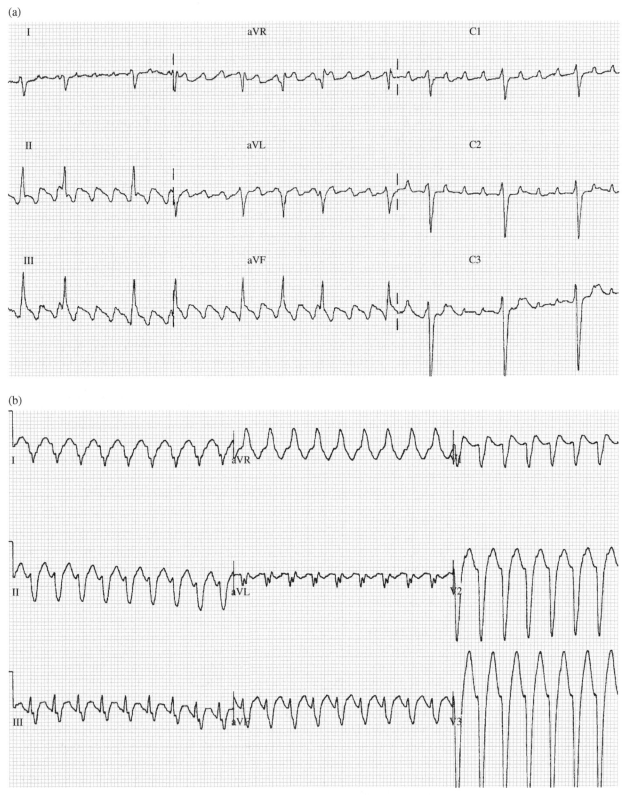

(b)

Figure 19.1 (a) Patient with atrial flutter with 2:1 AV conduction. (b) Same patient after flecainide: the drug slowed the atrial rate, facilitating 1:1 AV conduction and consequently a marked increase in ventricular rate.

Unwanted effects

Short-term treatment with intravenous amiodarone is unlikely to cause side effects, although a few cases of hepatitis associated with the drug have been described. It often causes phlebitis if administered via a peripheral vein.

Longer-term oral therapy is associated with a high incidence of side effects.

Amiodarone: main unwanted effects

Dermatological: photosensitivity and blue-grey pigmentation
Corneal microdeposits
Thyroid dysfunction: hyperthyroidism and hypothyroidism
Pulmonary fibrosis
Hepatitis
Neuropathy
Myopathy
Sleep disturbance: insomnia, vivid dreams and nightmares
Tremor
Alopecia
Torsade de pointes tachycardia
Warfarin potentiation

Dermatological

Skin photosensitivity to UVA radiation affects two-thirds of patients. Though only a minority experience severe photosensitivity, all patients should be warned about the possibility. If necessary, protective clothing, avoidance of prolonged sunlight and barrier creams containing zinc oxide may be recommended. Severe photosensitivity is the commonest reason for stopping the drug. Symptoms may persist for over a year afterwards. There appears to be no relation between skin type or dosage and this unwanted effect.

After prolonged usage a small number of patients develop marked blue-grey pigmentation of the skin, particularly the nose and forehead. This pigmentation will persist for many years after amiodarone is stopped.

Ophthalmic

Corneal microdeposits occur in virtually all patients, but permanent damage does not occur. The microdeposits disappear if the drug is stopped and are a useful sign of compliance. There have been a few reports of optic neuropathy.

Thyroid

Amiodarone contains very large amounts of iodine and causes moderate elevation of both serum thyroxine and reverse tri-iodothyronine, and depression of serum tri-iodothyronine. Thyroid-stimulating hormone (TSH) can be depressed. *These changes are compatible with normal thyroid function* during amiodarone therapy. However, amiodarone can cause both hypothyroidism and hyperthyroidism. Up to 15% of patients can be affected.

Hyperthyroidism can result from activation of pre-existing subclinical thyroid disease which results in increased thyroid hormone synthesis, or from thyroiditis developing in a previously normal thyroid gland and thus increased hormone release. If hyperthyroidism occurs, the patient will often become unwell with weight loss and other signs of thyroid overactivity. Previously controlled arrhythmia may recur. *Both* serum thyroxine and tri-iodothyronine will be increased. Hyperthyroidism may be very severe and sudden in its onset. *It may develop many months after amiodarone has been stopped*. Amiodarone should, if possible, be stopped, but in some cases continuation is essential to prevent frequent and dangerous ventricular arrhythmias. Large doses of carbimazole may be required. In severe cases short-term steroid therapy should be given. Referral to an endocrinologist is advisable. Thyroiditis may be self-limiting, and there are reports of reintroduction of amiodarone without further hyperthyroidism. Recurrence of hyperthyroidism may dictate the need for treatment with radio-iodine.

If hypothyroidism occurs, serum thyroxine will be low and TSH will be elevated. Sometimes there will be no clinical signs. Thyroid hormone replacement is indicated. It is not necessary to stop amiodarone. The presence of thyroid autoantibodies suggests pre-existing thyroid disease and that hypothyroidism might progress even if amiodarone is stopped.

Patients receiving long-term amiodarone should have thyroid tests every 6–12 months. *There should always be a high index of suspicion of hyperthyroidism* in a patient who is taking or who has taken amiodarone.

Other side effects

Other serious side effects include pulmonary fibrosis, hepatitis, neuropathy and myopathy. Sometimes several major unwanted effects occur together. Usually, but not invariably, serious side effects are associated with higher dosages of amiodarone.

Pulmonary fibrosis is the most common of these problems. It usually presents with dyspnoea, which may be severe, and widespread shadowing in the lung fields which can be mistaken for pulmonary oedema. The risk is not increased by pre-existing lung disease. Amiodarone should be stopped as soon as the diagnosis becomes evident and short-term therapy with steroids given. A reduction in total lung diffusing capacity without clinical manifestation is common.

Other unwanted effects include nausea, rash, alopecia, tremor, testicular dysfunction, insomnia and nightmares which can be very vivid.

The drug's class III action results in QT prolongation, often with prominent U waves. There are reports of the drug causing torsade de pointes tachycardia (Chapter 13). The drug commonly causes sinus bradycardia.

It is important to note that the drug potentiates oral anticoagulants, usually halving the required dosage. Amiodarone increases blood levels of digoxin, quinidine, verapamil, flecainide and cyclosporine.

With some arrhythmias, the major advantages of amiodarone – its efficacy, absence of important negative inotropic action and long duration of action – are outweighed by the formidable list of side effects. However, most of the side effects are reversible and the risk of them should not be a contraindication in patients with life-threatening arrhythmias, a short life expectancy or in whom other antiarrhythmic measures have failed.

Administration

The drug has a delayed onset of action. When given by mouth, it usually takes 3–7 days before it takes effect and it may take 50 days to achieve its maximal action. If necessary, delay can be minimised by giving very large doses (e.g. 600–1200 mg) daily for one or two weeks. The dose can then be reduced to 400 mg daily.

Once the arrhythmia is controlled, it is recommended that the dose be progressively reduced until the lowest effective dose is found. The usual maintenance dose is 200–400 mg daily. In a few patients, a dose as small as 200 mg on alternate days will suffice. In the author's experience, arrhythmias often recur if the dose in adults is reduced below 300 mg daily. With dangerous arrhythmias where a recurrence cannot be risked, it is best not to reduce the dose below 300 mg daily.

The drug is metabolised by the liver. It is not excreted by the kidneys. The main metabolite is desethylamiodarone, which may itself have an antiarrhythmic action.

Very high concentrations of amiodarone and its metabolite are achieved in the lungs, heart, liver and adipose tissue.

Intravenous administration will lead to an earlier effect than oral therapy, but unlike most drugs, an immediate antiarrhythmic effect does not often occur: an effect is usually seen within 1–24 hours. When an arrhythmia has been difficult to control, it is often worth resorting to intravenous amiodarone in spite of possible delay in action rather than to try further drugs which are less potent and which often cause unwanted effects.

The recommended intravenous dosage is 5 mg/kg body weight over 30 minutes to 1 hour followed by 15 mg/kg over 24 hours. In an emergency, the initial infusion can be given more rapidly, but its vasodilator action may cause marked hypotension. It is important to give the drug via a central venous line to avoid phlebitis. If this is not possible, frequent changes of peripheral infusion site will often suffice.

Dronedarone

Dronedarone is a derivative of amiodarone that has similar electrophysiological actions to amiodarone. It lacks the iodine radical that has been linked with amiodarone's thyroid, pulmonary, hepatic and dermatological unwanted effects. It has a shorter duration of action than amiodarone with a half-life of 1–2 days. Typical dosage is 400 mg twice daily. It can cause a rash, nausea and vomiting, and diarrhoea.

Studies have shown it to be moderately effective in preventing recurrences of atrial fibrillation, but less so than amiodarone. It can also slow the ventricular rate during atrial fibrillation. Unlike flecainide and propafenone, dronedarone is regarded as safe to administer to patients with coronary artery disease.

However, recently, it has been shown to worsen heart failure and increase mortality in patients with heart failure, and there are reports of the drug causing severe hepatic dysfunction and pulmonary fibrosis in spite of the absence of iodine. Current recommendations are that it is contraindicated if there is a history of pulmonary or hepatic toxicity caused by amiodarone, in patients with cardiac failure or left ventricular dysfunction, and in permanent atrial fibrillation. In fact, in spite of the original theoretical attractions of the drug, it is now *only recommended as a second-line drug for adult, clinically stable patients with paroxysmal or persistent atrial fibrillation for the maintenance of sinus rhythm after successful cardioversion.* Hepatic and renal function should be monitored and pulmonary investigations performed if dyspnoea occurs.

It should not be given together with class I or III antiarrhythmic drugs. It can be problematic when given with digoxin, beta-blockers, calcium antagonists, some statins, dabigatran and drugs associated with torsade de pointes tachycardia.

Celivarone, another derivative of amiodarone, is currently being assessed.

Dofetilide

Dofetilide is new class III antiarrhythmic drug that has been shown to be moderately successful in terminating and preventing atrial fibrillation and flutter. It does not have a negative inotropic effect.

Like amiodarone, it prolongs the QT interval. It causes torsade de pointes tachycardia in approximately 3% of patients. In spite of its proarrhythmic action, the drug was shown not to increase mortality in a large group of patients with heart failure. Torsade de pointes usually (but not always) occurs within the first few days of therapy, and in-hospital ECG monitoring and serial QTc measurements for at least three days are essential.

Orally, the usual dose is 500 mg twice daily, but dosage should be reduced if there is renal impairment. If the QT interval prolongs by more than 15% after the first dose, subsequent doses should be halved. The drug should be stopped if the QTc exceeds 500 ms.

The drug should not be given to patients who have a prolonged QT interval or who are receiving verapamil, cimetidine, ketaconazole, timethoprim or prochlorperazine.

A number of drugs, including amiodarone, diltiazem, metformin and amiloride, and grapefruit juice, may increase blood levels.

Vernakalant

Vernakalant is a member of a novel group of drugs that specifically affects the electrophysiology of atrial myocardium. Intravenously, it has been shown to restore normal rhythm within a few minutes in approximately 50% of patients with recent-onset atrial fibrillation, the success rate being higher if the arrhythmia started within the previous 72 hours. Side effects, which include hypotension, paraesthesiae and nausea, are brief.

Adenosine

Adenosine is a potent blocker of AV nodal conduction. It has an extremely short duration of action: 20–30 s. It is very effective in terminating supraventricular tachycardia due to an AV junctional re-entrant mechanism (Figure 19.2) and will transiently slow or interrupt the ventricular response to atrial fibrillation and flutter, making the respective f or F waves more easily identifiable (Figure 19.3). It will terminate some

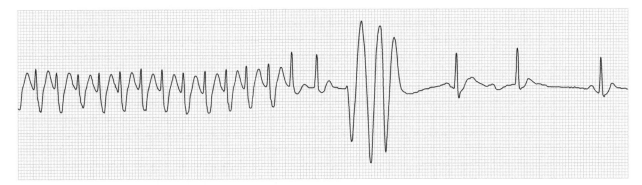

Figure 19.2 AV junctional re-entrant tachycardia with rate-related right bundle branch block. Adenosine slows the rate slightly, facilitating normal intraventricular conduction for two cycles, and then terminates the arrhythmia. After termination, as often occurs, there is a triplet of ventricular ectopic beats and a brief period of impaired AV conduction.

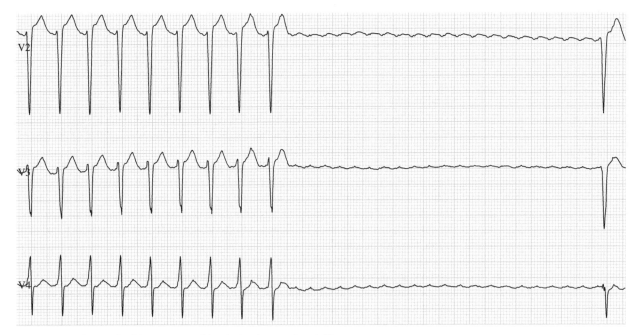

Figure 19.3 Adenosine 'briefly' interrupts AV nodal conduction, demonstrating atrial flutter.

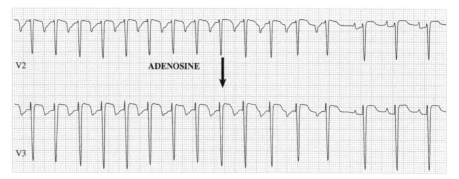

Figure 19.4 Adenosine terminates atrial tachycardia with 1:1 AV conduction.

atrial tachycardias (Figure 19.4). Because of its very short duration of action and its safety, it is the drug of choice for the termination of AV and AV nodal re-entrant tachycardias.

A positive response to adenosine points strongly towards a supraventricular origin to the tachycardia. However, a minority of supraventricular tachycardias will not respond to adenosine, perhaps because a dose in excess of the recommended upper limit is required, and the drug will terminate right ventricular outflow tract tachycardia. Thus response or lack of response to adenosine is a useful pointer towards the origin of a tachycardia but cannot be taken as an absolutely reliable guide.

Most patients will experience chest tightness, dyspnoea and flushing, but the symptoms last less than 60 s. There may be complete AV block for a few seconds following termination of the tachycardia. The drug does not have a negative inotropic action. It is a safe drug to give except perhaps to patients with asthma, in whom there is a possibility of bronchospasm. The drug is antagonised by aminophylline and potentiated by dipyridamole. Adenosine does cause sinus bradycardia and may briefly worsen sinus node function in patients with the sick sinus syndrome.

It should be given as a rapid (2 s) intravenous bolus, followed by a flush of saline. The initial dose in adults and in children is 3 mg and 0.05 mg/kg, respectively. If ineffective, further dosages of 6 mg (0.10 mg/kg) and, if necessary, 12 mg (0.20 mg/kg) can be given after 1.0 min intervals.

Adenosine abuse

Adenosine is often used in a 'knee-jerk' response to a broad complex tachycardia in patients with known myocardial infarction or cardiomyopathy. Ventricular tachycardia is highly likely and it is pointless to use adenosine in these situations unless there is a strong suspicion that the rhythm is atrial flutter or tachycardia with aberration, in which case the drug is being used for diagnostic purposes rather than for arrhythmia termination.

The drug is also commonly given to patients who present with atrial fibrillation. Even if the QRS complexes are broad, the diagnosis will be clear from the totally irregular ventricular rhythm. All adenosine will achieve is slowing of the ventricular response for a few seconds, which is clearly futile (Figure 19.5)!

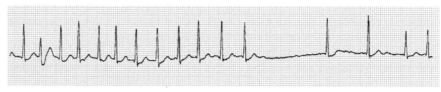

Figure 19.5 Adenosine abuse. The rhythm is totally irregular and clearly due to atrial fibrillation. The drug leads to a short pause in ventricular activity. So what?

Verapamil

Intravenous verapamil (5–10 mg over 30–60 s) quickly and effectively slows AV nodal conduction. It will terminate AV junctional re-entrant tachycardia and will promptly slow the ventricular response to atrial fibrillation and flutter.

Orally, verapamil is less effective in the treatment of AV junctional re-entrant tachycardias but will often control the ventricular response to atrial fibrillation. Because much of each dose is metabolised by the liver, large doses (120–360 mg daily), preferably given in a controlled-release preparation, are required.

The drug is recognised to be able to terminate right ventricular outflow tract tachycardia and fascicular tachycardia. However, when given orally it is not often effective in preventing the onset of these arrhythmias.

Intravenous verapamil is contraindicated if the patient has received an intravenous or oral beta-blocker: profound bradycardia or hypotension can result and may be fatal. Sometimes, the combination of oral verapamil and an oral beta-blocker will cause profound sinus or junctional bradycardia. Verapamil is contraindicated in patients with impaired sinus or AV node function or digoxin toxicity unless a ventricular pacing wire is *in situ* because of its depressant effects on the sinus and AV nodes.

Verapamil does have a significant negative inotropic effect and may cause hypotension in patients with very poor myocardial function. Two studies report that administration of intravenous calcium chloride immediately prior to intravenous verapamil prevents hypotension.

Diltiazem

The actions of diltiazem are similar to those of verapamil.

Orally, a controlled-release preparation, e.g. diltiazem LA, should be used, the dosage being 200–300 mg daily. Diltiazem can cause a skin rash. Intravenously, the dosage is 20 mg as a bolus, repeated after 15 minutes if necessary. A maintenance infusion of 5–15 mg hourly can be given if required.

Beta-adrenoceptor antagonists

Beta-blockers have antiarrhythmic properties by virtue of their principal action – antagonising the effects of catecholamines on the heart. They are most effective in arrhythmias caused by increased sympathetic nervous system activity (e.g. those caused by exertion, emotion, thyrotoxicosis, acute myocardial infarction and the hereditary QT prolongation syndromes).

Beta-blocking drugs slow AV nodal conduction and thus, like verapamil, are useful in arrhythmias of supraventricular origin, and in particular for reducing the ventricular rate during atrial fibrillation. Unwanted bradycardia caused by beta-blockade can usually quickly be reversed by atropine.

Intravenous esmolol has an extremely short half-life of only two minutes. Its beta-adrenoceptor antagonist action and any associated unwanted effects will therefore be brief.

Sotalol

Sotalol, in addition to its beta-blocking property, prolongs the duration of the action potential and hence QT interval: it has a significant class III or amiodarone-like action. Unlike other beta-blockers, sotalol has a marked effect upon the recovery periods of atrial and ventricular myocardium and accessory AV pathways.

It has a long half-life and can be given once daily. The oral dosage is 160–320 mg daily. The drug is excreted by the kidneys: dosage should be reduced if renal function is impaired. Intravenously, it should be given slowly up to a dosage of 1.5 mg/kg.

There are reports of the drug – usually in association with other drugs or hypokalaemia – causing torsade de pointes tachycardia. It should not be given to patients whose QT interval is already prolonged or if there is a family history of hereditary QT prolongation. It must be stopped if the QTc exceeds 500 ms.

Several but not all studies show that sotalol is more effective than other beta-blockers for prevention of atrial fibrillation and other supraventricular arrhythmias. It has been shown to be effective in the treatment of ventricular tachycardia, including in patients with implantable defibrillators.

Digoxin

Digoxin is widely used as an AV nodal blocking drug in the control of the ventricular rate during atrial fibrillation. *However, digoxin is often ineffective at rate control when the patient is active.*

The usual dose is 0.25–0.375 mg daily. A number of factors, such as hypokalaemia, renal impairment, age, dehydration (often caused by diuretics) and therapy with verapamil or amiodarone, predispose to digoxin toxicity and are an indication for dosage reduction.

Digoxin toxicity

Digoxin toxicity is a common problem. Over 10% of patients receiving the drug who are admitted to hospital have been found to have evidence of digoxin toxicity.

A number of symptoms suggest digoxin toxicity. These include anorexia, nausea, vomiting, diarrhoea, mental confusion, xanthopsia and visual blurring. However, none of these symptoms is specific to digoxin toxicity; in patients with severe congestive heart failure in particular, gastrointestinal symptoms are often caused by heart failure rather than digoxin.

Digoxin toxicity can cause a number of disorders of cardiac rhythm. These include atrial tachycardia with AV block (Figure 19.6), junctional tachycardia (Figure 19.7), ventricular ectopic beats (often bigeminy) (Figure 19.8), ventricular tachycardia, first-, second- and third-degree AV block, a slow ventricular response to atrial fibrillation (Figure 19.9) and sinoatrial block (Figure 19.10). A recent large study of anticoagulant therapy in atrial fibrillation found an increased mortality in those patients receiving digoxin.

Digoxin is often used to control the ventricular rate during atrial fibrillation. When a patient receiving digoxin for this purpose develops a regular pulse a number of possibilities should be considered. First, sinus rhythm may have returned. Second, an arrhythmia due to digoxin toxicity may have developed (e.g. atrial tachycardia with AV block, junctional tachycardia or atrial fibrillation with complete AV block).

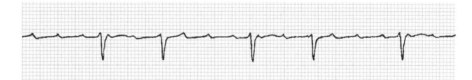

Figure 19.6 Atrial tachycardia with varying degrees of AV block.

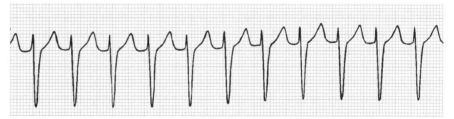

Figure 19.7 Junctional tachycardia.

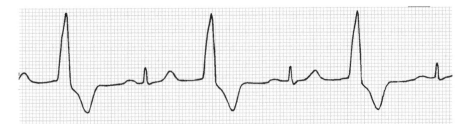

Figure 19.8 First-degree AV block with ventricular bigeminy.

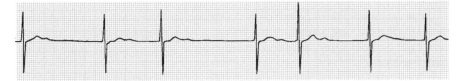

Figure 19.9 Slow ventricular response to atrial fibrillation.

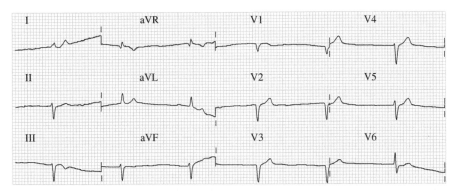

Figure 19.10 Junctional rhythm in a patient receiving digoxin for atrial fibrillation. Digoxin level 5.9 nmol/L.

Without an ECG it may be difficult to ascertain whether the regular rhythm is due to an arrhythmia or not.

Plasma digoxin levels can be measured but must be interpreted in conjunction with clinical features. Levels less than 1.5 ng/mL, in the absence of hypokalaemia, indicate that digoxin toxicity is unlikely. Levels in excess of 3.0 ng/mL indicate that toxicity is probable. With levels between 1.5 and 3.0 ng/mL digoxin toxicity should be considered a possibility, particularly if there are symptoms or arrhythmias attributable to digoxin toxicity or if there is renal impairment, or if the patient appears to be on an inappropriately large dose of digoxin. Blood for digoxin concentration estimation must be taken at least six hours after the last dose.

Usually, temporary discontinuation of the drug and correction of hypokalaemia, if present, are all that is required. *Serious toxicity can be treated with specific digoxin-binding antibodies raised in sheep.*

If high degrees of AV block occur, temporary cardiac pacing may be necessary. Cardioversion is dangerous in the presence of digoxin toxicity. If cardioversion is essential, low energy levels (e.g. 5–10 J), increasing gradually as necessary, should be used and lignocaine 75–100 mg should be given.

Lignocaine

Lignocaine is a first-line drug for ventricular arrhythmias but is ineffective in supraventricular arrhythmias. The drug is a vasoconstrictor and, unlike many drugs, rarely causes hypotension or heart failure.

A 100 mg bolus given intravenously over 2 minutes will often be successful. If not, a further bolus (50–75 mg) should be given after 5 minutes.

Several concentrations of lignocaine are available. Disasters have occurred because the wrong concentration has been used. Remember, 10 mL 1% lignocaine contains 100 mg.

Lignocaine may be used for short-term prevention of ventricular arrhythmias. The therapeutic effect of lignocaine is closely related to plasma levels, which fall rapidly after a bolus injection. Thus it is necessary to give a continuous infusion immediately after the bolus. There is, however, no point in giving a continuous infusion if the bolus has failed to work or, since lignocaine cannot be administered by mouth, if long-term prophylaxis is required.

It can be difficult to maintain therapeutic levels of lignocaine. With subtherapeutic levels, the patient is at risk from arrhythmias while toxic levels may cause symptoms related to the central nervous system, including light-headedness, confusion, twitching, paraesthesiae and epileptic fits. With conventional infusion rates (1–4 mg/min) subtherapeutic levels commonly occur in the first hour or two after the infusion is commenced.

Lignocaine is metabolised by the liver: where there is liver disease or where hepatic blood flow is reduced by heart failure or by shock, dosages should be halved to avoid toxicity. Hypokalaemia may impair lignocaine's efficacy.

Quinidine

Quinidine can cause torsade de pointes tachycardia. Several surveys have shown that it increases mortality, even in patients with non-dangerous arrhythmias. There are safer alternative drugs for many arrhythmias.

However, recently there have been reports about the value of this drug in treating the 'arrhythmia storms' that may occur in the Brugada syndrome and in the treatment of the rare short QT syndrome.

Disopyramide

Disopyramide has been widely used for both supraventricular and ventricular arrhythmias. However, it is only moderately effective and does have significant unwanted effects.

The intravenous dose is 1.5–2.0 mg/kg up to a maximum of 150 mg, given over no less than 5 minutes. The injection should be stopped if the arrhythmia is terminated. Therapy can be continued by intravenous infusion at 20–30 mg/hour up to a maximum of 800 mg daily, or the patient can be transferred to oral therapy. The oral dose is 300–800 mg daily in three or four divided doses. If necessary, a loading dose of 300 mg can be given.

Given intravenously, the drug is more likely to cause hypotension and heart failure than lignocaine and related drugs, and its use can be disastrous if the recommended minimum period of administration is ignored.

Orally, the drug's side effects are mainly related to its anticholinergic (atropine-like) action, which often causes a dry mouth, blurred vision, urinary retention and, by enhancing AV nodal conduction, an increase in the ventricular response to atrial flutter and fibrillation. The drug may precipitate heart failure in patients with impaired myocardial function. It may occasionally induce torsade de pointes tachycardia and should not be given to patients with QT interval prolongation. Disopyramide may worsen impaired sinus node function and is contraindicated in the sick sinus syndrome. The drug is partially excreted by the kidneys, and dosage should be reduced in renal disease.

Procainamide

Procainamide has similar antiarrhythmic properties to quinidine. It is not widely used and is now never used by the author. It has a short half-life, necessitating very frequent dosage when given by mouth. Even with a slow-release preparation, eight-hourly administration is necessary. Furthermore, unwanted effects such as systemic lupus syndrome, gastrointestinal symptoms, hypotension and agranulocytosis make it unsuitable for long-term use. Impaired renal function and a slow acetylator status both reduce procainamide requirements. *N*-Acetyl-procainamide, a metabolite of procainamide, has been shown to have a longer duration of action and not to cause systemic lupus.

Ranalozine

Recently, there has been interest in the antiarrhythmic properties of the antianginal drug ranalozine. It has effects on both sodium and potassium channels. It appears to be well tolerated, and small studies have indicated that it may be effective in treating arrhythmias due to ischaemia, in atrial fibrillation, in ventricular arrhythmias and, even though it may prolong the QT interval, in the hereditary long QT syndromes.

Grapefruit

Grapefruit juice and fresh segments have been shown to inactivate the hepatic cytochrome P450 system and can lead to increased levels of a wide variety of cardiac medications: antiarrhythmic drugs including verapamil, amiodarone, quinidine, disopyramide and propafenone and other cardiac medications, including carvedilol, atorvastatin, simvastatin and nifedipine.

Grapefruit juice alone has been shown to slightly prolong the QT interval.

Antiarrhythmic drugs during pregnancy

No antiarrhythmic drug is completely safe during pregnancy. Concerns include a teratogenic effect when given during the first eight weeks of pregnancy, impaired intrauterine growth, and secretion in breast milk. Where possible, drugs should be avoided in patients with well-tolerated arrhythmias, particularly in the first trimester.

Of the commonly used drugs, adenosine, beta-blockers and flecainide (which has been shown to be very effective in treating fetal supraventricular tachycardia) have been used quite widely and appear relatively safe. Digoxin crosses the placental barrier and has been reported to cause fetal death. Amiodarone has been reported to cause congenital abnormalities including hypothyroidism.

20 Sudden Cardiac Death

Sudden cardiac death is most commonly due to ventricular tachycardia or fibrillation caused by poor ventricular function resulting from coronary artery disease or from dilated cardiomyopathy. Other causes include the hereditary long QT syndromes, arrhythmogenic right ventricular cardiomyopathy, the Brugada syndrome and hypertrophic cardiomyopathy.

Patients resuscitated from sudden cardiac death not due to acute infarction or reversible cause are likely to experience a recurrence: investigation and treatment, which often includes an implantable defibrillator, should be undertaken.

Sudden death due to cardiac disease is common. The annual incidence in the United Kingdom is estimated to be 100 000 and in the United States, 300 000 – i.e. in the order of 1–2 per thousand of the general population. The risk is higher in those with known heart disease, for example past myocardial infarction – especially those with poor left ventricular function. It is reported that recently there has been a modest decline in the rate of sudden cardiac death, presumably due to better coronary prevention measures.

Definition

Sudden cardiac death can be defined as unexpected death due to a cardiac cause occurring within 60 minutes of the onset of symptoms. Many sudden deaths are unwitnessed and few occur during ECG monitoring. Thus it cannot be assumed that sudden death is synonymous with arrhythmic death: there are other possible causes such as valvular and congenital heart diseases, cardiac tumours, electromechanical dissociation (EMD), cerebrovascular accident, pulmonary embolism and massive haemorrhage, e.g. from a ruptured aortic aneurysm. Furthermore, even a documented episode of ventricular fibrillation might be a terminal event resulting from a cardiovascular catastrophe such as massive myocardial infarction. Nevertheless, most sudden cardiac deaths are caused by an arrhythmia, usually ventricular tachycardia or fibrillation (Figure 20.1).

Bennett's Cardiac Arrhythmias: Practical Notes on Interpretation and Treatment, Eighth Edition. David H. Bennett.
© 2013 John Wiley & Sons, Ltd. Published 2013 by John Wiley & Sons, Ltd.

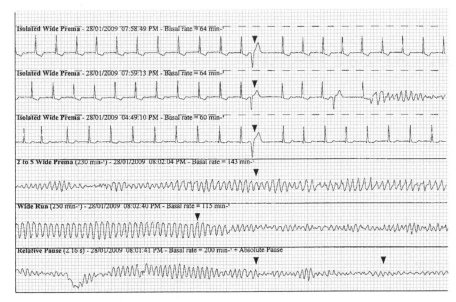

Figure 20.1 Ventricular fibrillation following a series of unifocal ventricular ectopic beats.

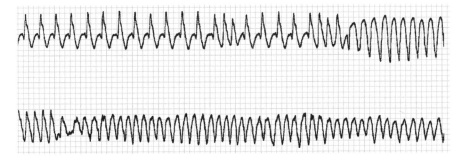

Figure 20.2 Continuous recording as monomorphic ventricular tachycardia deteriorates into ventricular fibrillation.

Causes of arrhythmic sudden death

Ventricular fibrillation often results from degeneration from ventricular tachycardia, rather than being the primary arrhythmia (Figure 20.2). A minority of arrhythmic deaths are caused by bradycardia.

Coronary heart disease is by far the most common cause of sudden cardiac death. Though acute myocardial infarction commonly leads to ventricular fibrillation, it accounts for less than one-third of patients presenting with sudden death. The majority have been found to have extensive coronary disease and poor left ventricular function but not acute infarction. The main causes are included in the table, and are discussed elsewhere in this book.

Genetically determined causes

If an inheritable cause of sudden cardiac death is identified, then relatives should be recommended to undergo cardiological and/or genetic examination. In the young, where no evidence of structural heart disease has been found in spite of a thorough autopsy, there is a strong possibility of cardiac ion 'channelopathy' being responsible. It should be borne in mind that relatives can carry an abnormal gene and yet have a normal ECG.

Causes of arrhythmic sudden cardiac death

Acute myocardial infarction
Acute myocardial ischaemia
Myocardial damage due to coronary heart disease
Congenital coronary artery abnormalities
Dilated cardiomyopathy
Hypertrophic cardiomyopathy
Arrhythmogenic right ventricular cardiomyopathy
Myocarditis
Atrioventricular block
Hereditary and acquired long QT syndromes
Brugada syndrome
Wolff–Parkinson–White syndrome
Idiopathic ventricular fibrillation
Catecholaminergic polymorphic ventricular tachycardia
Short QT syndrome
Electrolyte abnormalities
Proarrhythmic drugs (including cocaine)
Commotio cordis

Aborted sudden cardiac death

Several centres have shown that facilities for out-of-hospital cardiopulmonary resuscitation do save lives. However, it should be appreciated that only 8–10% of those resuscitated in the community survive to leave hospital. Patients who are resuscitated and who have not sustained acute infarction remain at risk. There is a recurrence rate of up to 60% within two years.

Patients resuscitated from cardiac arrest not caused by acute infarction or by a correctable cause must be investigated to assess the need for myocardial revascularisation, drug therapy and/or implantation of an automatic defibrillator before discharge from hospital.

It should be noted that hypokalaemia is commonly found after resuscitation. It is usually the result of the stress of collapse and resuscitation and cannot be assumed to be the cause of a ventricular arrhythmia.

Impaired ventricular function

In patients whose arrest was a consequence of poor ventricular function, the worse the ejection fraction the more likely is a recurrence. Additional factors pointing to a poor prognosis include left bundle branch block and non-sustained ventricular tachycardia.

Amiodarone has little or no effect on mortality, and other antiarrhythmic drugs have been shown to increase mortality.

Beta-blockers, angiotensin-converting enzyme inhibitors, spironolactone or eplerenone, and statins have all been shown to improve prognosis whether by antiarrhythmic or by other actions. The most important treatment to consider is defibrillator implantation (Chapter 24).

Athletic activities

Sudden cardiac death can occasionally occur during sporting activities. In the young, common causes include hypertrophic cardiomyopathy, arrhythmogenic right ventricular cardiomyopathy, the long QT syndrome and dilated cardiomyopathy. In the older male, the commonest cause is coronary artery disease. In patients known to have any of these conditions, competitive strenuous sporting activities should be avoided.

'Pre-participation' screening prior is recommended by several authorities with the aim of preventing sudden cardiac death during competitive sports. However, there is in fact little objective evidence that lives are saved, and concern has been voiced that screening is not cost-effective. Another problem is differentiating between 'athlete's heart' and cardiac disease: physical training can lead to left ventricular hypertrophy, non-specific ST-T wave ECG changes, and first-degree and Wenckebach atrioventricular block due to high vagal tone. Difficulty can also arise where the evidence for cardiac disease is marginal, e.g. a QTc in the range of 440–470 ms.

Commotio cordis

A rare cause of sudden cardiac death during sporting activities is commotio cordis: ventricular fibrillation is caused by a blunt, non-penetrating blow to the precordium that coincides with the upstroke of the T wave. It occurs in young people during ball games and other contact sports. The sooner defibrillation can be carried out, the greater the chance of survival.

21 Cardioversion

Electrical cardioversion is the delivery of a direct current shock to the heart of brief duration and high energy to terminate a tachyarrhythmia. The usual positions for the defibrillator paddles or self-adhesive electrodes for transthoracic cardioversion are the cardiac apex and to the right of the upper sternum. Except for ventricular fibrillation, shock delivery should be synchronised to the R or S wave of the ECG. Initial energy levels (biphasic) should be 50 J for atrial flutter and 150 J for ventricular fibrillation. 150–200 J is usually required to cardiovert atrial fibrillation. Digoxin toxicity is a contraindication.

In atrial fibrillation or flutter, anticoagulation should precede cardioversion.

Damage to an implanted pacemaker or defibrillator can be prevented if the electrodes are placed at least 15 cm from the generator. Enzyme measurements have shown that cardioversion may affect skeletal but not cardiac muscle. Transvenous cardioversion for atrial fibrillation may be more effective than transthoracic, especially in large patients.

Electrical cardioversion is the use of an electric shock of brief duration and high energy to terminate a tachyarrhythmia (Figure 21.1). The shock depolarises the myocardium, thus interrupting the tachycardia and allowing the sinus node to resume control of the heart rhythm.

Chemical cardioversion is the restoration of normal rhythm by antiarrhythmic drugs, and it is discussed elsewhere.

Transthoracic cardioversion

Cardioversion is usually carried out by delivering a shock between two electrodes placed on the chest.

Procedure

Facilities for monitoring the ECG and for cardiopulmonary resuscitation must be available.

The rhythm should be checked immediately before cardioversion to ensure that spontaneous reversion has not occurred.

Bennett's Cardiac Arrhythmias: Practical Notes on Interpretation and Treatment, Eighth Edition. David H. Bennett.
© 2013 John Wiley & Sons, Ltd. Published 2013 by John Wiley & Sons, Ltd.

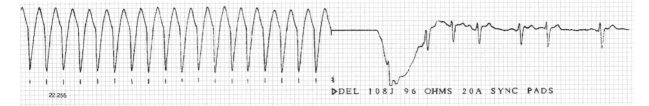

Figure 21.1 Termination of ventricular tachycardia by delivery of 100 J shock.

Anaesthesia

The patient should fast for four hours before elective cardioversion.

A conscious patient should receive a short-acting general anaesthetic, or alternatively intravenous drugs to achieve deep but brief sedation. Small incremental doses of intravenous midazolam (total 1–10 mg) in combination with fentanyl (50 mg) are very effective. It is essential that the patient's airway and oxygen saturation are carefully monitored and that drugs to reverse fentanyl (i.e. naloxone) and midazolam (i.e. flumazenil) are immediately available in the unlikely event of respiratory depression.

Delivery of shock

The shock is delivered between two electrodes. Correct positioning is important. Usually one electrode is placed at the level of the cardiac apex, close to the mid-axillary line, and the other is positioned to the right of the upper sternum.

Alternatively, a flat paddle, if available, can be placed beneath the patient's back, behind the heart, and a second paddle positioned over the precordium. If a flat paddle is unavailable, standard electrodes can be applied anteroposteriorly if the patient is turned onto his or her side: one paddle is placed over the precordium and the other paddle below the left shoulder to the left of the spine.

To achieve good electrical contact and to avoid burning the skin, electrode jelly must be applied to the areas beneath metal paddles. However, it is essential to avoid spreading jelly between the two paddles. Pads impregnated with electrode gel prevent jelly being spread over inappropriate areas, including the operator!

The defibrillator is charged to the desired energy level (see below), which takes a few seconds. The charge is usually delivered by pressing the button(s) on the defibrillator paddle(s). Metal paddles should be applied with firm pressure to reduce the electrical resistance of the thorax.

Before discharge it is essential to ensure that no one is in contact with the patient.

If cardioversion is unsuccessful, depending on the circumstances, further shocks with higher energy levels may be tried.

It is important to become thoroughly familiar with the controls of defibrillators that one might be required to use.

Synchronisation

Ventricular fibrillation may be initiated if a shock coincides with the ventricular T wave. Therefore, defibrillators have a mechanism whereby discharge is triggered to coincide with the R or S wave. This mechanism should be used during cardioversion for all arrhythmias except ventricular fibrillation. With ventricular fibrillation there will be no detectable R wave and thus, if the mechanism is in operation, the defibrillator will not discharge.

Before synchronised cardioversion, the operator should check that the synchronising signal coincides with the onset of the QRS complex. Sometimes, the amplitude of the ECG has to be increased to enable synchronisation.

Biphasic waveform

Modern defibrillators deliver a biphasic rather than a monophasic shock. With biphasic shocks the direction of current flow is reversed approximately halfway through the discharge. Biphasic defibrillation allows delivery of greater energy at lower voltage. A biphasic 150J shock is roughly equivalent to a monophasic 200J shock.

Complications

Complications are rare.

Cardioversion often causes marked elevation in creatinine kinase but does not significantly elevate troponin levels. Thus, cardioversion may affect skeletal muscle but does not cause myocardial damage. Biphasic shocks are less likely to affect skeletal muscle. Skin burns can sometimes result from cardioversion. This complication has been shown to be less likely with biphasic shocks.

Transient arrhythmias occasionally occur, but these are rarely a problem unless there is digoxin toxicity.

In patients with the bradycardia–tachycardia syndrome cardioversion may cause a major bradycardia: temporary pacing may be required to cover cardioversion.

Systemic embolism may occur when cardioversion is carried out for atrial fibrillation (see below).

Digoxin toxicity

Cardioversion in the presence of digoxin toxicity can produce dangerous ventricular arrhythmias. For this reason cardioversion should be a last resort and should be preceded by lignocaine 75–100 mg. When digoxin toxicity is likely, very low energy levels should be used, starting at 5–10J.

Because of the dangers of digoxin toxicity, it has become common practice to stop digoxin for 24–48 hours before cardioversion. However, cardioversion in the presence of therapeutic levels of digoxin is safe. There is no need to postpone cardioversion provided the patient is receiving standard doses of digoxin, renal function and plasma electrolytes are normal and there are no symptoms or ECG findings suggestive of digoxin toxicity (Chapter 19).

Implanted pacemakers and defibrillators

Cardioversion may cause pacemaker or defibrillator damage unless the electrodes are placed at least 15 cm from the device and preferably are positioned so they are at right angles to the line between the device and the heart.

Indications
Ventricular fibrillation

Immediate cardioversion is necessary. The initial energy level should be 150–200J (biphasic). If unsuccessful, further 200J (360J if monophasic) shocks should be given.

Sequential or simultaneous shocks, delivered by means of two defibrillators with separate pairs of electrodes, should be considered in any patient who is not defibrillated with repeated 360J shocks.

Ventricular tachycardia

Cardioversion is indicated if the arrhythmia causes shock or cardiac arrest, or if drug therapy has failed. With very fast ventricular tachycardias it may be difficult to synchronise delivery of the shock and it may be necessary to deliver an unsynchronised shock. Energy levels as for ventricular fibrillation should be used.

Atrial fibrillation

Sinus rhythm can be restored by cardioversion in most patients with atrial fibrillation. However, not infrequently the arrhythmia returns.

High-energy shocks are usually required. The first shock should be 150 200 J biphasic. If necessary, 200 J shocks can be repeated. A shock applied between anterior and posterior electrodes may be successful in resistant cases.

Anticoagulation

Cardioversion can result in systemic embolism because of dislodgement of pre-existing thrombus. New atrial thrombus can develop after cardioversion because atrial mechanical activity often does not return for up to three weeks after the procedure and because cardioversion itself can increase blood hypercoagulability. Hence embolism can occur in the few weeks following cardioversion. It is therefore recommended that non-urgent cardioversion in patients who have been in atrial fibrillation for more than 24–48 hours is preceded by warfarin for at least three weeks and that anticoagulation is continued for at least four weeks after restoration of normal rhythm. In patients who are at high risk of embolism long-term anticoagulation should be considered, because there is a significant possibility of further atrial fibrillation, either paroxysmal or sustained.

If urgent cardioversion is required before anticoagulation can be established, transesophageal echocardiography should be used to exclude left atrial thrombus or stasis. The echocardiographic signs of left atrial stasis are spontaneous echo contrast and reduced left atrial appendage flow velocity. If cardioversion has to be carried out urgently, heparin should be given until adequate anticoagulation is achieved with warfarin.

Recurrence of atrial fibrillation

While cardioversion only leads to long-term sinus rhythm in a minority of patients, an attempt at restoring sinus rhythm should be considered in those patients with recent atrial fibrillation (less than 12 months) where no cause has been identified or in whom the disorder which has caused the arrhythmia has resolved or is self-limiting. Cardioversion should also be considered in patients with atrial fibrillation which has been present for more than 12 months if symptoms due to the arrhythmia are severe, even when there is only a small chance of long-term normal rhythm.

If there is a recurrence, a further attempt at cardioversion, after initiation of antiarrhythmic therapy, should only be undertaken in those with troublesome symptoms attributable to the arrhythmia. Several drugs, such as disopyramide, flecainide, sotalol, and especially amiodarone, reduce the relapse rate after cardioversion and ideally should be prescribed prior to cardioversion.

Atrial flutter

This arrhythmia, which is often difficult to treat with drugs, responds to low-energy shocks (50 J). The risk of embolism is lower than with atrial fibrillation. However, flutter and fibrillation can sometimes coexist so some recommend the same anticoagulant regime as for atrial fibrillation. Anticoagulation is definitely indicated if there is myocardial or valve disease, or a history of embolism.

Cardioversion is almost always successful, but atrial flutter will recur in half of cases – though it many be many months before the arrhythmia does recur.

Atrioventricular junctional re-entrant tachycardia

Cardioversion is indicated on the very few occasions when other measures, such as vagal stimulation or intravenous adenosine or verapamil, have failed.

Transvenous cardioversion

Transvenous cardioversion is now an established technique for terminating atrial fibrillation. A low-energy shock (15–30 J) is delivered between transvenous electrodes

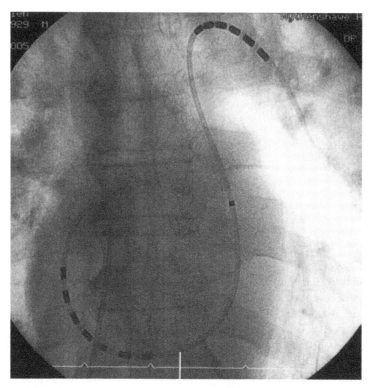

Figure 21.2 Transvenous cardioversion. There is a single lead with a multipolar cathode in the left pulmonary artery and a multipolar anode in the right atrium.

positioned in the right atrium and either the coronary sinus or pulmonary artery. Though energy levels are lower, sedative or anaesthetic requirements are the same as for transthoracic cardioversion.

A single-lead, balloon-guided system is available which also facilitates atrial and ventricular pacing, if required (Figure 21.2).

Success rates are higher than for transthoracic cardioversion, especially in very large patients.

This approach should be considered in patients where transthoracic cardioversion has failed but restoration of normal rhythm is thought to be of great importance, and as a first-line strategy in large patients.

22 Ambulatory ECG Monitoring

Ambulatory electrocardiography enables monitoring of the heart rhythm for long periods and is invaluable in the investigation of syncope, near-syncope, palpitation and other symptoms thought to be due to an arrhythmia when routine electrocardiography has not provided a diagnosis. Artefacts can produce apparent arrhythmias but can be recognised by careful inspection of the recording.

Studies in apparently normal subjects have demonstrated that some rhythms detected by ambulatory electrocardiography are not of pathological significance, e.g. ventricular ectopic beats in the setting of a structurally normal heart, nocturnal sinus bradycardia and nocturnal atrioventricular Wenckebach block.

For patients with infrequent, non-disabling palpitation, provision of a handheld event recorder is the best method of investigation. An implantable loop recorder, a very small device, can facilitate ECG monitoring for more than one year in patients with episodes that are few and far between.

The standard resting 12-lead ECG records the heart rhythm for no more than 30s and is therefore not suitable for detecting intermittent disturbances in heart rhythm. Ambulatory ECG monitoring is an invaluable diagnostic tool. The ECG can be continuously or intermittently recorded for long periods.

Continuous ECG recording

The ECG can be continuously recorded, usually for 24–120 hours, using a portable battery-operated recorder that is usually worn around the neck or waist. The ECG is recorded in digital form in a solid state recording system. If appropriate, the patient can be fully ambulant, carrying out his or her normal day-to-day activities.

The ECG is recorded by means of adhesive electrodes applied to areas of thoroughly cleaned skin. Usually one electrode is placed over the upper sternum and the other electrode over the V5 chest lead position. As an alternative, a modified V1 lead can be obtained by placing one electrode over the V1 chest lead position and the other electrode beneath the lateral part of the left clavicle.

Bennett's Cardiac Arrhythmias: Practical Notes on Interpretation and Treatment, Eighth Edition. David H. Bennett.
© 2013 John Wiley & Sons, Ltd. Published 2013 by John Wiley & Sons, Ltd.

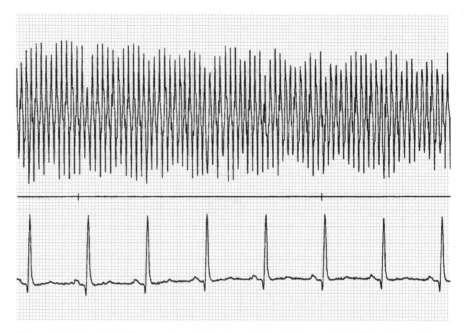

Figure 22.1 The artefact in the upper trace might have been misinterpreted as ventricular fibrillation had not the lower trace been recorded simultaneously.

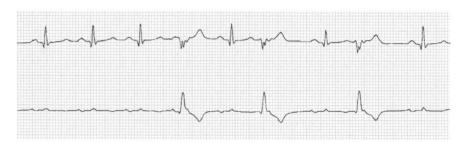

Figure 22.2 The lower trace suggests AV block but the simultaneous upper trace clearly shows that the small complexes in the lower trace are not P waves.

Most systems allow simultaneous recording of two or more leads. This increases diagnostic accuracy and aids in the detection of artefacts, which are unlikely to appear on both leads at the same time (Figure 22.1). Furthermore, sometimes one lead does not reveal important diagnostic information while the other does (Figure 22.2).

The recording is analysed by replaying it at 60–100 times real-time. Playback systems have facilities for printing out selected portions of the recording on ECG paper at standard speed. Most recording systems can automatically detect bradycardias, tachycardias and ectopic beats, though in practice an operator has to supervise the analysis.

Artefacts

Several technical problems during ambulatory electrocardiography can result in what appear to be arrhythmias to the unwary.

Not infrequently, a lead will become disconnected during a recording: because no activity is being recorded the ECG will appear as a straight line and mimic sinus arrest. Furthermore, sometimes an electrical connection can intermittently fail, resulting in repeated episodes of apparent sinus arrest. However, if a lead becomes disconnected it may do so at any point in the cardiac cycle, and it is unlikely the onset of 'asystole' will arise after the ventricular T wave as it would if sinus arrest were real.

(a)

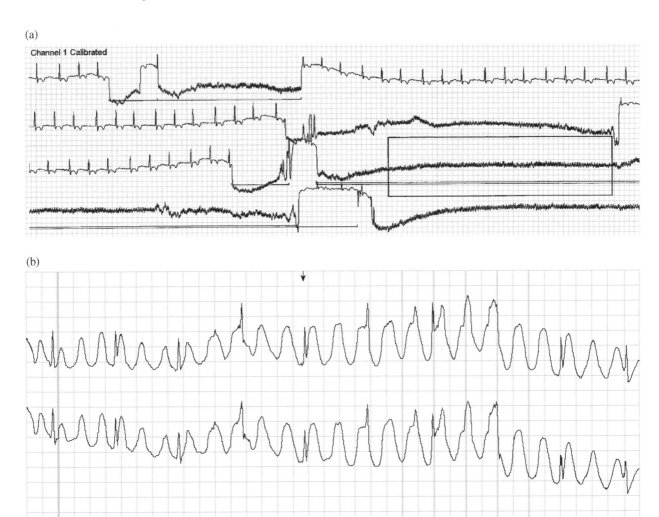

(b)

Figure 22.3 (a) Artefact due to intermittent lead disconnection: apparent asystole can be seen to start during inscription of a T wave. (b) On close inspection narrow QRS complexes (indicated by letters N and A at the bottom of the trace) can be seen walking through apparent ventricular arrhythmia.

If the onset of sinus arrest occurs during the inscription of an atrial or ventricular complex, artefact can be assumed (Figure 22.3a).

Occasionally, artefact can produce an apparent tachycardia, but close inspection will reveal that normal QRS complexes are 'walking through' the tachycardia (Figure 22.3b).

If the recording speed slows for any reason, complexes will appear closer together and mimic tachycardia. However, the duration of each ventricular complex will be shorter than normal and this should alert the observer to the likelihood of artefact. Conversely, if the recording runs too fast, apparent bradycardia with broader than normal complexes will result.

Clinical applications

Ambulatory ECG monitoring enables the detection and diagnosis of intermittent disorders of cardiac rhythm and may thus reveal the cause of symptoms such as syncope, near-syncope, palpitation and chest pain (Figures 22.4–22.9).

It may be of value in ascertaining whether paroxysmal atrial fibrillation has been responsible for a patient's stroke. Other indications include the assessment of rate

(a)

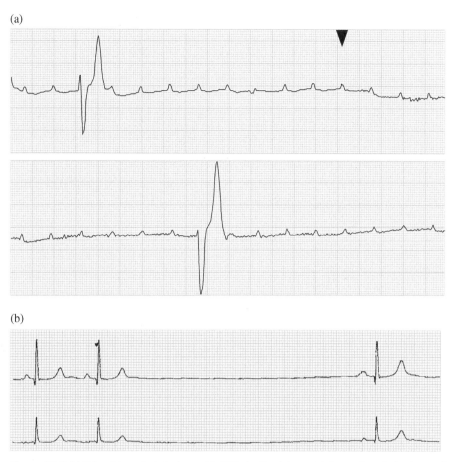

(b)

Figure 22.4 (a) Stokes–Adams attack due to complete AV block with only two ventricular complexes. During the rest of the 24-hour tape recording the patient was in sinus rhythm. (b) Near-syncope due to sinus arrest.

control in atrial fibrillation, the identification of ventricular arrhythmias which may have prognostic significance in patients with hypertrophic cardiomyopathy (Figure 22.9) or who have sustained myocardial infarction, the assessment of pacemaker function, and ensuring an antiarrhythmic drug does not have a proarrhythmic effect.

The technique is most valuable when the patient experiences his or her usual symptoms during an ECG recording. The patient should be instructed to record the time of onset and nature of the symptoms so these can be correlated with the heart rhythm. With most recorders the patient can operate an event marker that indicates the time of symptoms on the tape.

Even when the patient does not experience symptoms during a recording, rhythm abnormalities of diagnostic significance may be detected. Obviously, if the patient does not experience symptoms during the recording and no rhythm abnormalities are found, an arrhythmic cause for the patient's symptoms is not excluded. Conversely, if a patient experiences his or hers *typical* symptoms during the recording and yet no arrhythmia is found then it can be concluded that symptoms are not due to a disturbance of heart rhythm. In the absence of typical symptoms, the finding of a minor abnormality of rhythm does not rule out a more major rhythm disturbance being responsible for the patient's complaints.

It is important to analyse the heart rate immediately prior to the onset of an arrhythmia. For example, sinus bradycardia prior to the onset of an atrial arrhythmia points to the possibility that atrial pacing may prevent the tachyarrhythmia. Sinus tachycardia

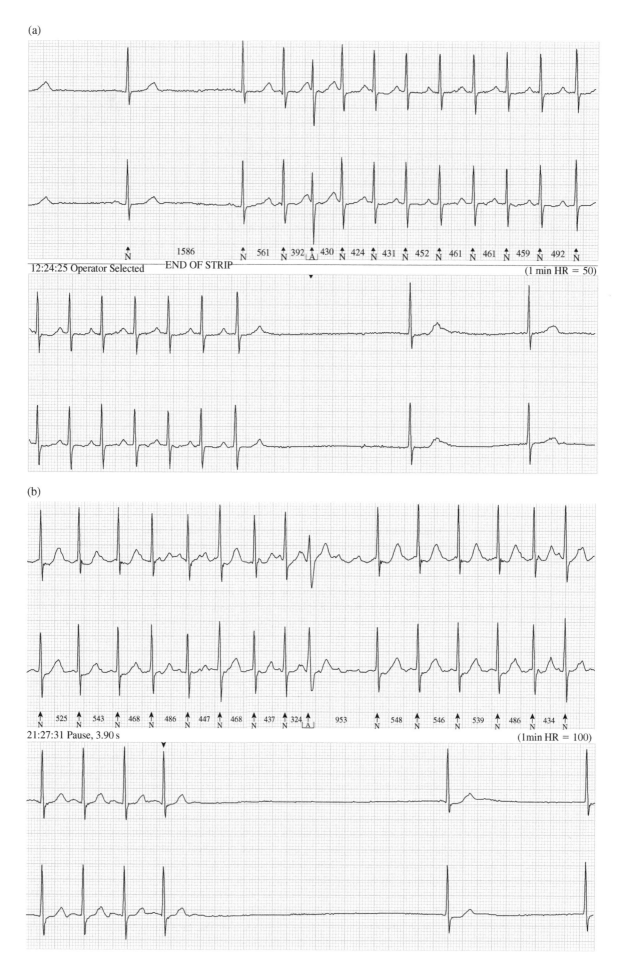

(a)

12:24:25 Operator Selected   END OF STRIP   (1 min HR = 50)

1586   N 561   N 392   A 430   N 424   N 431   N 452   N 461   N 461   N 459   N 492   N

(b)

21:27:31 Pause, 3.90 s   (1min HR = 100)

N 525 N 543 N 468 N 486 N 447 N 468 N 437 N 324 A 953 N 548 N 546 N 539 N 486 N 434 N

Figure 22.5 (a) Palpitation due to paroxysmal atrial tachycardia, preceded by sinus bradycardia and succeeded by a junctional escape rhythm i.e. bradycardia–tachycardia syndrome. (b) Paroxysmal atrial fibrillation followed by sinus arrest. Recordings from the same patient.

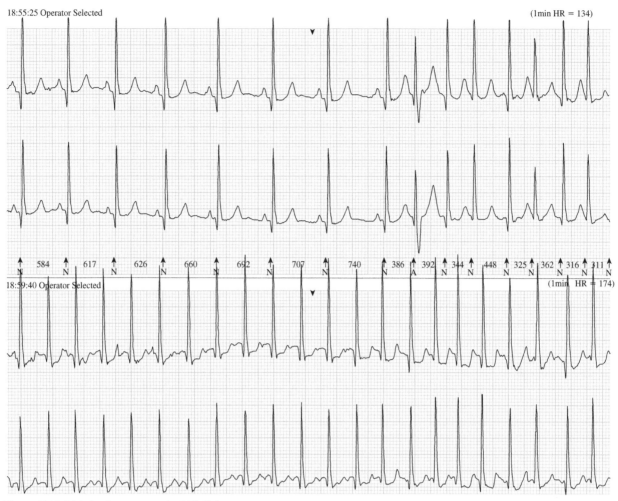

Figure 22.6 Palpitation due to paroxysmal atrial fibrillation.

before the onset of a tachyarrhythmia points to the possibility that the rhythm disturbance was initiated by catecholamines and that beta-blockade may prevent it.

Normal findings

Sinus bradycardia, short pauses (up to 2 s) due to sinoatrial block, first-degree and AV Wenckebach block (Figures 22.10, 22.11) can occur in normal people during sleep and should not be regarded as evidence of conduction tissue disease. These rhythms may also occur during the day in young people with high vagal tone.

Sinus tachycardia will of course also be seen in recordings from people with normal hearts at times of exertion.

Whereas a routine 12-lead ECG records approximately 60 heart beats, a normal 24-hour tape recording is likely to contain at least 90 000 beats. Thus ambulatory electrocardiography is a much more sensitive tool than a standard recording. For example, the finding of a single ventricular ectopic beat on a routine ECG suggests a much higher frequency than a hundred ectopic beats on a 24-hour tape. In fact, studies of apparently normal people using ambulatory electrocardiography have shown that unifocal ventricular extrasystoles occur commonly, as do supraventricular ectopic beats. The frequency of ventricular ectopic beats increases with age. Some studies have also found short runs of relatively slow ventricular tachycardia in apparently normal young subjects.

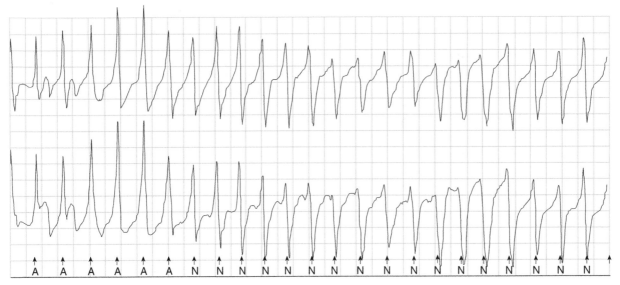

22:26:27

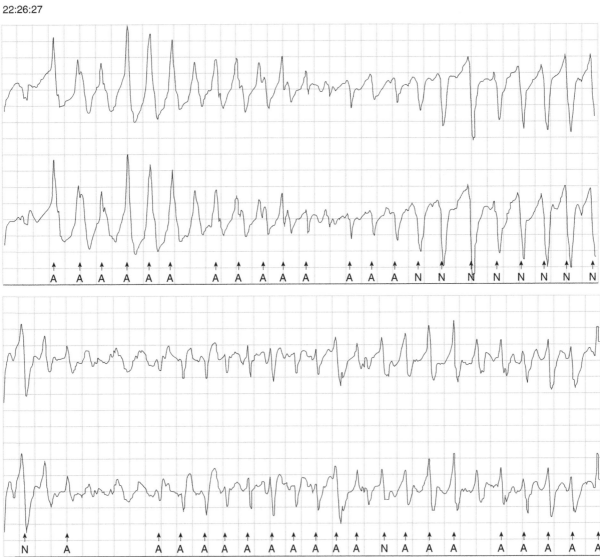

Figure 22.7 Syncope due to torsade de pointes tachycardia (NB: recorded at slow paper speed).

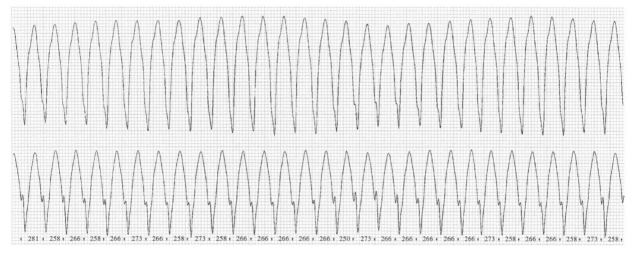

Figure 22.8 Ventricular tachycardia in a patient with cardiomyopathy.

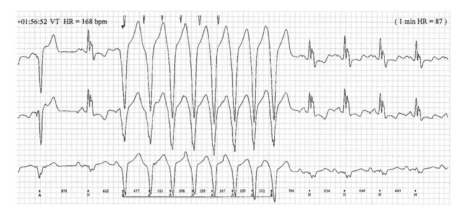

Figure 22.9 Non-sustained ventricular tachycardia in a patient with hypertrophic cardiomyopathy.

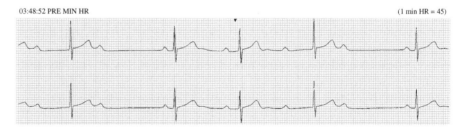

Figure 22.10 Nocturnal sinus bradycardia conducted with AV Wenckebach block in a young person: a normal finding.

Non-sustained ventricular tachycardia only rarely occurs in subjects without structural heart disease, but if it does it is not associated with risk.

Intermittent ECG recording

Event recorders

Patients with symptoms occurring at intervals of less than one week are unlikely to experience an episode during the 24–120 hours of continuous ambulatory electrocardiography. A hand-held event recorder is a very useful and inexpensive device that enables a patient to record his or her ECG for 30s during symptoms. The patient can

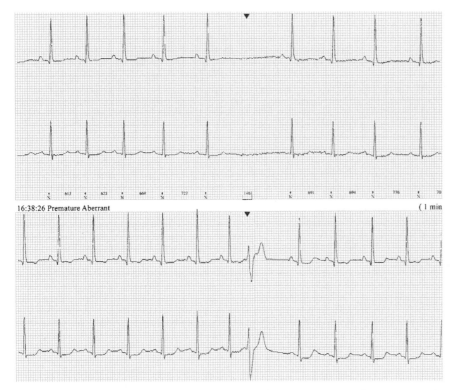

16:38:26 Premature Aberrant (1 min

Figure 22.11 Single nocturnal pause due to sinoatrial block and a daytime ventricular ectopic beat in a subject with a structurally normal heart: normal findings.

carry the device around until an episode occurs. He or she then applies the device to the chest wall and initiates a recording that is stored in a memory and can be replayed directly or transmitted via the telephone into an ECG machine (Figure 22.12). Some devices enable several recordings to be made.

It is very important to explain to the patient precisely when and how to use the recorder. Clearly, these devices are not suitable for the investigation of episodes that disable the patient to the extent that he or she cannot activate the recorder.

Sometimes patients will record sinus tachycardia. It may well be that this rhythm was responsible for the patient's symptoms. However, another possibility is that sinus tachycardia resulted from a tachyarrhythmia which had stopped by the time the recorder was activated.

More recently, a small device has become available which can be worn for up to seven days. Arrhythmias that the device detects and rhythms when the patient activates an event marker can be stored in memory. Importantly, the heart rhythm immediately prior to a symptomatic or detected event is also saved.

Implantable loop recorders

The implantable ECG loop recorder is a very small device (only 15 g) that can easily be implanted subcutaneously. It facilitates ECG monitoring for up to three years and is therefore ideal for diagnosis in patients with infrequent symptoms.

It is usually positioned a few inches beneath the left clavicle, lateral to the sternum in a semi-vertical position with its two electrodes facing the under-surface of the skin. *It is important to ensure that the subcutaneous pocket created to accommodate the device is tight: if the recorder is mobile within the pocket signal loss can result, which could be misdiagnosed as asystole.*

After the patient experiences typical symptoms, he or she can hold an external device over the implanted recorder that triggers storage of the ECG before, during

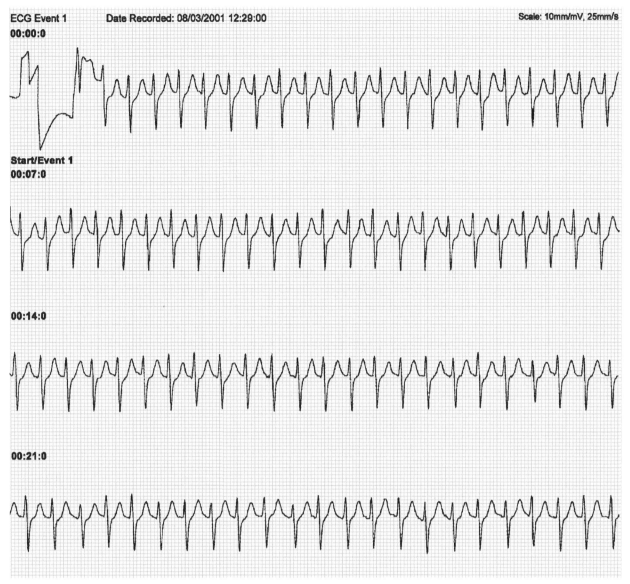

ECG Event 1   Date Recorded: 08/03/2001 12:29:00   Scale: 10mm/mV, 25mm/s
00:00:0

Start/Event 1
00:07:0

00:14:0

00:21:0

Figure 22.12 Recording during palpitation demonstrating paroxysmal supraventricular tachycardia.

and after the event (Figures 22.13, 22.14). Depending on how many episodes the device is programmed to record, the patient may have up to 30 minutes after the event to initiate the recording. Thus, the ECG of an arrhythmia that has caused temporary incapacity can be saved. The data can then be downloaded into a computer for analysis.

The device can be programmed to automatically identify and record bradycardia, atrial fibrillation and tachycardia, and ventricular tachycardia. Though this facility will ensure that major arrhythmias are stored even if the patient fails to use the external activating device, there is the disadvantage that arrhythmias may be recorded which do not coincide with symptoms and may be of uncertain clinical significance. The number and recording duration of patient-activated and auto-activated events can be programmed.

Patient safety will not be endangered by airport and other security systems, MRI or CT scanning, diathermy, electrosurgical cautery, therapeutic radiation, external defibrillation (the defibrillation paddle must not be placed directly over the recorder),

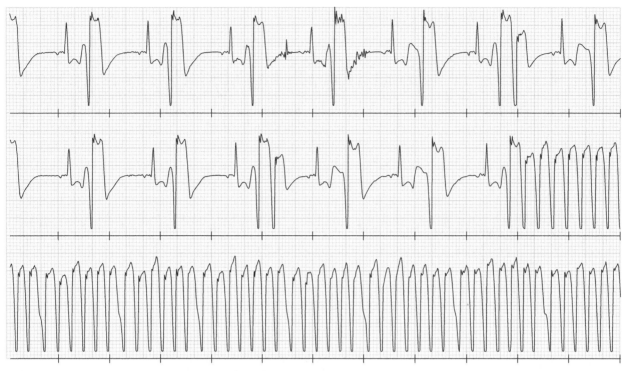

Figure 22.13 Recording of ventricular bigeminy and then polymorphic ventricular tachycardia stored by patient with implanted loop recorder on recovering consciousness.

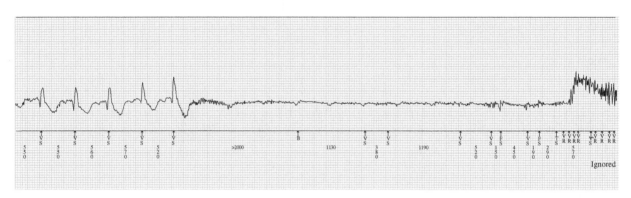

Figure 22.14 Recording of complete AV block and ventricular asystole stored by patient with implanted loop recorder on recovering consciousness.

lithotripsy, transcutaneous electrical nerve stimulators or radiofrequency ablation but electrical reset of the device and/or corruption of ECG data may result. Magnetic resonance imaging (MRI) should be avoided during the first six weeks after implantation while the wound heals.

Long-term pacing is indicated in cases of symptomatic bradycardia whether due to atrioventricular (AV) block or sick sinus syndrome, and should be considered in asymptomatic patients with high-degree AV block or long pauses in sinus node activity.

Dual-chamber pacing (DDD) preserves the haemodynamic benefit of normal AV synchronisation and facilitates a chronotropic response to exercise provided sinus node function is normal. In patients with impaired sinus node function, rate-responsive systems (DDDR/VVIR) can increase the stimulation rate in response to a physiological parameter that alters with exercise.

The modern pacemaker is small, reliable and has a long battery life. It is usually implanted over the pectoral muscle. The pacing lead(s) are introduced via the subclavian or cephalic vein. Infection is the commonest complication.

Electromagnetic interference from household devices and from electronic surveillance equipment is unlikely to affect the modern pacemaker. Caution is required with cardioversion, diathermy, MRI scanning and radiotherapy.

Long-term cardiac pacing

An artificial cardiac pacemaker generates electrical stimuli that can initiate myocardial contraction. The stimuli are delivered to the heart by transvenous leads or much less commonly via epicardial electrodes. (Currently, a *leadless* miniature pacemaker inserted percutaneously into the cavity of the right ventricle is being developed!)

The first pacemaker was implanted in 1958. Rapid progress in technology and an increasing awareness of the benefits of pacing have led to pacemakers being widely used. People of all ages, from the newborn to patients over 100 years old, have been paced.

Common indications for long-term pacing

There are international guidelines for the indications for pacemaker implantation, some of which the author has found somewhat difficult to interpret! The indications below are largely in accordance with those guidelines.

Bennett's Cardiac Arrhythmias: Practical Notes on Interpretation and Treatment, Eighth Edition. David H. Bennett.
© 2013 John Wiley & Sons, Ltd. Published 2013 by John Wiley & Sons, Ltd.

Complete atrioventricular block

Syncope

The most common reason for pacemaker implantation is to prevent recurrence of syncope or near-syncope due to complete atrioventricular (AV) block. A single episode is a sufficient indication, and since the next blackout may cause injury or be fatal, delay should be minimal. Even in patients with a short life expectancy, pacing should be considered if by preventing syncope independence may be preserved and injury avoided.

Dyspnoea and heart failure

Complete heart block can reduce cardiac output and thereby cause exertional dyspnoea and sometimes cardiac failure.

Prognosis

Without pacing, the prognosis in patients with complete heart block is poor. With an artificial pacemaker, life expectancy closely approaches that of the general population, though those with overt coronary heart disease or with heart failure have a less good outlook.

Pacemaker implantation should be considered in *asymptomatic* patients with complete AV block, particularly when the ventricular rate is 40 beats/min or less, on purely prognostic grounds. Furthermore, by preventing a first syncopal episode, pacing may well prevent major injury to the patient.

QRS breadth

Narrow ventricular complexes during complete AV block suggest that interruption in conduction is at the AV nodal level and that, in contrast to infranodal block, a subsidiary pacemaker within the bundle of His will discharge reliably at a relatively rapid ventricular rate. However, in practice, patients with narrow ventricular complexes during complete heart block often experience syncope and impaired exercise tolerance and do require pacing.

Congenital heart block

Congenital heart block, i.e. complete AV block that is discovered when the patient is a neonate or child and is not caused by acquired disease, is widely regarded as benign. This is incorrect. Patients do develop symptoms and can die suddenly. If heart block has caused symptoms then pacing is indicated.

In young *asymptomatic* patients the risks of not implanting a pacemaker have to be weighed against the possibility of complications associated with several decades of pacing. There are a number of documented risk factors: day-time ventricular rate less than 50 beats/min, broad QRS complexes, pauses more than 3.0 s, frequent ventricular ectopic beats and poor chronotropic response to exercise. Unpaced patients should undergo ambulatory and exercise electrocardiography at regular intervals. In older patients who present with congenital heart block, the threshold for implanting a pacemaker should be low.

Neuromuscular diseases

Pacing is indicated in neuromuscular diseases such as myotonic muscular dystrophy, limb-girdle muscular dystrophy and peroneal muscular atrophy, if there is high-degree AV block, because of the risk of sudden death. Indeed, pacing should be considered with any form of AV block with or without symptoms, because of the high risk of rapid progression to complete AV block.

Second-degree atrioventricular block

Mobitz II AV block often progresses to complete AV block. The management of Mobitz II is the same as that for complete AV block.

A study has refuted the previously held view that Mobitz I (Wenckebach) AV block is benign, in that the incidence of symptoms, prognosis and benefits of pacing were the same as for patients with Mobitz II block. However, Mobitz I block in young people with transient and often nocturnal Wenckebach block is due to high vagal tone. It is benign and pacing is *not* indicated. Adult patients who are found to have sustained periods of AV Wenckebach block during the *daytime* should be considered for pacing unless they undertake a lot of physical training, in which case their AV block may be attributable to high vagal tone.

First-degree atrioventricular block

First-degree AV block is not usually an indication for cardiac pacing. If a patient presents with first-degree block and syncope it is quite possible that the symptoms are due to transient second- or third-degree AV block, but a pacemaker should not be implanted without proof of this, e.g. by ambulatory electrocardiography.

Exceptionally, the PR interval is so long that the P wave immediately follows the preceding QRS complex. This may lead to the equivalent of the 'pacemaker syndrome' (see below), in which case dual-chamber pacing is indicated.

Bundle branch and fascicular blocks
Bundle branch block

The risk of high-degree AV block developing in an asymptomatic patient with either left or right bundle branch block is relatively small (Chapter 4), and pacing is not indicated. In patients who present with syncope or near-syncope, confirmation of intermittent high-degree AV block should be sought.

Bifascicular block

In bifascicular block the remaining functioning fascicle may fail to conduct, intermittently or persistently, and cause high-degree AV block. In patients with a *typical history* of Stokes–Adams attacks, pacemaker implantation is indicated to prevent syncope without further investigation. With atypical symptoms, high-degree AV block must be documented first. It should be borne in mind that some patients with bifascicular block have been shown to be prone to ventricular tachycardia.

In *asymptomatic* bifascicular block, the chances of progression to complete AV block is in the order of 2% per year, and the major determinants of prognosis are the presence of coronary artery or myocardial disease; prophylactic pacing is generally not indicated. Additional first-degree AV block or bundle of His electrographic evidence of prolonged infranodal (HV) conduction suggests that conduction in the functioning fascicle is also impaired. Guidelines do recommend that patients with bifascicular block who are found to have a markedly prolonged HV interval at His bundle electrography (Chapter 25) are considered for pacing.

Alternating bundle branch block

'Alternating bundle branch block', i.e. alternating patterns of left and right bundle branch block or, in patients with right bundle branch block, alternating left anterior and posterior fascicular block, is an indication for pacing.

Atrioventricular and bundle branch block after myocardial infarction

AV block due to inferior myocardial infarction usually resolves within a few days and almost always by three weeks. When anterior infarction is complicated by high-degree AV block, there is usually extensive myocardial damage and hence the prognosis is poor. Though block may persist, it is prudent to ensure that the patient is going to survive before implanting a pacemaker. Thus, pacemaker implantation should not be considered unless second- or third-degree AV block is present three weeks after either inferior or anterior myocardial infarction.

Bifascicular block persisting after acute anterior infarction complicated by a period of AV block raises the possibility that complete AV block might recur. However, there is little evidence that prophylactic pacing reduces mortality.

When a patient is admitted to hospital with heart block, there is often an *unnecessary* delay before referral for long-term pacing while myocardial infarction is excluded. Unless the patient has experienced typical cardiac pain or there are typical ECG changes of recent infarction, it is very unlikely that AV block has been caused by acute infarction, and delay should be avoided.

Sick sinus syndrome

Syncope

Sick sinus syndrome accounts for more than one-third of pacemaker implantations. Pacing is indicated when syncope or near-syncope are caused.

It should be remembered that sinus bradycardia and pauses in sinus node activity for up to 2.0 s, particularly if nocturnal, can be physiological.

Bradycardia–tachycardia syndrome

In patients with the bradycardia–tachycardia syndrome, pacing may be required to avoid severe bradycardia caused by antiarrhythmic drugs. Atrial tachyarrhythmias which start during bradycardia may be prevented by atrial pacing.

Prognosis

Pacing for sick sinus syndrome is not usually indicated in the absence of symptoms. However, daytime pauses in cardiac activity for several seconds might be considered an indication for pacing in those who operate machinery, including a motor car, to avoid an accident should syncope occur.

Hypersensitive carotid sinus and malignant vasovagal syndromes

Pacing will improve symptoms in these syndromes provided there is a significant cardioinhibitory component (Chapter 17).

Hypertrophic cardiomyopathy

Dual-chamber pacing with a short AV delay has been shown to reduce symptoms and left ventricular outflow tract gradient in some patients with hypertrophic cardiomyopathy who have a significant pressure gradient across the left ventricular outflow tract.

Resynchronisation therapy

Biventricular pacing can improve symptoms and also prognosis in patients with poor left ventricular function who have marked prolongation of QRS duration and impaired left ventricular function. Ventricular 'resynchronisation' is achieved by near-simultaneous delivery of stimuli conducted via right and left ventricular leads, usually resulting in significant shortening of QRS duration.

Left ventricular pacing is achieved by passing a lead into a lateral branch of the coronary sinus (Figure 23.24b). It can be technically challenging to introduce the lead into a suitable branch of the coronary sinus, achieve a satisfactory stimulation threshold and avoid diaphragmatic stimulation. Biventricular pacing is primarily to deal with cardiac failure rather than arrhythmia and therefore is not discussed in detail in this book.

Pacing modes

The first generation of pacemakers functioned in a fixed-rate mode. The pacemaker stimulated the ventricles repeatedly, usually at 70 beats/min, irrespective of any

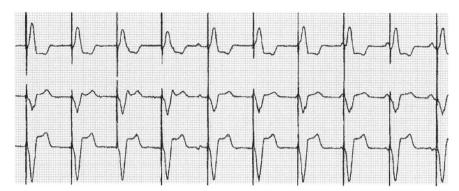

Figure 23.1 Fixed-rate ventricular pacing (leads I, II, III). A large pacing stimulus precedes each ventricular complex. P waves dissociated from ventricular complexes can be seen.

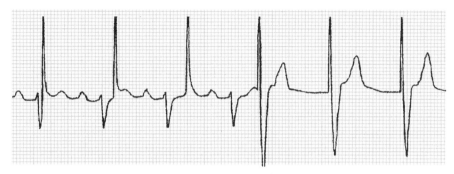

Figure 23.2 Fixed-rate ventricular pacing in a patient with first-degree AV block. The first three stimuli fall during the refractory period and are ineffective. The fourth causes a premature contraction.

(a)

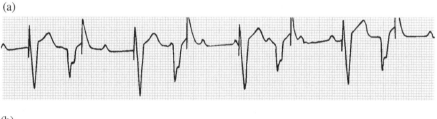

(b)

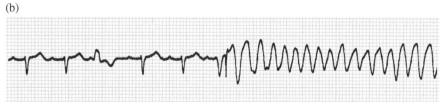

Figure 23.3 Examples of failure to sense. (a) Failure to sense in a demand ventricular pacemaker. The first, third, fifth and seventh pacing stimuli capture the ventricles. The second, fourth, sixth and eighth stimuli fall on the T waves of spontaneous ventricular beats. (b) Failure to sense the sixth ventricular complex, resulting in a pacemaker stimulus coinciding with the T wave and initiating ventricular fibrillation.

spontaneous cardiac activity (Figure 23.1). Competition with a spontaneous rhythm could cause irregular palpitation (Figure 23.2), and stimulation during ventricular repolarisation could possibly initiate ventricular fibrillation (Figure 23.3).

Subsequent developments enabled sensing of spontaneous activity via the stimulating lead to facilitate demand pacing. A sensed event resets the timing of delivery of the next pacemaker stimulus to avoid competition with spontaneous activity (Figure 23.4).

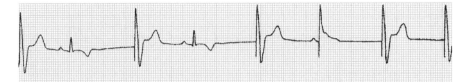

Figure 23.4 Demand ventricular pacemaker. The pacemaker is inhibited by the sinus beats (second and fourth complexes). The sixth complex is a fusion beat. A P wave can be seen to precede the pacing stimulus: by chance, a sinus impulse has arisen at the instant when the pacemaker was set to discharge and the ventricles have been activated by both the sinus node impulse and the pacemaker. Fusion beats should not be confused with failure to pace.

With the advent of reliable atrial transvenous pacing leads it became straightforward to pace and sense in the atrium as well as the ventricle, thus allowing atrial 'single-chamber' pacing and also 'dual-chamber' pacing, whereby stimulation and/ or sensing can take place at both atrial and ventricular levels. These developments have facilitated a physiological approach to cardiac stimulation.

Pacing system code

A five-letter code is widely used to describe the various pacing modes, as shown in the table.

Pacing system codes

The first character identifies the chamber or chambers that are paced: A for atrium, V for ventricle and D (for dual) if both atrium and ventricle can be stimulated.

The second character indicates the chamber or chambers whose activity is sensed. In addition to the use of A, V and D, O indicates that the pacemaker is insensitive.

The third character denotes the response to the sensed information. I indicates that pacemaker output is inhibited by a sensed event, T that stimulation is triggered by a sensed event and D that ventricular sensed events inhibit pacemaker output while atrial sensed events trigger ventricular stimulation. O indicates that there is no response to sensed events.

A fourth character, R, is used if there is a rate-responsive facility whereby the pacing rate is adjusted by a sensor that detects a physiological variable such as physical activity or respiration.

The fifth character only relates to multisite pacing: O indicates none, while A, V and D indicate a second atrial lead, a second ventricular lead and additional atrial and ventricular leads, respectively.

Single-chamber pacing

Ventricular demand pacing (VVI)

In the absence of spontaneous ventricular activity, a ventricular demand pacemaker, like a fixed-rate unit, delivers stimuli to the ventricles at a regular rate. However, if spontaneous activity is sensed via the ventricular lead, the timing of delivery of the next pacemaker output is reset to avoid competition.

In ventricular inhibited pacemakers (VVI) a sensed event terminates the current stimulation cycle, thus inhibiting pacemaker output, and starts a new cycle (Figure 23.4). The pacemaker is rendered insensitive immediately after a paced or sensed event for an interval which approximates the duration of myocardial activation plus recovery, to prevent sensing the ventricular electrogram which is produced by the event. This interval (250–300 ms) is referred to as the refractory period.

Ventricular demand pacing is a commonly employed mode, but its use has diminished now its disadvantages – the inability to facilitate the normal sequence of cardiac chamber activation and to provide a chronotropic response to exercise – are widely appreciated (see below).

Indications for ventricular demand pacing include bradycardia associated with persistent atrial fibrillation, second- and third-degree AV block in patients who are

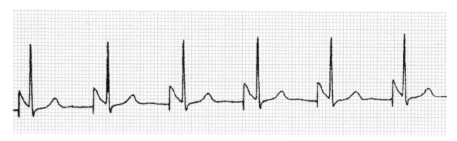

Figure 23.5 Atrial pacing. A pacing stimulus precedes each P wave. AV conduction is normal and hence each paced P wave is followed by a normal QRS complex after a normal PR interval.

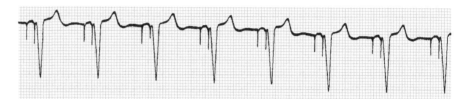

Figure 23.6 AV sequential (DVI) pacing. Pacing stimuli precede both atrial and ventricular complexes.

limited by impaired cerebral or locomotor function, and infrequent bradycardia when the pacemaker will be mainly on 'standby'.

Atrial demand pacing (AAI)

The timing cycles of atrial inhibited (AAI) are the same as for ventricular demand pacing, as described above (Figure 23.5). With atrial pacing, the refractory period is usually longer, to avoid inappropriate inhibition of the pacemaker by sensing the 'far field' ventricular electrogram via the atrial lead.

Atrial pacing is indicated for treatment of the sick sinus syndrome unless AV conduction is impaired. By stimulating the atria rather than the ventricles, the normal sequence of cardiac chamber activation is maintained, loss of which can reduce cardiac output by up to one-third.

In patients with sick sinus syndrome, atrial pacing (including dual-chamber pacing, see below) has been shown to reduce the incidence of atrial fibrillation, heart failure and the pacemaker syndrome (see below) as compared with those patients in whom only the ventricles are paced.

Sick sinus syndrome can sometimes be associated with impaired AV conduction. However, if there is no evidence of it at the time of pacemaker implantation the subsequent development of impaired AV conduction is uncommon. Nevertheless, it is common practice to implant a dual-chamber pacemaker even though the risk of subsequent AV block is small. A dual-chamber pacemaker *should* be implanted if there is also bifascicular or bundle branch block, or if during pacemaker implantation, atrial pacing at a rate of 120 beats/min causes second-degree AV block.

Dual-chamber pacing
AV sequential pacing (DVI and DDI)

In AV sequential (DVI) pacing, the atria are stimulated first and then, after a delay that approximates the normal PR interval, the ventricles are stimulated (Figure 23.6). The pacemaker is inhibited by spontaneous ventricular activity but no sensing occurs in the atrium. As with other dual-chamber modes, both atrial and ventricular electrodes are required.

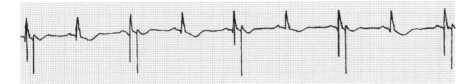

Figure 23.7 DVI pacing: fusion beats.

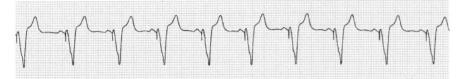

Figure 23.8 Atrial synchronised pacing. Each P wave triggers a paced ventricular beat.

Fusion beats (Figure 23.7) are commonly seen during DVI pacing and are sometimes misinterpreted as pacemaker malfunction. Whereas the pacemaker is inhibited by an event sensed in the ventricles, the first chamber to be stimulated is the atrium. Pacemaker output may therefore occur at the same time as spontaneous atrial activation because its resultant ventricular depolarisation has not yet occurred.

Subsequently, DDI pacing was introduced, superseding DVI pacing. Sensing occurs at atrial as well as ventricular levels, thus avoiding competitive atrial pacing.

Unlike DDD pacing, sensed atrial events do not trigger ventricular stimulation, and thus DVI and DDI pacing will not facilitate endless loop tachycardia (see below).

The main indications for DVI and DDI pacing are sick sinus syndrome associated with impaired AV conduction, and carotid sinus and malignant vasovagal syndromes.

Atrial synchronised ventricular pacing (VDD)

In this mode, ventricular stimulation is *triggered* by a sensed atrial event after an interval similar to the normal PR interval (Figure 23.8). Thus the normal sequence of cardiac chamber activation is maintained and, provided sinus node function is normal, an increase in sinus node rate during exercise will lead to an increase in ventricular stimulation rate, i.e. a chronotropic response to exercise is facilitated.

If an atrial event is not sensed, ventricular stimulation continues at a fixed cycle length – otherwise atrial standstill might lead to ventricular asystole. To avoid atrial tachycardia or fibrillation triggering inappropriately fast ventricular pacing rates, there is an atrial refractory interval: the atrial channel is rendered insensitive during the AV delay and for a period after ventricular stimulation. Sensed atrial activity at a cycle length shorter than this period will not trigger ventricular stimulation.

The upper atrial rate that can trigger ventricular output is determined by the 'total atrial refractory period', which consists of the AV delay plus the post-ventricular stimulus refractory period. For example, if the AV delay is 125 ms and the atrial refractory period is 250 ms, the upper rate limit will be 60 000/375 = 160 beats/min.

In earlier years, sensing only took place in the atrium and pacing only in the ventricle (VAT). Thus, atrial activation would trigger ventricular activation irrespective of ventricular ectopic beats or ventricular rhythms faster than the sinus node rate. Subsequently, VDD pacing was introduced whereby sensing takes place in the ventricles as well so that spontaneous ventricular activity will inhibit the pacemaker (Figure 23.9).

VDD ventricular pacing is indicated in second- and third-degree AV block when sinus node function is normal. It is contraindicated in the sick sinus syndrome or when there are atrial tachyarrhythmias.

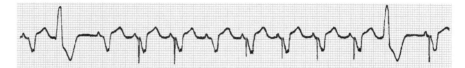

Figure 23.9 VDD pacing, showing chronotropic response to exercise (pacing rate = 98 beats/min) and inhibition of ventricular pacing by ventricular ectopic beats.

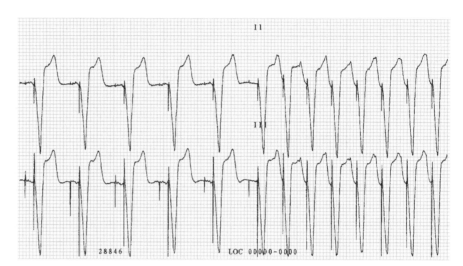

Figure 23.10 Pacemaker-mediated tachycardia after six cycles of dual-chamber pacing.

Endless loop tachycardia

If a ventricular stimulus is conducted retrogradely to the atria via either the AV junction or, if present, an accessory AV pathway, and the timing of the resultant atrial activation is outside the pacemaker's atrial refractory period, it will trigger ventricular stimulation and hence initiate an 'endless loop tachycardia' (Figure 23.10), also referred to as 'pacemaker-mediated tachycardia'.

Ventriculoatrial conduction is present in approximately two-thirds of patients with the sick sinus syndrome and one-fifth of those with complete AV block. Endless loop tachycardia can usually be prevented by prolongation of the atrial refractory period, but at the expense of reduction of the upper rate limit for ventricular stimulation. *Endless loop tachycardia can be avoided in 90% of patients by setting the AV delay to 125 ms and the post-ventricular atrial refractory period to 300 ms.*

Most pacemakers can automatically detect endless loop tachycardia and terminate it, for example by prolonging the atrial refractory period for one cycle.

Atrioventricular universal pacing (DDD)

In this mode (DDD), which all modern dual-chamber pacemakers can facilitate, both sensing and pacing can take place at atrial and ventricular levels, allowing the pacemaker to function in atrial demand (AAI), AV sequential (DDI) or atrial synchronised (VDD) modes, depending on the spontaneous heart rhythm (Figure 23.11).

If there is sinus bradycardia it functions as an atrial demand pacemaker. If there is impaired AV conduction, ventricular pacing is triggered either by spontaneous atrial activity or by delivery of an atrial stimulus. When sinus node function is normal, it functions in the atrial synchronised mode, thus providing a chronotropic response to exercise. The pacemaker is inhibited by both atrial and ventricular ectopic beats. Endless loop tachycardia may occur if there is retrograde AV conduction.

DDD pacing is indicated in second- and third-degree AV block.

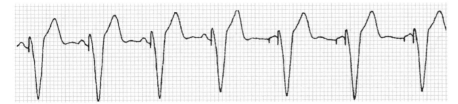

Figure 23.11 Universal (DDD) pacing. In the first four beats, spontaneous P waves arising from the sinus node trigger ventricular stimulation. There is then sinus node slowing to which the pacemaker responds by pacing the atria as well as the ventricles (pacing stimuli can be seen preceding both the P waves and the QRS complexes).

'Physiological pacing'

Physiological pacing systems facilitate a chronotropic response to exercise by maintaining AV synchronisation as the sinus node rate varies, and/or by a rate-adaptive mechanism.

Atrial synchronised ventricular pacing (VDD, DDD)

VDD and DDD modes both maintain AV synchronisation and facilitate a chronotropic response to exercise.

Exercise capacity has been measured on a double-blind basis in patients with complete AV block during ventricular pacing (i.e. VVI) at 70 beats/min and during atrial synchronised ventricular pacing. The latter mode was shown to increase exercise capacity by approximately 30%.

Atrial synchronised pacing improves parameters in addition to exercise tolerance. Shortness of breath, dizziness and palpitation are less frequent, whereas fixed-rate pacing tends to impair the normal blood pressure response to exercise and leads to a higher respiratory rate and perceived exertion during submaximal exercise. The advantages of atrial synchronised pacing have been shown to be maintained long-term.

There are limitations to atrial synchronised ventricular pacing. First, normal or at least near-normal sinus node activity is required. Second, the ventricular stimulation rate may increase in response to an atrial tachyarrhythmia.

Rate-responsive systems

Several pacing systems are available that can facilitate a chronotropic response *independent of* atrial activity: a change in stimulation rate is achieved in response to a parameter that alters with exercise (see below). In contrast to atrial synchronised pacing, normal sinus node activity is not required.

In terms of exercise capacity, the ability to increase heart rate is far more important than maintaining AV synchronisation. This has been demonstrated by measuring exercise tolerance in patients with complete AV block during three pacing modes: fixed rate, atrial synchronised and ventricular pacing at a rate equal to but not synchronised with atrial activity. Both the latter forms of chronotropic pacing increased exercise performance to a similar degree as compared with fixed-rate pacing. Thus rate-responsive ventricular pacemakers can enable an enhanced exercise tolerance without AV synchronisation and in patients with atrial fibrillation.

Some patients with the sick sinus syndrome have chronotropic incompetence: there is little increase in sinus node rate in response to exercise. A rate-responsive system will facilitate an appropriate rate response.

According to the pacemaker code, atrial demand, ventricular demand and dual-chamber pacemakers with rate-response facilities are termed AAIR, VVIR and DDDR, respectively. All modern dual-chamber pacemakers can facilitate DDDR pacing.

Activity sensor

Vibration resulting from physical activity is sensed by a piezoelectric crystal attached to the inside of the pacemaker can or an accelerometer bonded to the circuitry within the pacemaker. The stimulation rate increases in parallel with the level of sensed activity. An accelerometer is regarded as more physiological, since it will respond to motion primarily in the anteroposterior direction.

The systems have been criticised because they are not truly physiological. For example, the same levels of vibration and hence the same heart rate will be generated by ascending and descending a flight of stairs, though less work is required for the latter. There will be no response to non-exertional stresses such as emotion or illness. In addition, in the case of a piezoelectric crystal, the pacemaker rate may increase in response to pressure on the pacemaker can itself. However, in contrast to systems using other sensors, a very prompt and reliable chronotropic response to exercise is achieved and this is the most widely used sensor.

It is possible to modify how the sensor determines the pacing rate by externally programming a number of parameters. These include the reaction time, i.e. the time during which the initial increase in sensor-driven pacing rate occurs; the recovery time, which is the time taken to return to standby rate after activity; and the slope, which determines the relation between sensor activity counts and pacemaker rate.

Evoked QT response

Though it has been known for many years that the QT interval decreases with increasing heart rate, it has only relatively recently been appreciated that sympathetic nervous system activity is a major independent determinant of QT interval duration (QT interval shortens during exercise even during fixed-rate pacing).

The pacemaker senses, via a conventional ventricular pacing electrode, the interval between pacing stimulus and apex of the elicited T wave; a decrease in the interval results in an increase in stimulation rate.

Since this system responds to sympathetic nervous system activity, it will increase the heart rate in response to emotion as well as exertion.

Respiration

There is a close relation between minute volume and heart rate. The system's discharge rate is governed by changes in intravascular impedance, a measure of respiratory minute volume, which is monitored by means of a conventional bipolar pacing lead.

Blood temperature

Skeletal muscle activity generates heat, which is transferred to the blood. There is a relation between level of exercise and right ventricular blood temperature. One problem, however, is that there is a latency in the system due to the delay of 1–2 minutes before blood temperature rises after the start of exercise.

Multisensor pacing

Dual-chamber pacemakers are available which, in addition to sensing atrial activity, will respond to parameters related to exercise such as activity or QT interval (DDDR). Thus, normal AV synchrony can be maintained and a chronotropic response to exercise can be provided even if sinus node function is impaired or if an intermittent atrial arrhythmia occurs.

Some newer pacing systems incorporate not one but two types of physiological sensor so that the limitations of each system can be minimised: for example, an activity sensor to provide a prompt response and a QT sensor to ensure the rate response is proportional to the workload.

Automatic mode switching

This very important facility allows implantation of DDD pacemakers in patients prone to paroxysmal atrial fibrillation and other atrial tachyarrhythmias. When rapid

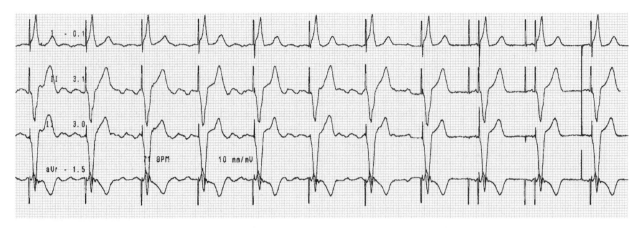

Figure 23.12 Automatic mode switching. During atrial fibrillation, there is VVIR pacing. DDDR pacing (pacemaker stimuli can be seen preceding both the P waves and the QRS complexes) returns on termination of atrial fibrillation.

abnormal atrial activity is sensed through the atrial lead, the pacing mode automatically switches from DDDR to DDIR or VVIR. Thus, tracking of atrial activity ceases and an inappropriately fast ventricular pacing rate is thereby avoided *but a chronotropic response to exercise is still possible*. Dual-chamber pacing resumes on termination of the atrial arrhythmia (Figure 23.12).

'Pacemaker syndrome'

It is at rest or during standing that the disadvantage of loss of AV synchrony caused by single-chamber ventricular pacing (VVI) may be most apparent. Loss of properly timed atrial systole reduces cardiac output by up to one-third and may cause hypotension; near-syncope and syncope can result (Figure 23.13). Other symptoms include weakness, dizziness and dyspnoea.

Hypotension is likely to be more marked whilst standing. It is most severe during the first few seconds of ventricular pacing (Figure 23.14), before reflex vasoconstrictor compensatory mechanisms can come into play, so ventricular pacing is particularly unsuitable for patients who are mainly in sinus rhythm but who often develop bradycardia at a rate less than the cycle length of the ventricular pacemaker (i.e. those with sick sinus or carotid sinus syndrome). This has been demonstrated by recording ambulatory blood pressure in patients with ventricular demand pacemakers. The onset of ventricular pacing was followed by hypotension, which was greater in those who had complained of syncope and near-syncope.

Ventriculoatrial conduction (Figure 23.15) of ventricular paced beats causes even greater haemodynamic upset; the resultant atrial distension may initiate a reflex vasodepressor effect. AV sequential pacing or, when AV conduction is not impaired, atrial pacing will avoid these problems.

Pacemaker syndrome does not occur in every patient with a VVI pacemaker but it does occur in a significant minority, as demonstrated in several clinical trials. Furthermore, less severe forms of the pacemaker syndrome are probably not recognised. The syndrome can be avoided by dual-chamber pacing. In the author's opinion, in patients other than those with persistent atrial fibrillation, VVI (Figure 23.16) rather than DDD pacing should only be undertaken in exceptional circumstances.

Right ventricular apical pacing may cause heart failure

Several studies have shown that long-term pacing with the pacing lead tip positioned at the apex of the right ventricle, the conventional site in past years, can impair ventricular function and cause heart failure in some patients; it can also increase the incidence of atrial fibrillation. Right ventricular apical pacing results in a delay and an

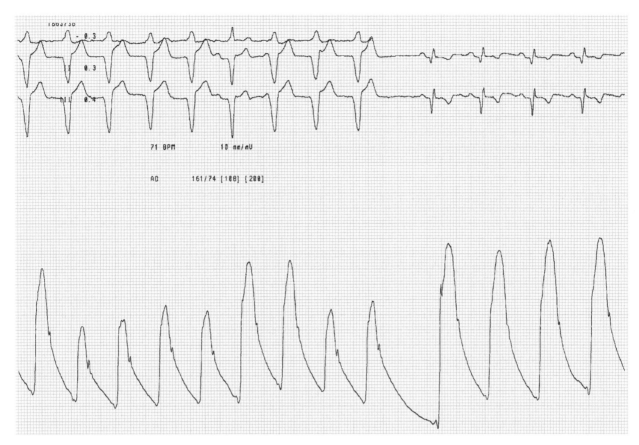

Figure 23.13 The peak arterial pressure and the pulse pressure (which is a measure of cardiac output) are lower during ventricular pacing (left side of panel) than during sinus rhythm (right side of panel). During ventricular pacing, the pressure varies depending on the relation between paced beats and dissociated P waves.

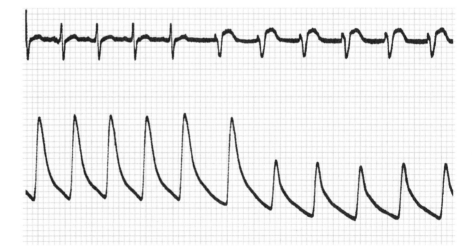

Figure 23.14 Pacemaker syndrome. Symptomatic hypotension (see lower blood pressure trace) developed at onset of ventricular pacing which occurred after the first four sinus beats.

abnormal sequence of electrical and hence mechanical ventricular activation similar to that which occurs in left bundle branch block. The incidence of failure is related to the proportion of pacing compared with spontaneous ventricular activation. Furthermore, myocardial perfusion imaging has shown that apical pacing can cause perfusion defects even in patients with normal coronary arteries.

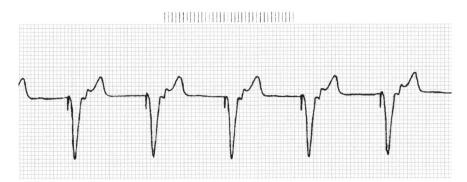

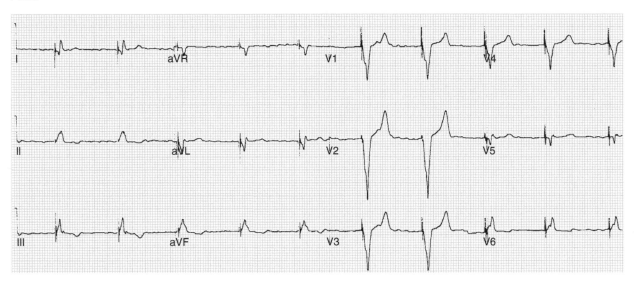

Figure 23.15 Ventricular pacing with retrograde activation (lead III). Each ventricular complex is followed by an inverted P wave.

Figure 23.16 VVIR pacing in a patient with persistent atrial fibrillation.

An option that is now being widely adopted is to pace the right ventricular outflow tract (Figure 23.17b) or the ventricular septum rather than apex. Whereas there is good evidence of the deleterious effect of apical pacing, there is to date none with regards to outflow tract pacing, and there is evidence of haemodynamic advantage.

In patients with right ventricular apical leads who have developed heart failure, improvement can be achieved by upgrading to a biventricular system.

In patients with dual-chamber systems who have no or only intermittent impaired AV conduction, the AV delay should if possible be increased to facilitate normal ventricular activation and thereby minimise ventricular pacing (e.g. program the AV interval up to 250ms). A sophisticated algorithm has been developed to keep ventricular pacing to a minimum: AV conduction is assessed after every atrial event (paced or sensed); occasional non-conducted atrial events are permitted but if two out of four consecutive P waves are not followed by QRS complexes the pacemaker changes to DDD pacing. During DDD pacing, at intervals the device returns to AAI mode to test if normal AV conduction has returned.

Pacemaker hardware

Pulse generator

A pulse generator consists of a power source together with electronic circuits to control the timing and characteristics of the impulses that it generates.

(a)

(b)

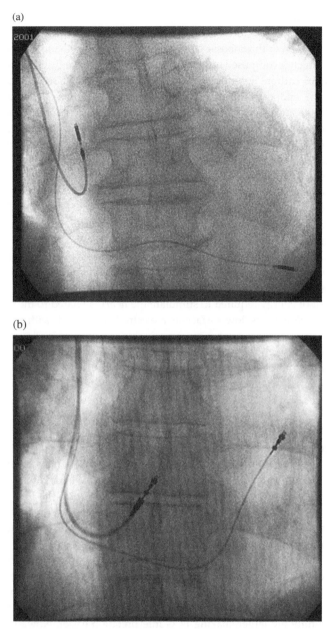

Figure 23.17 (a) X-ray showing 'screw-in leads' positioned in right ventricular apex and right atrial appendage. (b) X-ray showing 'screw-in leads' positioned in right ventricular outflow tract and on low atrial septum.

In the past, several power sources have been used, including mercury zinc cells, rechargeable nickel cadmium cells and nuclear energy. Now, lithium iodide cells are used almost exclusively. Lithium pacemakers have a lifespan of 4–15 years and predictable, progressive discharge behaviour. They are contained in a hermetically sealed titanium can, 35–50 g in weight, and generally have a maximum diameter of no more than 50 mm and a thickness of as little as 6 mm.

Pacemaker leads
Stimuli produced by the pulse generator are conducted to the heart via a lead or leads consisting of an insulated wire with an electrode at its tip that is attached to the heart.

Transvenous leads are used in virtually all pacemaker implantations. A modern lead consists of a multifilar, helically coiled wire insulated by a material that does not cause tissue reaction or thrombosis: silicone rubber or polyurethane. At the lead tip is the cathode, which is composed of an inert material such as platinum-iridium, elgiloy, steel or vitreous carbon. For effective stimulation, this must be securely and closely attached to the endocardium. If fibrous tissue, which is non-excitable, develops between cathode and endocardium the amount of energy required to stimulate the heart will increase and may exceed the output capability of the pacemaker.

To achieve secure endocardial attachment and a low threshold for stimulation, several 'fixation devices' have been employed. 'Passive' fixation devices include tines, flanges or fins positioned proximal to the lead tip, which can become entrapped in the myocardial trabeculae. 'Active' devices involve a metal screw, usually retractable, that can be screwed into the endomyocardium (Figure 23.17). 'Porous' metal or carbon electrodes are now widely used; the surface of the cathode consists of many microscopic pores that promote rapid tissue ingrowth and hence very secure fixation. Movement between electrode and endocardium and thus generation of fibrous tissue is minimised. Many types of electrode elute dexamethasone to minimise local tissue reaction and hence stimulation threshold.

The amount of energy required to stimulate the heart is related to the surface area of the cathode. Nowadays, low-surface-area electrodes are used, with a surface area of 6–12 mm^2.

Leads that are sewn onto the epicardium or screwed into the myocardium necessitate thoracotomy and are now, with the advent of reliable transvenous leads, rarely used unless pacemaker implantation is undertaken at the time of open heart surgery, or if venous thrombosis or a tricuspid valve prosthesis preclude a transvenous approach.

Unipolar versus bipolar pacing

In unipolar pacing the anode is remote from the heart; it is usually the can that contains the pulse generator. In bipolar pacing, both anode and cathode are within the cardiac chamber to be paced, the anode positioned along the lead near to its cathodal tip. A commonly held view is that an electrogram sensed by a unipolar lead is larger than that from a bipolar lead. There is in fact usually no difference between bipolar and unipolar electrograms or stimulation thresholds.

Bipolar pacing has the advantage that inappropriate sensing of electromagnetic interference and skeletal muscle electromyograms is much less likely, as is extracardiac stimulation. Reasons for favouring unipolar pacing were that in the past bipolar electrodes have been less reliable and larger in calibre, and surface ECG unipolar pacemaker stimuli are larger, making ECG interpretation easier. Nowadays, bipolar pacing leads are reliable, enable better sensing of cardiac events, and are to be preferred.

Costs

In the United Kingdom, the current approximate costs of a pulse generator plus leads for single-chamber and dual-chamber rate-responsive pacing systems are £800 and £1500, respectively.

Pacemaker implantation

For pacemaker implantation, facilities for fluoroscopy, ECG monitoring and cardiopulmonary resuscitation are required. The procedure is usually carried out under local anaesthesia and takes less than 45 minutes. Conscious sedation, as discussed in Chapter 21, is often used. Strict aseptic technique is essential. Thorough hand-washing is necessary: surgical gloves have been shown to be imperfect barriers.

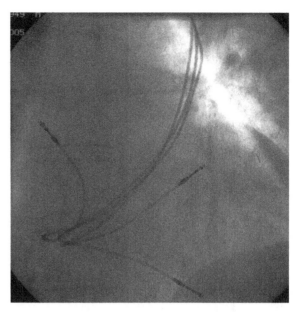

Figure 23.18 Leads to right atrial appendage, right ventricular outflow tract and right ventricular apex (i.e. 'bifocal pacing') via persistent left-sided superior vena cava.

Subclavian approach

This approach is widely used. The pacemaker lead(s) are introduced via infraclavicular subclavian vein puncture and are connected to the pulse generator which is implanted in a subcutaneous pocket fashioned over pectoralis major.

Usually, the left subclavian vein is used. Occasionally, however, a persistent left-sided superior vena cava, which will drain into the coronary sinus, will be encountered, dictating that the atrial and/or ventricular leads will have to be positioned via the coronary sinus. This is usually possible but can be technically challenging (Figure 23.18). A left-sided superior vena cava is most commonly encountered in a patient with congenital heart disease, particularly atrial septal defect. If a patient is known to have congenital heart disease, the right subclavian vein is to be preferred.

An incision is made 2 cm below the junction of the middle and inner thirds of the clavicle and is extended in a lateral and inferior direction for approximately 6 cm. A subcutaneous pocket large enough to accommodate the pulse generator is created by blunt dissection. Puncture of the subclavian vein is much easier if the vein is distended: a slight head-down position will help or, alternatively, the legs should be raised. Dehydration, which can markedly reduce venous pressure and thereby make puncture more difficult, should be avoided or corrected.

A needle is introduced just below the inferior border of the clavicle at the junction of its middle and inner thirds and directed towards the sternoclavicular joint so that it passes behind the posterior surface of the clavicle. As the needle punctures the vein, venous blood will be aspirated easily; only a trickle suggests that the needle is not in the vein. Aspiration of air or bright pulsatile blood indicates puncture of the pleura or subclavian artery, respectively. If the patient has a 'deep' chest, and particularly if the clavicle bows anteriorly, it may be necessary to introduce the needle more laterally and to point it slightly posteriorly.

Cannulation of the vein is then achieved by introducing a flexible guidewire with a J-shaped tip through the needle. Resistance to its passage indicates that the wire is not in the vein. The wire is passed into the superior vena cava and its position checked by fluoroscopy. (If screening demonstrates that the wire is in the centre of the chest it is likely that the subclavian artery has been entered and the tip of the wire is in the

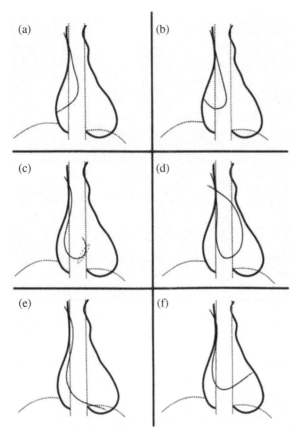

Figure 23.19 Insertion of a transvenous pacing lead. (a and b) A loop is formed in the right atrium. (c) The loop is positioned near the tricuspid valve, indicated by the oval of dashes. (d) Entry into the right ventricle can be confirmed by passing the wire into the pulmonary artery. (e) The pacing lead is then positioned in the apex of the right ventricle. (f) The characteristic appearance of a pacing lead in the coronary sinus.

aorta.) The needle is then withdrawn and a sheath, within which is a vessel dilator, is passed over the wire into the vein. The guidewire and dilator are then removed and the pacing lead inserted into the sheath.

If it is planned to introduce a second or third lead, then two or three guidewires can be introduced into the vein via the sheath. The sheath can then be removed and individual dilators and sheaths advanced over each guidewire. 'Peel-away' sheaths are used so that removal is not prevented by the connector at the proximal end of the lead.

Cephalic vein approach

An alternative to subclavian vein puncture is to cut down onto the cephalic vein in the deltopectoral groove. This approach avoids the risks of subclavian vein puncture but sometimes the vein is not big enough. It can sometimes be difficult to advance a lead from the cephalic into the subclavian vein. However, use of a hydrophilically coated guidewire, over which introducer and sheath are advanced, makes negotiation of the bends between the cephalic and subclavian veins very much easier.

Ventricular lead positioning

To facilitate manipulation of a long-term pacing lead, which is very flexible, a wire stylet is passed down the body of the lead. Bending the distal part of the stylet or its slight withdrawal will often aid positioning.

The lead is passed into the right atrium (Figure 23.19). Sometimes the lead can then be directly advanced through the tricuspid valve to the right ventricle. More often, it is necessary to form a loop in the atrium by impinging the lead tip on the atrial wall and then advancing the lead a little further. By rotating the lead its tip can then be positioned near the tricuspid valve. Slight withdrawal of the lead will allow it to 'flick' through the valve into the ventricle. Ventricular ectopic beats are always provoked as the valve is crossed. *If ventricular ectopics do not occur then it is highly probable that the tricuspid valve has not been crossed and the coronary sinus has been entered.*

Entry into the ventricle can be confirmed by advancing the lead into the pulmonary artery. Once in the right ventricle, the lead tip is positioned in or near the ventricular apex or right ventricular outflow tract by a process of lead rotation, advancement and withdrawal. A stable position should be ensured by checking for continuous pacing and for absence of excessive lead tip movement during deep inspiration and coughing. Additional measures to ensure lead stability include brief partial withdrawal of the lead so that there is only a little slack and then temporarily advancing the lead so that there is excessive slack in the body of the lead.

Once a satisfactory position has been achieved both in terms of stability and measurements (see below), it is essential that the lead is secured by placing a short sleeve around it near its point of entry into the vein and fixing it to the underlying muscle with a non-absorbable suture. It is important to check that the lead is *securely fixed* within the sleeve – otherwise lead displacement may occur.

Atrial lead positioning
The right atrial appendage is the usual site for atrial pacing. If necessary, atrial pacing may be performed by using a 'screw-in' lead to pace from the septal or free right atrial walls.

For pacing the right atrial appendage, the lead tip is advanced to near the tricuspid valve using a straight stylet. A stylet whose terminal 5 cm has been shaped into a tight J-shaped curve is then used to position the lead in the atrial appendage: as the lead is slowly withdrawn from the tricuspid valve position it will 'flick' into the atrial appendage. Correct positioning will be demonstrated by the lead tip moving from side to side with atrial systole. Lateral screening will demonstrate that the lead is pointing anteriorly. Lead stability should be confirmed by twisting the lead 45 degrees in either direction; the lead tip should not turn. It is important that there is the correct amount of slack in the lead. During inspiration the angle between the two limbs of the J should not exceed 80 degrees.

Measurement of stimulation and sensing thresholds
Low stimulation and sensing thresholds are essential for satisfactory long-term pacing. High thresholds suggest that the cathode is not in close apposition to excitable tissue. Thresholds rise after pacemaker implantation, usually peaking three weeks to three months after surgery. If they become high they may exceed the stimulation and sensing capabilities of the pulse generator. Thresholds are measured with a pacing systems analyser (PSA).

Stimulation threshold
The stimulation threshold is the smallest electrical stimulus (delivered by the cathode outside the ventricular effective and relative refractory periods) that will consistently activate the myocardium.

To measure the stimulation threshold, the analyser is usually set to deliver impulses 10–20 beats/min in excess of the spontaneous rate with an impulse duration similar to that which the implanted pulse generator will deliver (often 0.5 ms) and a voltage output of 5 V. The threshold is then established by progressively reducing the output until failure of capture occurs. If the patient has no spontaneous rhythm, pacemaker output will have to be promptly increased to avoid asystole. It is important to know that the stimulation threshold is substantially greater when increasing output from a

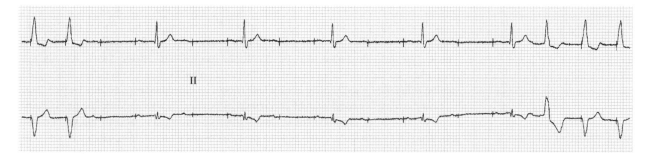

Figure 23.20 Wedensky phenomenon. The stimulation threshold is measured by progressively reducing the ventricular output by 0.1 V decrements until after the second paced beat there is failure to capture. The output is then increased by 0.1 V increments. Only after 10 increments is ventricular capture achieved. Had there not been a spontaneous rhythm while there was failure to capture there would have been an embarrassing and probably symptomatic period of asystole! The output should have been immediately increased by at least 2 V as soon as the stimulation threshold had been established.

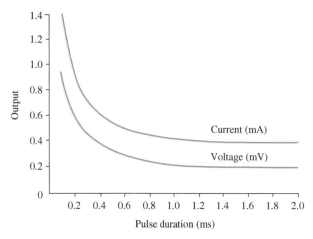

Figure 23.21 Typical strength–duration curve. The stimulation threshold is measured at different pulse widths. There is no significant reduction in stimulation threshold when the pulse duration is increased above 1.0 ms.

sub-threshold level. This phenomenon is known as the Wedensky phenomenon (Figure 23.20). *Therefore, as soon as there is a failure to capture, pacemaker output should be immediately increased by at least 2 V.*

At a pulse duration of 0.5 ms, a voltage threshold of less than 1 V is satisfactory; often the threshold will be less than 0.5 V. It should be noted that with screw-in leads the threshold can initially be quite high but will fall within 3–4 minutes after fixation.

It is important that the distal and proximal poles of the electrode are connected to the pacemaker cathode (−) and anode (+), respectively. If the poles are reversed, the measured stimulation threshold will be significantly higher. The longer the duration of the pacing stimulus the more energy is delivered and hence the lower the stimulation threshold. However, the relationship is not linear: the range of efficient impulse duration, in terms of energy consumption, is 0.25–1.0 ms (Figure 23.21). (The output at which a further increase in pulse duration does not reduce the stimulation threshold is called the rheobase. Twice this value is termed the chronaxie.)

When measuring the stimulation threshold of a unipolar lead the distal pole of the electrode is connected to the pacemaker cathode (−) and the proximal electrode (+) is connected to a metal object such as a self-retaining retractor which is placed in the wound. It is important that the surface area of the anode approximates that of the pacemaker can; otherwise a falsely high threshold will be obtained.

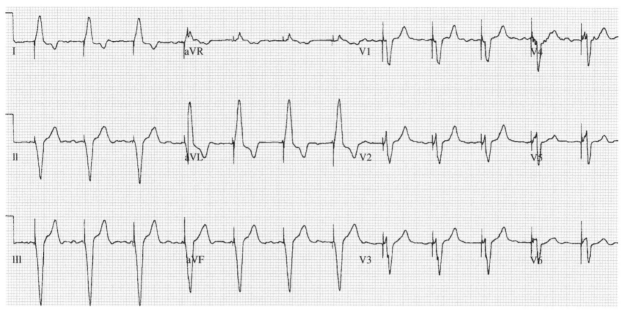

Figure 23.22 Right ventricular apical pacing: left axis deviation and left bundle branch block configuration.

Sensing threshold

To ensure satisfactory sensing it is important that the intracardiac electrogram resulting from spontaneous activity of the cardiac chamber to be paced is of sufficient amplitude. It is usually measured with a pacing systems analyser. Ventricular and atrial electrograms should be greater than 4 mV and 2 mV, respectively. In 'borderline' cases the slew rate (i.e. the rate of change of signal voltage) is also important: low rates may result in failure to sense.

Lead impedance

The pacing systems analyser can also be used to measure lead impedance, which is a measure of resistance to flow of current in the lead. It varies with lead type but is usually in the order of 400–1000 ohms.

A low impedance suggests a break in insulation and hence leakage of current, whereas a high impedance points to lead fracture.

Paced ventricular electrogram

Pacing the right ventricular apex will lead to a ventricular complex with left axis deviation and left bundle branch block configuration (Figure 23.22). Right ventricular outflow tract pacing results in right axis deviation and left bundle branch block configuration (Figure 23.23) as would occur with right ventricular outflow tract tachycardia (Chapter 12). Inadvertent pacing of the left ventricle via a patent foramen ovale leads to a paced complex with right bundle branch block configuration.

Biventricular pacing for resynchronisation therapy typically results in a relatively narrow ventricular complex (Figure 23.24a,b).

Fashioning a pacemaker pocket

It might appear that creating a pocket for the pacemaker is the least challenging part of the implantation procedure. However, unless it is done well, wound complications are likely; often, they develop some months after implantation.

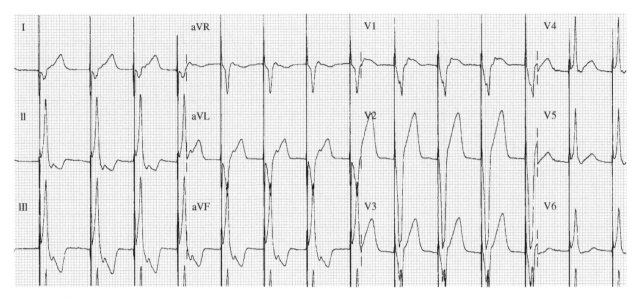

Figure 23.23 Right ventricular outflow tract pacing: right axis deviation and left bundle branch block configuration.

A subcutaneous space to accommodate the pacemaker is usually fashioned by blunt dissection. Extensive infiltration with local anaesthesia is required, and even then some patients experience discomfort during the minute or so that the pocket is created. It is important that the wound is sufficiently deep that the pacemaker is placed on the surface of the pectoral muscle. A common mistake is to site the pocket close to the clavicle where there is little subcutaneous tissue – inviting pacemaker erosion. The pocket should be positioned more inferiorly, enabling it to be covered by a thicker layer of 'flesh'.

Fashioning of a generator pocket that is too large may allow spontaneous or intentional repeated rotation of the pulse generator, which can cause dislodgement or fracture of the pacing lead – the 'twiddler's syndrome'. Too small a pocket, and the skin over the pacemaker will be tense and erosion is likely.

In very thin patients or in those who are anxious for the generator to be as inconspicuous as possible, the device should be positioned beneath the pectoral muscle.

Complications of pacemaker implantation
Bleeding
Bruising is not uncommon but occasionally a haematoma will result: if tense, it must be evacuated without delay. Evacuation can be achieved without reopening the wound by making a 1–2 cm incision over the site of maximal fluctuation. Blood clot can be removed by repeated expression through this incision. A pressure bandage *must be applied* to prevent re-accumulation.

Not infrequently, patients requiring pacemaker implantation are on anticoagulant drugs. If warfarin is prescribed for atrial fibrillation it should be temporarily stopped four days before the procedure and restarted following implantation. In patients with prosthetic metallic valves or in whom lifelong anticoagulants were prescribed following pulmonary embolism or coagulopathy, warfarin should be stopped two or three days beforehand, aiming for an INR ≤ 2.5. A small dose of *oral* vitamin K (2–3 mg) can be very effective at reducing the INR if it is markedly prolonged. Heparin should be avoided: it often leads to major haematoma formation. Clopidogrel and similar antiplatelet drugs can also often cause this complication but it many not be possible to stop them, e.g. within the first year of coronary artery stenting. Whenever there is

(a)

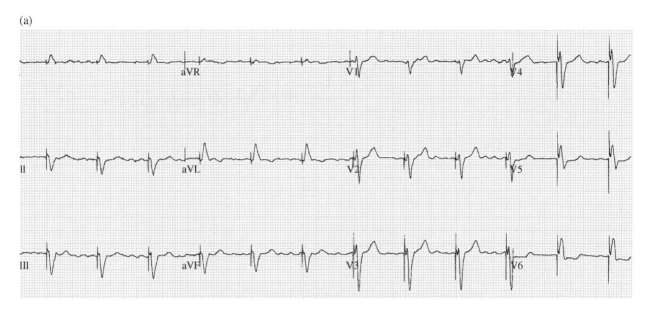

(b)

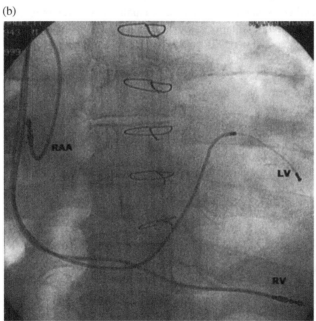

Figure 23.24 (a) Biventricular pacing resulting in shorter QRS duration than occurs with single lead stimulation. (b) Biventricular pacing leads: radiograph showing leads in right atrial appendage (RAA), apex of right ventricle (RV), and lateral branch of coronary sinus (LV).

concern about the risk of haematoma formation a pressure bandage should be applied immediately after implantation.

Lead displacement
Lead displacement was once a common problem, but with modern leads it occurs in less than 1% of implantations.

Subclavian vein puncture
Complications of attempted subclavian vein puncture are infrequent. They include pneumothorax, haemothorax, air embolism, brachial plexus damage and puncture of the subclavian artery. Surprisingly, inadvertent subclavian artery puncture rarely leads to problems.

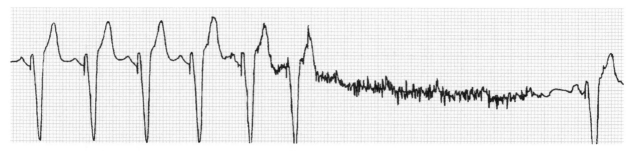

Figure 23.25 Electromyographic inhibition of a DDD pacemaker. Activities such as washing hands caused near-syncope. Corrected by decreasing pacemaker sensitivity.

Infection

Infection is reported to occur in 1–2% of implantations and is virtually always staphylococcal. Several studies have shown that antibiotic cover, usually with flucloxacillin, significantly reduces the risk of infection. A large recent study showed an 80% reduction in infection with intravenous cefazolin.

Unless infection is only superficial, explantation will usually be required even if antibiotics appear to help initially. Ideally, the pacing lead(s) should be removed, and this is very desirable if there has been systemic infection. It is usually easy to remove leads within the first year or so after implantation by moderate, sustained traction. Clearly, with screw-in leads the metal tip needs to be retracted before removal. However, removal late after implantation can be difficult, particularly if the leads have a passive fixation device such as fins. Use of extraction devices such as 'locking stylets' or laser sheath are often effective and reduce the risk of cardiac tamponade. Rarely, it is necessary to resort to thoracotomy. If extraction is not carried out, the lead should be shortened so that it no longer lies in or close to the infected area. The proximal end should be capped and fixed with a suture. However, there is a risk of persistent infection and bacteraemia.

Transoesophageal echocardiography may sometimes reveal a mass on a pacemaker lead. It should be noted that a study has shown that many such masses are not in fact infected, and lead removal should only be considered if there is evidence of systemic infection.

Erosion

Erosion of the skin overlying the pacemaker is a late complication but is often a consequence of implantation technique. Factors that predispose to erosion include creation of a pacemaker pocket that is too tight or too superficial, a very thin patient, and use of a generator with sharp corners. The skin will be found to be thinned around the site of erosion. Infection is often present but it is secondary to erosion. If the skin is broken, explantation will be necessary.

Thinned, reddened skin over the generator is a sign of 'threatened' erosion: *the generator should be re-sited without delay before the skin breaks down.*

Complications related to pulse generator
Electromyographic interference

This common problem is virtually confined to unipolar pacing systems. Myopotentials generated from the underlying muscle are sensed by the pacemaker as spontaneous cardiac activity (Figure 23.25). In systems where sensed events inhibit output, inappropriate cessation of pacing will occur. Short periods of electromyographic inhibition are common and usually asymptomatic. Longer periods may cause syncope and necessitate adjustment to sensitivity, pacing mode or polarity.

Susceptibility to electromyographic inhibition can be demonstrated by asking the patient to extend his or her arms and then to press the hands firmly together.

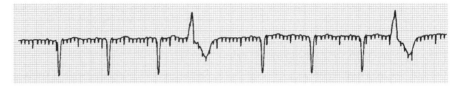

Figure 23.26 A runaway pacemaker. Fortunately, in this case the stimuli were sub-threshold.

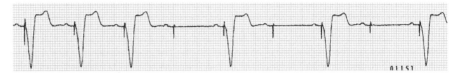

Figure 23.27 DDD pacing. After three paced ventricular complexes, there is intermittent exit block: pacing stimuli are not followed by ventricular complexes.

Inhibition is only significant if it lasts for several seconds, particularly if the patient's symptoms are reproduced.

Muscle stimulation

This complication can be caused by unipolar pacing and is a consequence of the pacemaker can being the anode: stimulation of the underlying pectoral muscle occurs. It can also result from left ventricular pacing in patients with biventricular pacemakers.

Generator failure

Premature generator failure does occur occasionally. Very rarely, a device can malfunction such that it delivers pacing stimuli at an extremely fast rate with the risk of initiating ventricular fibrillation – a 'runaway pacemaker' (Figure 23.26).

Complications related to pacing lead

Exit block

The development of excessive fibrous tissue, which is non-excitable, around the cathode may increase the stimulation threshold to a level higher than the pacemaker's output. The result will be intermittent or persistent failure to pace without evidence of lead displacement (Figure 23.27). Exit block is most likely to occur in the first three weeks to three months after implantation, when stimulation threshold is at its highest. Sometimes exit block is transient; otherwise lead repositioning will be required unless generator output can be increased by reprogramming (see below). Modern leads with low surface area, porous-surfaced electrodes and positive fixation devices rarely cause this complication.

Lead fracture and insulation breakdown

With modern leads, fracture is rare. If it occurs it is usually at the point where the lead enters the venous system, at the site of a fixation suture or wherever there is excessive angulation of the lead. Lead fracture will cause intermittent or persistent failure to pace and sense. Lead impedance will be very *high*.

Lead fracture can often be detected radiographically but should not be confused with 'pseudofracture', in which the pressure of a tight ligature directly applied to the lead compresses the insulation and spreads the coils of wire inside without interfering with lead function.

Insulation breakdown will allow leakage of current, which may cause stimulation of adjacent muscles, and hence premature battery depletion. *Lead impedance will be markedly reduced (≤ 200 ohms).*

Lead fracture and insulation breakdown are less common with a cephalic vein approach.

Phrenic nerve and diaphragmatic stimulation

The phrenic nerve or diaphragm can sometimes be stimulated through the intervening thin myocardial walls by atrial and ventricular (especially left ventricular) leads, respectively. Lead repositioning will be required unless, in programmable pacemakers, cessation of extracardiac stimulation can be achieved by output reduction.

Venous thrombosis

Clinically apparent subclavian vein thrombosis is rare and pulmonary embolism even rarer. Anticoagulant therapy is indicated. Angiographic studies have reported that asymptomatic venous thrombosis is not infrequent: in pacemaker patients requiring a new or an additional lead, a subclavian vein angiogram should be carried out by introducing x-ray contrast into an arm vein.

Pacemaker programmability

A programmable pacemaker can be non-invasively adjusted in one or more of its functions by radiofrequency signals emitted from an external programming device. Programmability enables achievement of optimal pacemaker function for the individual patient and can also be used in the diagnosis and treatment of certain pacemaker complications.

A wide variety of parameters can be adjusted. Examples are listed below, together with typical options:
1. Lower rate limit (30–150 beats/min)
2. Output (2.5–7.5 V)
3. Pulse duration (0.1–1.0 ms)
4. Sensitivity (0.25–8 mV)
5. Pacing mode (e.g. AAI, VVI, DDD, rate-responsive, mode switching)
6. Refractory period (200–500 ms)
7. Pacing polarity (unipolar or bipolar)
8. Upper rate limits for dual-chamber and rate-responsive pacemakers (100–180 beats/min)
9. AV delay for dual-chamber pacemakers (0–300 ms)
10. Maximum tracking rate
11. Maximum sensor rate
12. Hysteresis rate
13. Stored EGM (atrial, ventricular or both)

Pacemakers have the facility of rate hysteresis. The interval after a sensed event which would trigger delivery of a pacemaker stimulus can be greater than the interval between paced beats. For example, a pacemaker can be programmed to stimulate the heart at 70 beats/min or higher only if the spontaneous rate falls below 40 beats/min, thus helping to avoid problems that might occur with loss of AV synchrony.

Whereas a slow heart rate at rest may be optimal for many pacemaker patients, it may not be appropriate if there is an episode of heart failure or major haemorrhage. It is sometimes forgotten that a pacemaker can be temporarily programmed to a higher rate to deal with such an event.

Automatic capture management

Some pacemakers have the facility to verify on a beat-to-beat basis whether a pacemaker stimulus has led to myocardial activation. This facility enables pacemaker algorithms that can achieve myocardial stimulation using outputs just above the stimulation threshold. If a stimulus fails to capture the myocardium then the pacemaker immediately delivers a high output stimulus. Automatic

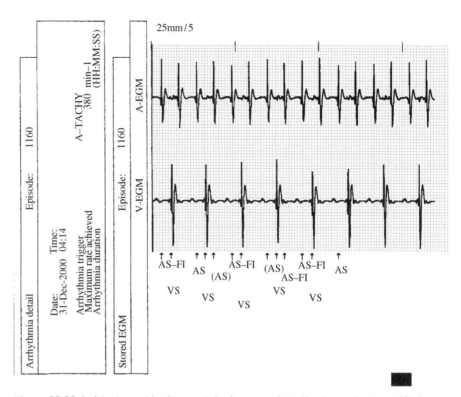

Figure 23.28 Real-time intra-atrial and intraventricular electrograms obtained by telemetry, showing atrial fibrillation in a patient with a mode-switching pacemaker.

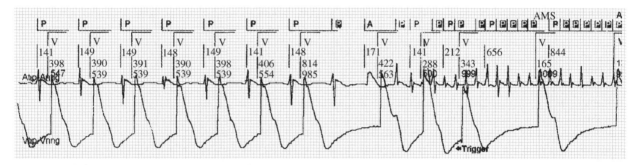

Figure 23.29 Stored electrogram showing intracardiac atrial (AtipAring) and ventricular (VtipVring) electrograms at the onset of an episode of atrial fibrillation resulting in almost immediate mode switching (AMS).

capture management thereby maximises battery longevity and provides a safety feature in that pacemaker output automatically adapts should the stimulation threshold rise.

Telemetry data

With most modern pacemakers, real-time and stored intracardiac electrograms can be obtained by telemetry (Figures 23.28, 23.29).

Other telemetered information includes how the pacemaker has been programmed; lead impedance; battery impedance and status; the percentages of time during which there has been pacing or inhibition; and range of paced and sensed heart rates that have occurred. These latter data can be helpful in programming rate-responsive systems to ensure that the sensor facilitates an appropriate chronotropic response.

Basic parameters

	Initial	Present	
Mode	DDI	DDI	
Base Rate	70	70	min[21]
A-V Delay	150	150	ms
Vent Pulse Configuration	Unipolar	Unipolar	
V. Pulse Width	0.4	0.4	ms
V. Pulse Amplitude	3.0	3.0	V
V. Sense Configuration	Unipolar Tip	Unipolar Tip	
V. Sensitivity	2.0	2.0	mV
V. Refractory	250	250	mV
Atrial Pulse Configuration	Unipolar	Unipolar	
A. Pulse Width	0.4	0.4	ms
A. Pulse Amplitude	2.5	2.5	V
A. Sense Configuration	Unipolar Tip	Unipolar Tip	
A. Sensivity	0.50	0.50	mV
A. Refractory	275	275	ms
Blanking	38	38	ms
Vent. Safety Option	Enabled	Enabled	
Rate Resp. A -V Delay	Disabled	Disabled	
Magnet Response	Off	Off	

Sensor parameters

Sensor	Off	Off	
Max Sensor Rate	140	140	min[21]
Threshold	2.0	2.0	
Meas Average Sensor	2.4	2.4	
Slope	8 Normal	8 Normal	
Reaction Time	Fast	Fast	
Recovery Time	Medium	Medium	

Measured data

Measured Rate	62.9	min[21]
Ventricular		
Pulse Amplitude	2.9	V
Pulse Current	5.3	mA
Pulse Energy	5	mJ
Pulse Charge	2	mC
Lead Impedance	552	V
Atrial		
Pulse Amplitude	2.1	V
Pulse Current	3.9	mA
Pulse Energy	3	mJ
Pulse Charge	1	mC
Lead Impedance	538	V
Battery Data .... (W.G. 8077 - nom. 1.8 Ah)		
Voltage	2.26	V
Cuttent	11	mA
Impedance	21	kV

Warning: The Elective Replacement Indicator has been reached.

Figure 23.30 Telemetered pacemaker data indicating how the pacemaker has been programmed and satisfactory lead impedances. The battery voltage is very low and the battery impedance exceptionally high, indicating that generator change should have been performed several months previously!

Pacemaker clinic

Follow-up

Patients with implanted pacemakers should regularly attend a follow-up clinic. The purposes are to check that the pacemaker is working satisfactorily; to ensure that there are no pacing complications; to detect impending battery depletion so that generator replacement can be carried out before the patient is at risk; to adjust pacemaker output to at least twice stimulation threshold; and to maintain a record of patients' locations should a recall of a particular generator or lead be necessary.

Occasionally, a manufacturer reports that a fault has occurred in some of its pacemakers. Usually the failure rate is very low, but regulations dictate that a report is made and those suspect pacemakers monitored more closely. Sometimes a recommendation is made that generator replacement should be considered. One has to balance the risk of pacemaker failure against the not insignificant morbidity (especially infection) associated with generator change. Clearly the case is more compelling in a pacemaker-dependent patient.

Battery depletion

Pulse generators have the facility to transmit data to the programmer (i.e. telemetry). Marked reduction in battery voltage and increase in battery internal resistance are indicators of imminent battery depletion (Figure 23.30). There are two stages towards the end of battery life: 'recommended replacement time' (RRT) and 'end of life' (EOL). Some pacemakers will automatically revert to the VVI mode when EOL is reached, in order to minimise battery consumption.

Because of the likelihood of a delay before a patient can be admitted to hospital for generator change, it is desirable to make a decision based on careful analysis of battery data as to the timing of generator replacement before RRT is reached and certainly before EOL is reached.

Some pacemakers provide conflicting and confusing data so that it may be difficult to predict when generator change should be undertaken. It is important that pacemaker clinics are thoroughly familiar with the types of pacemaker implanted in their centre and that they are able to receive prompt advice from the manufacturer if there is any doubt as to data obtained.

Prior to generator replacement, timely reassessment of the pacing system and pacing requirements should take place. For example, a patient may have developed permanent atrial fibrillation, in which case a VVIR rather than DDDR generator would be indicated. A patient may have suffered left ventricular failure and would benefit from an upgrade to biventricular pacing. There may be a patient who has never benefited from pacing, or who has been paced for sinus node disease and who has developed atrial fibrillation with satisfactory ventricular rates, who no longer requires a pacemaker. The occasional patient will have a suspect pacing lead, for example with rising threshold or abnormally low or high impedance, necessitating a decision as to whether lead change should be undertaken at the time of generator replacement.

Electromagnetic interference

External electromagnetic interference may affect pacemakers and cause either inhibition or reversion to the fixed-rate mode, reprogramming or damage to the pacemaker circuitry. In practice, because pacemakers are well shielded and because of the use of appropriate filters, very few problems are encountered and patients should be reassured that the risks are minimal.

Electronic article surveillance systems (EAS) and metal detectors

These could transiently inhibit or possibly reprogram a pacemaker. However, there are only a few reports of adverse incidents and no patient has been harmed. Current advice to patients is:

1. It is sufficient to pass the system at an ordinary pace. Do not stay near an EAS system or metal detector longer than is necessary and do not lean against the system.

2. Be aware that EAS systems may be hidden or camouflaged in entrances, and exist in many commercial establishments.

3. If scanning with a hand-held metal detector is necessary, warn the security personnel that you have an electronic medical device and ask them not to hold the metal detector near the device any longer than is absolutely necessary; or you may wish to ask for an alternative form of personal search. In fact, a recent large study showed that modern handheld metal detectors used for security screening do not interfere with implanted devices.

Transcutaneous electrical nerve stimulation (TENS)

Unipolar pacemakers can be inhibited, and it is recommended that the heart rhythm is monitored during initial TENS application in patients with bipolar systems.

Cellular phones

Mobile telephones may possibly cause transient interference of pacemaker function. It is recommended that a mobile telephone is kept at least 15 cm from the pacemaker and that when the phone is in use it should be put to the ear opposite to the implant site. In fact, a number of manufacturers have indicated that their devices are 'phone-proof'.

Magnets

A magnet held directly over a pacemaker can activate its reed-switch and thereby make it function in a fixed-rate mode. The effect should only last as long as the magnet is applied. Patients should be advised to avoid clothing and accessories that contain magnets.

Headphones used with personal music players contain magnets. Studies have shown that interference with device function can occur if headphones are within 3 cm distance: they should not be worn around the neck or placed in a pocket over the device but are otherwise safe to use.

Diathermy

Diathermy may possibly damage a pacemaker, cause inappropriate inhibition or precipitate ventricular fibrillation. The pacemaker should be checked prior to surgery: some pacemakers are more prone to external interference when the batteries are approaching their end of life. If possible, a bipolar diathermy system should be used. If a unipolar system has to be used, output should be kept as low as possible. The active electrode should be kept at least 15 cm from the generator and the indifferent electrode sited as far away as possible so that its dipole is perpendicular to the pacing system. The pulse should be monitored so that diathermy can be interrupted if prolonged inhibition occurs. A pacemaker check should be performed soon after surgery.

Radiotherapy

Radiation for therapeutic use may cause damage to an implanted device if directly in the radiation beam: the CMOS circuitry in a modern pacemaker is particularly sensitive. If necessary, re-siting of the generator should be considered. Device function should be checked before and after treatment.

Magnetic resonance imaging

Limited experience with magnetic resonance imaging (MRI) indicates that some pacemakers will revert to fixed-rate mode and some may pace at a dangerously fast rate. There has also been concern about tissue damage, heating at the lead tip, and cessation of therapy. General advice is that pacemaker patients should not undergo MRI. However, there are a now a number of reports that patients with pacemakers have undergone MRI scanning without significant problem. *If a scan is performed the pacemaker's sensor and magnet responses should both be programmed off.*

Recently, 'MRI safe' pacing systems have become available.

Arc welding

Arc welders should wear non-conductive gloves, should not work in a wet area, should avoid high current settings and never exceed 400 A, and connect the ground clamp to the metal as close as possible to the welding point.

Neurostimulators

Serious interaction can occur between implanted cardiac devices and neurostimulators. If both systems are required they should be implanted on opposite sides of the body, they should function in bipolar mode, and there should be extensive testing to ensure there is no interaction. Manufacturer's advice should be sought.

Devices that are safe

The following will not affect a pacemaker: microwave ovens, electric blankets, electric shavers, metal detectors, television remote controls, electric toothbrushes, ham or CB radios, computers, acupuncture, laser surgery, dental drills and ultrasonic scaling, electroconvulsive therapy (ECT) and diagnostic x-rays.

Other precautions

Cardioversion and defibrillation

Pacemaker damage can be prevented if the elecrodes are at least 15 cm from the generator and preferably are positioned so they are at right angles to the pacing system. Pacemaker function should be checked after the procedure.

Lithotripsy

Shocks should not be focused directly over the pacemaker. The pacemaker should be programmed to non-rate-responsive VVI mode.

Driving

In the United Kingdom, driving must cease if a patient has sinoatrial disease or AV block and the arrhythmia has caused or is likely to cause incapacity. Patients may resume driving ordinary motor cars and motor cycles one week after implantation of a pacemaker or generator change provided there is no other disqualifying condition.

Heavy goods and public service vehicle drivers are disqualified from driving for six weeks after pacemaker implantation. Licensing may be permitted thereafter provided there is no other disqualifying condition.

Diving

The increased hydrostatic pressure under water can compress pacemaker cans and cause device failure. Many pacemakers are affected at depths of 11 m. Manufacturer's advice should be sought.

Cremation

A pacemaker must be explanted before cremation to avoid explosion, which might well lead to structural damage. Relevant staff need to be aware that occasionally the patient will have more than one pulse generator *in situ*, and occasionally generators migrate to unusual locations!

Temporary cardiac pacing

The transvenous route is usually used for temporary pacing but, in emergencies, a transcutaneous approach is a possible short-term alternative.

Temporary transvenous pacing is a simple procedure. However, complications are common because circumstances are such that it is often carried out by inexperienced, unsupervised operators. The need for temporary transvenous pacing should be carefully considered before proceeding.

Indications
Myocardial infarction
1. Second- and third-degree AV block due to acute anterior myocardial infarction.
2. Second- and third-degree AV block caused by acute inferior infarction only when complicated by hypotension, ventricular tachyarrhythmia or a ventricular rate less than 40 beats/min.
3. Symptomatic sinus arrest or junctional bradycardia due to acute myocardial infarction.

Chronic conduction tissue disease
Temporary pacing may be necessary as a first measure in patients with recent syncope caused by chronic disease of the sinus node or AV junction who are to be referred for long-term pacing. Patients with infrequent bradycardias should not receive a temporary pacemaker while awaiting implantation of a long-term pacemaker.

Tachycardias
Pacing is useful in terminating AV re-entrant tachycardia, atrial flutter and ventricular tachycardia. In the bradycardia–tachycardia syndrome temporary pacing should be used to cover cardioversion if required for the termination of supraventricular arrhythmias.

Methods
The method for insertion of a temporary ventricular pacing lead is similar to that for long-term pacing as described above but there is no stylet in a temporary pacing lead and a peel-away sheath is not required. The electrode is connected to an external battery-powered pulse generator.

An alternative to pacing via the subclavian vein is femoral vein puncture. This method is very easy and quick, provided that pulsation of the adjacent femoral artery is easily palpable. However, it should be reserved for short-term emergency purposes because electrode stability is poor and there is a risk of venous thrombosis. The femoral vein is *medial* to the femoral artery. Pressure on the abdomen causes distension of the femoral vein and makes venepuncture much easier.

Pacing
When a stable electrode position has been achieved, the distal and proximal poles of the electrode should be connected to the pacemaker cathode (–) and anode (+), respectively. If the poles are reversed, the stimulation threshold will be substantially higher.

The pacing threshold should then be measured. It should be less than 1.0 V, assuming the pulse generator delivers impulses whose duration is 1 or 2 ms. Some

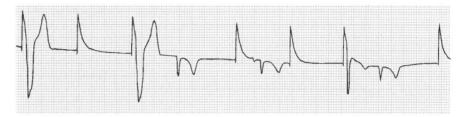

Figure 23.31 Intermittent failure to pace (lead II). Only the first and third pacing stimuli capture the ventricles.

temporary pacemakers allow adjustment of the pulse width: shorter pulse durations lead to a higher threshold and are not indicated for temporary pacing. Sometimes, in an emergency, a pacing threshold or electrode position which is less than optimal has to be accepted. Occasionally a patient may become dependent on the pacemaker, making adjustment of the electrode position risky. In these circumstances it may be necessary to insert a second pacing electrode (e.g. via the femoral vein) to cover the period of repositioning.

To avoid lead displacement, it is essential to *securely* suture the electrode to the skin at its point of entry. The pacing threshold often rises to 2–3 V during the first few days after electrode insertion. The threshold should be checked *daily* and the output set to at least twice the measured threshold. Battery and electrical connections should also be checked daily. *It is surprising how often the connections between pacemaker and pacing lead, on which a patient's life may depend, are found to be loose or insecure!*

Pacing complications
Electrode displacement
Electrode displacement may cause intermittent or complete failure to pace (Figure 23.31). The electrode may fall back into the right atrial cavity and lead to atrial rather than ventricular pacing.

Myocardial perforation
Temporary pacing leads are rather stiff, and occasionally the electrode tip may perforate the thin right ventricular myocardium. Failure to pace, diaphragmatic stimulation, pericardial friction rub and pericardial pain may result. Cardiac tamponade is rare.

Exit block
Sometimes pacing failure occurs without electrode tip displacement or other cause. In these cases failure is attributed to 'exit block', which is caused by excessive tissue reaction at the junction between electrode tip and endocardium.

Electrical fracture
A break in the electrical connection or in the electrode itself can be the cause of intermittent or complete pacing failure. In contrast to exit block, no pacing stimuli will appear on the ECG.

Inappropriate inhibition
External inhibition of a demand pacemaker from electromagnetic waves being emitted from electrical equipment can occasionally inhibit a pacemaker and will result in absent pacing stimuli. This problem can be quickly solved by changing the pacemaker to fixed-rate mode.

Failure to sense
Pacemakers are most often used in the demand mode, whereby the pacemaker senses spontaneous cardiac activity and only discharges a stimulus if a spontaneous beat has

not occurred within a pre-set period. In some patients, those with myocardial infarction, the signal generated by spontaneous activity may be too small for the pacemaker to sense. As a result, the pacemaker will function in a fixed-rate mode and pacing stimuli will be discharged at inappropriate times, and may fall on the T wave of a spontaneous beat This is undesirable in acute myocardial infarction because of the risk of precipitating ventricular fibrillation (Figure 23.3b).

Infection

Infection can occur at the site of entry of a transvenous pacing electrode. Bacteraemia can result in serious infection, often staphylococcal. If there is valve disease, endocarditis could develop. Infection will not clear unless the pacing lead is removed.

Temporary pacing leads should be removed as soon as it is possible to do so in order to minimise the risk of infection.

Temporary transcutaneous and oesophageal pacing

Transcutaneous cardiac pacing was first attempted many years ago but was usually unsuccessful and caused severe discomfort due to skeletal muscle stimulation. Recently, considerable success with less discomfort has been achieved by using large-surface-area skin electrodes and stimuli of much longer duration than are used for endocardial stimulation (20–40 ms).

The latest generation of transcutaneous pacemakers function in the demand mode and have a maximum output in the region of 150 mA. One electrode is applied to the front of the chest and the other to the back over the right scapula. Pacing is likely to stimulate the atria at the same time as the ventricles. It is not always possible to ascertain from the ECG that the heart is being stimulated: monitoring of an arterial pulse may be necessary.

With oesophageal pacing, long impulse duration is necessary (10 ms). Atrial stimulation is more successful than ventricular stimulation.

As with transvenous pacing, transcutaneous and oesophageal pacing are unlikely to be successful after a prolonged period of cardiac arrest.

The implantable cardioverter defibrillator (ICD) can automatically terminate ventricular tachycardia or fibrillation by delivering an appropriate therapy: either a train of rapid ventricular pacing stimuli or a DC shock. The device can also act as a pacemaker. Indications are considered in terms of primary and secondary prevention.

Primary prevention is for conditions associated with a high risk of death from ventricular tachycardia or fibrillation when these arrhythmias have not yet occurred, e.g. poor left ventricular function caused by myocardial infarction or by cardiomyopathy, or cardiac conditions which carry a high risk of sudden death, including the hereditary long QT syndromes and hypertrophic cardiomyopathy.

Secondary prevention is therapy for patients who have experienced cardiac arrest, syncope or shock due to a ventricular tachyarrhythmia not caused by a reversible condition or within six weeks of myocardial infarction, or who have had ventricular tachycardia and have a left ventricular ejection fraction $\leq 35\%$.

Possible complications include infection, inappropriate shock delivery, psychological distress, and lead and device malfunction.

The implantable cardioverter defibrillator (ICD) is a device that can recognise and automatically terminate ventricular tachycardia or fibrillation by delivering an appropriate electrical therapy.

The therapies are:

1. Brief, rapid train(s) of ventricular pacing stimuli to terminate ventricular tachycardia (see Figures 12.7, 24.6).

2. Low-energy (0.5–10J) DC shock to terminate ventricular tachycardia, i.e. cardioversion (Figure 24.1).

3. Higher-energy (10–35J) DC shock to terminate ventricular tachycardia or fibrillation (Figure 24.2).

In addition, the device can act as a pacemaker to prevent bradycardia and to provide a chronotropic response to exercise.

Bennett's Cardiac Arrhythmias: Practical Notes on Interpretation and Treatment, Eighth Edition. David H. Bennett.
© 2013 John Wiley & Sons, Ltd. Published 2013 by John Wiley & Sons, Ltd.

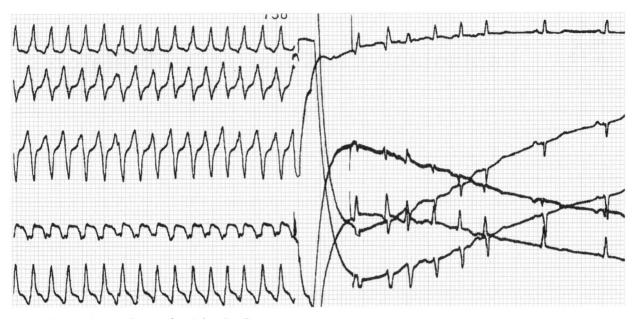

Figure 24.1 Transvenous cardioversion of ventricular tachycardia.

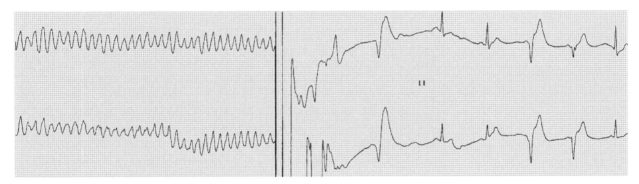

Figure 24.2 Termination of ventricular fibrillation by an ICD.

The first defibrillator was implanted in 1980. Early devices were very large, necessitating implantation abdominally in the rectus sheath, and employed epicardial leads.

Current devices are somewhat larger than a pacemaker and are usually implanted subcutaneously over pectoralis major (in thin patients the device can be implanted beneath the pectoral muscle). Therapy is delivered via a right ventricular lead introduced via the cephalic or subclavian vein. Like a pacing lead, there is an electrode at its tip for pacing and sensing. Just proximal to the tip is a coil that acts as the cathode so a DC shock can be delivered between it and the device case or 'can', which is the anode. 'With 'dual-coil' leads there is an additional coil located a few centimetres more proximally so that it lies in the superior vena cava. It also acts as an anode together with the can. In theory, a dual-coil lead may enable lower energy requirements for shock delivery, but most studies show no significant advantage of dual-coil as compared with single-coil leads.

In patients without persistent atrial fibrillation, dual-chamber systems are often employed, requiring the addition of an atrial pacing lead. Dual-chamber devices provide the same benefits as dual-chamber pacemakers for the management of bradycardia. Additionally, atrial sensing enables better discrimination between supraventricular and ventricular arrhythmias.

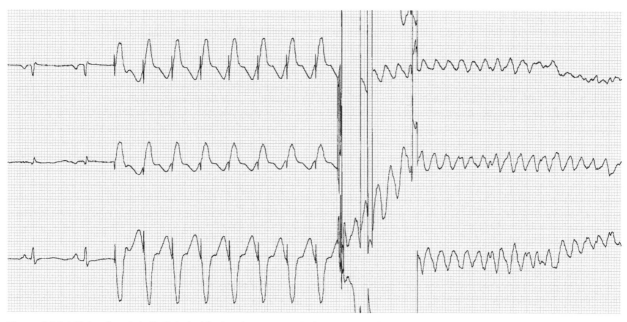

Figure 24.3 Initiation of ventricular fibrillation by delivering a low-energy DC shock on the T wave of the eighth paced beat.

Defibrillator implantation

The implantation procedure for a transvenous system is similar to that for a pacemaker and is usually carried out under local anaesthesia. The risks of complication are the same as for pacemaker implantation. Infection and hematoma are the commonest: these are also not infrequently encountered at ICD generator replacement.

Defibrillation threshold

Routine practice was to ensure that the device could terminate ventricular fibrillation by measuring the defibrillation threshold (DFT): after hefty intravenous sedation, ventricular fibrillation was initiated by delivering via the implanted device a DC shock coincident with the T wave (Figure 24.3), or by a burst of alternating current (50 or 60 Hz), or by a brief, very rapid train of ventricular stimuli. It was desirable to establish that an output at least 10 J less than the device's maximum output, which is in the region of 35 J, was effective. Usually, the initial output would be set to 18 J. The device was programmed to deliver a 24 J shock if the first one failed: if the second shock failed, immediate external defibrillation would be carried out. It was interesting that sometimes ventricular fibrillation terminated spontaneously while the device was charging! If a high DFT was encountered then sometimes programming reversal of polarity such that the distal coil acted as the anode could lead to a lower DFT; otherwise lead repositioning was required.

However, with modern devices the DFT is almost always found to be satisfactory, and studies have shown the DFT not to be a predictor of long-term survival. Furthermore, there are risks in DFT measurement. If in atrial fibrillation, defibrillation might restore sinus rhythm and lead to left atrial thrombus dislodgement. Occasionally, prolonged resuscitation may be needed and very occasionally it might not be successful. The argument against routine DFT testing is greater in patients receiving a device for primary prevention (see below), in that risks have to be weighed against the possibility that ventricular fibrillation might never spontaneously occur. Many centres do not now routinely measure the DFT. Testing should, however, be carried out in patients with hypertrophic cardiomyopathy, where high DFTs are often encountered.

Subcutaneous ICD

Recently, an entirely subcutaneous ICD system has been introduced which obviates the challenges of venous access and complications associated with transvenous leads. It consists of a lead that has a shocking coil and sensing electrodes positioned subcutaneously parallel to the left edge of the sternum together with a pulse generator implanted subcutaneously in the region of the left anterior axillary line. It is suitable for patients at risk of sudden death who do not have indications for cardiac pacing.

Indications for ICD implanation

Indications are considered in terms of primary and secondary prevention. Primary prevention is therapy for patients who are at high risk of death from ventricular tachycardia or fibrillation who have *not yet* sustained these arrhythmias. Secondary prevention is therapy to deal with patients who have experienced ventricular tachycardia or fibrillation.

UK guidelines (National Institute for Health and Clinical Excellence)
Secondary prevention

> An implantable defibrillator should be considered for patients who present with the following, provided the arrhythmia is not due to acute myocardial infarction and there is no correctable cause:
> (1) Survivors of sudden cardiac death caused by ventricular fibrillation or tachycardia
> (2) Spontaneous sustained ventricular tachycardia causing syncope or significant haemodynamic compromise
> (3) Sustained ventricular tachycardia without syncope or cardiac arrest in patients who have a left ventricular ejection fraction <35% but are no worse than class III of the New York Heart Association functional classification of heart failure

Several major clinical trials have demonstrated that in the above groups of patients, an ICD reduces mortality as compared with antiarrhythmic drug therapy. Overall, these studies have shown a reduction in death due to cardiac causes of approximately 50% and a reduction in 'all-cause mortality' of approximately 24%. A survey has shown that over a three-year period one life is saved for every 4–5 defibrillators implanted.

Primary prevention

> Defibrillator implantation should be considered for patients with:
> (1) Previous myocardial infarction (more than four weeks) with symptoms no worse than class III of the New York Heart Association and
> All of the following:
>   (i) Non-sustained ventricular tachycardia on ambulatory electrocardiography
>   (ii) Inducible ventricular tachycardia at electrophysiological testing
>   (iii) Left ventricular ejection fraction <35%
> Or:
> Left ventricular ejection fraction <30% and QRS duration ≥120 ms

These recommendations are based on studies that have shown that mortality in patients with the above characteristics is reduced by an ICD as compared with antiarrhythmic drug therapy, mainly amiodarone.

(2) A cardiac condition in which it is recognised that the patient is at high risk of sudden death, including:
(i) Long QT syndrome
(ii) Hypertrophic cardiomyopathy
(iii) Brugada syndrome
(iv) Arrhythmogenic right ventricular cardiomyopathy
(v) Following surgical repair of congenital heart disease

The main indicators of high risk in conditions (i)–(iv) are discussed in chapters 12 and 13. Following repair of Fallot's tetralogy, prolonged QRS duration and ventricular dysfunction have been reported to be predictors of sudden death.

Further indications for primary prevention relevant to UK guidelines

Three recent studies have shown that in patients with poor left ventricular function (ejection fraction < 35%), whether due to coronary artery disease or to cardiomyopathy, and New York Heart Association class II or III heart failure, prognosis can be improved by ICD implantation even without there being non-sustained ventricular tachycardia or a positive ventricular stimulation study.

Analysis of these studies has shown that a policy of ICD implantation in patients with poor ventricular function will prolong life, on average, by 2–6 years and is 'cost-effective'. These studies have also clearly shown that antiarrhythmic therapy, mainly amiodarone, though it may reduce the incidence of ventricular arrhythmia, does not improve prognosis.

Recent myocardial infarction

In the studies referred to above, patients who had recently sustained a myocardial infarction were excluded. A study of patients early after myocardial infarction with an ejection fraction < 35% and indicators of higher risk of ventricular arrhythmia failed to show that ICD implantation within six weeks of acute myocardial infarction improved prognosis.

American College of Cardiology and American Heart Association guidelines

The main (i.e. class I) guidelines are:

ICD therapy is indicated in patients (class I indications):
(1) Who are survivors of cardiac arrest due to VF or haemodynamically unstable sustained VT after evaluation to define the cause of the event and to exclude any completely reversible causes.
(2) With structural heart disease and spontaneous sustained VT, whether haemodynamically stable or unstable.
(3) With syncope of undetermined origin with clinically relevant, haemodynamically significant sustained VT or VF induced at electrophysiological study.
(4) With LVEF (left ventricular ejection fraction) ≤ 35% due to prior MI who are at least 40 days post-MI and are in NYHA (New York Heart Association) functional class II or III.
(5) With non-ischaemic dilated cardiomyopathy who have an LVEF ≤ 35% and who are in NYHA functional class II or III.
(6) With LV dysfunction due to prior MI who are at least 40 days post-MI, have an LVEF ≤ 30%, and are in NYHA functional class I.
(7) With non-sustained VT due to prior MI, LVEF ≤ 40%, and inducible VF or sustained VT at electrophysiological study.

Reservations concerning defibrillator implantation for primary prevention

Before applying the conclusions from clinical trials to the individual, one has to discuss with the patient the negative aspects of defibrillator implantation as well as the significant benefits.

Disadvantages include the acute and long-term complications of ICD implantation, the possibility of inappropriate shock delivery, possible psychological effects and also motor vehicle driving restrictions (see below).

The patient needs to understand that though clinical trials have shown a significant prognostic benefit with ICD implantation, only approximately one in 11 recipients is going to receive lifesaving therapy from their device within the first three years of implantation. A recent review over an eight-year follow-up period found the number of patients need to be treated to save one life was eight.

With increasing age, patients are progressively more susceptible to non-cardiac diseases that may shorten life such as stroke and cancer. Thus, the elderly patient with poor ventricular function may be less likely to benefit in terms of life expectancy. Recently it has been shown that patients with 3 or more factors i.e. Age >70 years, NYHA class >II, blood urea >26mg/dl, QRS duration >120ms and atrial fibrillation were unlikely to benefit from primary ICD therapy.

Defibrillator function

Arrhythmia recording

Intra-atrial and intraventricular ECGs prior to and immediately after the device has delivered therapy can be recorded and stored. Thus it is possible to ensure that appropriate therapy was initiated and that the device had not responded to a supraventricular tachycardia (Figures 24.4, 24.5). The device can store data indicating the number of episodes of arrhythmia that have occurred, and the number of therapies that have been delivered and whether they were successful or not.

Tiered therapy

Ventricular tachycardias can often be terminated by 'antitachycardia pacing', i.e. 6–12 ventricular stimuli in rapid succession. Ventricular fibrillation can only be terminated by a high-energy shock. The advantages of terminating ventricular tachycardia by antitachycardia pacing are that it is painless and battery energy is conserved. However, antitachycardia pacing is not always effective and may sometimes accelerate the tachycardia such that shock delivery is required.

Detection of ventricular tachycardia and fibrillation is based primarily on the rate and duration of events sensed via the right ventricular lead. Other criteria such as rate stability, sudden onset of tachycardia and relation between sensed atrial and ventricular activity can be used to help distinguish between supraventricular and ventricular tachycardia.

Rate criteria are used to place the arrhythmia in one of three zones:

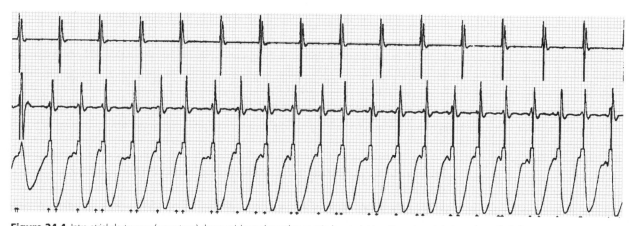

Figure 24.4 Intra-atrial electrogram (upper trace) shows atrial rate slower than ventricular rate (mid and lower traces) during tachycardia, indicating ventricular origin.

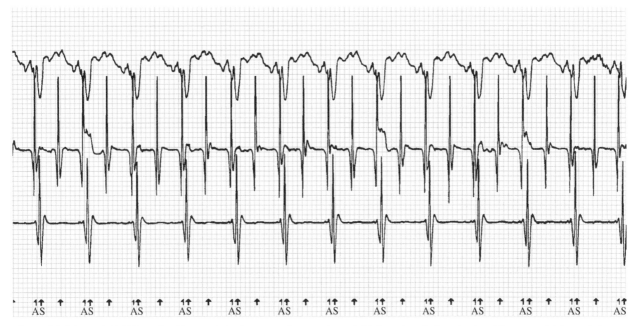

Figure 24.5 Intra-atrial (middle trace) and intraventricular electrograms (lower trace) recorded during tachycardia show that the atrial rate exceeded the ventricular rate, indicating an atrial arrhythmia.

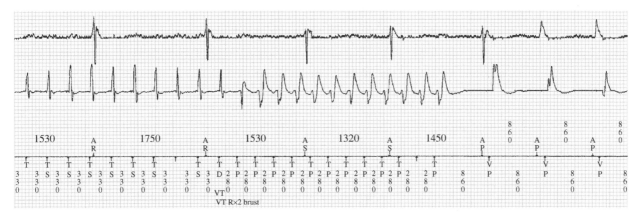

Figure 24.6 Lower electrogram shows ventricular tachycardia with a cycle length of 330 ms interrupted by a train of ventricular stimuli at a cycle length of 280 ms. Upper electrogram shows independent atrial activity during tachycardia.

Slow ventricular tachycardia zone

Ventricular tachycardia at a rate of 130–170 beats/min is termed 'slow'. There is a good chance that antitachycardia pacing will be effective (Figure 24.6).

Either 'burst' or 'ramp' pacing can be used. With the former, the interval between stimuli is constant, whereas with the latter, the interval between successive stimuli is decreased by approximately 8–10 ms. For most patients, burst and ramp pacing are in fact equally effective. Initial attempts at pacing typically employ a train of six impulses at 84% of the tachycardia cycle length. If ineffective, the device will then deliver more aggressive therapies, e.g. up to 12 impulses with shorter cycle lengths, 78–84% of tachycardia cycle length.

It is usual to program the device to attempt to terminate the tachycardia several times before proceeding to cardioversion. Though low-energy shocks (5–10 J) are effective they are as painful as high-energy shocks so most program the device to deliver a high-energy shock (35 J) if one is required.

It is important to ensure that the lower limit of the range of tachycardia detection does not overlap with a heart rate that the patient is likely to achieve during exertion when in sinus rhythm – otherwise the device will deliver therapy inappropriately.

Fast ventricular tachycardia zone

'Fast ventricular tachycardia' is usually defined as a rate between 170 and 200 beats/min. There is a moderate chance that it can be terminated by pacing but often little time can be allowed for pacing because it is likely that a tachycardia in this range will cause collapse. It is usual to program the device to attempt antitachycardia pacing up to four times. If unsuccessful the device will then proceed to deliver a shock (Figure 24.7).

Ventricular fibrillation zone

A rate in excess of 200 beats/min is assumed to be ventricular fibrillation. Electrograms during ventricular fibrillation are of low amplitude. To avoid failure to detect ventricular fibrillation, only a proportion of sensed electrograms are required to meet the rate criterion, e.g. 18/24. (Recently, an increase to 30/40 has been shown to reduce the incidence of inappropriate shocks). A high-energy shock (35 J) will be discharged after approximately 7–9 s (Figures 24.8, 24.9). If fibrillation is re-detected, further shocks will be delivered.

It has been shown that antitachycardia pacing may be effective even with very fast ventricular tachycardias. If within the ventricular fibrillation zone *each* cycle length is more than 240 ms, then ventricular tachycardia rather than fibrillation is diagnosed. A single burst of eight paced beats at 88% of the measured cycle length has been reported to terminate the arrhythmia in 80% of cases, thereby avoiding a painful DC shock. No time is wasted, in that the pacing therapy can be given while the device is charging.

Pacing mode

Choice of pacing mode is as for implanted pacemakers (Chapter 23). As with pacemakers, unnecessary ventricular pacing should be avoided to prevent right ventricular apical pacing causing heart failure. Where possible, DDIR pacing with a long AV delay should be employed.

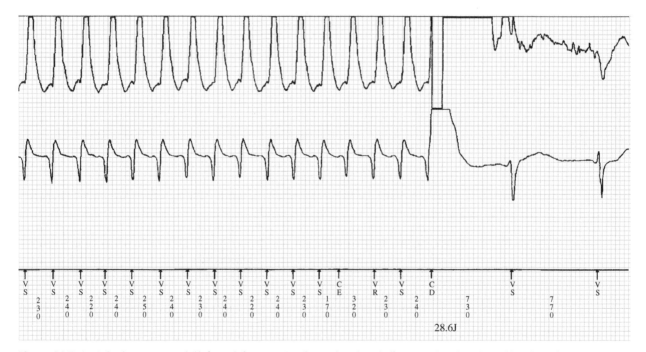

Figure 24.7 Ventricular electrograms recorded before and after termination of ventricular tachycardia (fast ventricular tachycardia zone) by delivery of a 28.6 J shock.

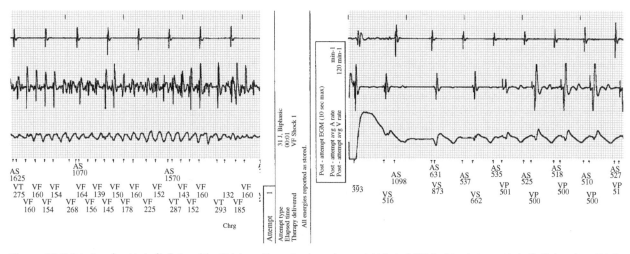

Figure 24.8 Detection of ventricular fibrillation while atrial channel (upper trace) records normal atrial rate. A 31 J shock terminates ventricular fibrillation, after which the device paces the ventricles to prevent bradycardia.

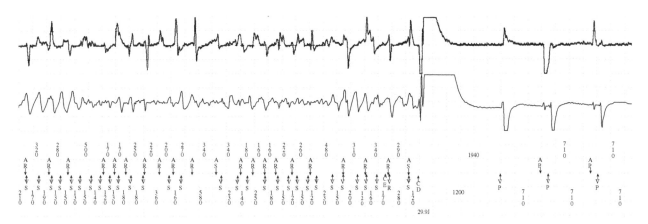

Figure 24.9 Delivery of 29 J shock terminates ventricular fibrillation (lower channel) and also fortuitously atrial fibrillation (upper channel).

Defibrillator clinic

Patients are usually seen every 3–6 months. Device function is checked and battery status measured in terms of battery voltage and capacitor charge time. Devices need to be replaced after 5–8 years.

Recently remote monitoring of ICD function has been developed so that ICD lead and battery function and heart rhythm can be monitored at home on a frequent basis, thereby reducing the need for clinic visits.

Audible alert alarms

Most devices can be programmed to deliver an audible alarm if lead impedance becomes abnormal (suggesting lead fracture or insulation breakdown) or if there is abnormal battery function. On hearing such an alarm, the patient should contact his or her cardiology centre. One manufacturer's device provides an alarm by periodically vibrating.

Limitations

The limitations of the implantable defibrillator should be appreciated.

Discharge of a DC shock in a conscious patient usually results in sudden, marked chest discomfort and may cause considerable distress! Patients describe experiencing sensations such as 'a blow to the chest' or 'a spasm making the whole body jump'. The device therefore is clearly not suitable for patients with frequently recurrent or incessant arrhythmias.

An ICD is often regarded as an alternative to antiarrhythmic drugs. However, to almost lose consciousness from ventricular fibrillation and then be defibrillated is not a pleasant experience. Ideally, the ICD should act as a 'backup' device. Often, antiarrhythmic drugs are required to minimise the frequency of ventricular arrhythmia (see below). Recently, it has been shown that, for whatever reason, patients receiving a shock, whether appropriate or inappropriate, have a poor prognosis.

Inappropriate discharges, which are often multiple, may occur in response to a rapid ventricular rate during atrial fibrillation or other supraventricular tachycardia, or as a result of lead malfunction. A recent study showed that 15% of patients received inappropriate therapy.

Many patients benefit psychologically from the peace of mind that the potentially lifesaving facility of an ICD offers, but some patients' mental well-being is adversely affected by the need for and reliance on an ICD. Patients who have received inappropriate or frequent shocks often dread further shocks and are psychologically disturbed as a consequence.

Device or lead malfunctions occur in a minority of patients. The rate is higher than is encountered with pacemakers.

Drug therapy in patients with defibrillators
Prognosis
There are a number of drugs that have been shown to improve prognosis in patients with poor ventricular function which clearly should, unless contraindicated, be prescribed whether or not an ICD has been implanted: beta-blockers, angiotensin-converting enzyme inhibitors, eplerenone and statins.

Arrhythmia reduction
Often, amiodarone, beta-blockers or sotalol are required to reduce the frequency of ventricular arrhythmias that might lead to shock delivery, or to prevent supraventricular arrhythmias.

These drugs, if not effective in preventing ventricular tachycardia, may prolong the cycle length and may therefore increase the chances of success with antitachycardia pacing. However, occasionally, antiarrhythmic drugs, especially amiodarone, may slow the rate during tachycardia such that it is below the device's detection rate and antitachycardia pacing is not delivered (Figure 24.10).

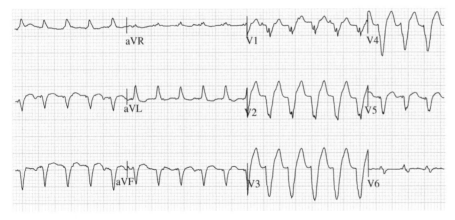

Figure 24.10 Symptomatic but relatively slow ventricular tachycardia (130 beats/min) which did not meet the ICD's detection criterion to initiate antitachycardia pacing.

Atrial arrhythmias

A very rapid ventricular response to atrial fibrillation and less commonly to atrial flutter and tachycardia can sometimes lead to inappropriate shock delivery (Figure 24.11). It is important to ensure that the ventricular rate is controlled by AV nodal blocking drugs. Sometimes these drugs are ineffective and catheter ablation of the atrioventricular (AV) node is required.

Defibrillation threshold

It should be noted that amiodarone may raise the defibrillation threshold and possibly render the device ineffective if the threshold was already high. Sotalol has been reported to reduce the defibrillation threshold. Other drugs that are reported to sometimes increase defibrillation threshold include lignocaine, mexiletine and flecainide.

Arrhythmia storms

Occasionally, patients experience periods when there are frequent episodes of ventricular arrhythmia necessitating defibrillation. Causes include hypokalaemia, worsening ventricular dysfunction, myocardial ischaemia and proarrhythmic drugs. Clearly, the cause should be dealt with if possible. Intravenous amiodarone, beta-blockers and occasionally mexiletine may be effective. Recently, ranolazine has been reported to be useful in arrhythmia storms.

A similar situation of frequent shock delivery, though not strictly an arrhythmia storm, can be precipitated by supraventricular arrhythmias, by sinus tachycardia due to hyperthyroidism (a possible consequence of amiodarone therapy) and by lead malfunction (Figure 24.12).

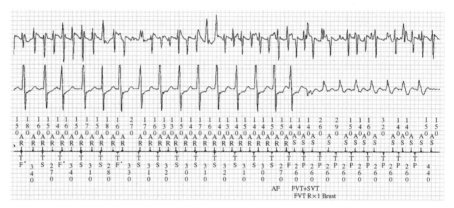

Figure 24.11 Intra-atrial (upper) and intraventricular (lower) electrograms demonstrating atrial fibrillation. The annotations at the bottom of the trace indicate that the rapid ventricular rate has led to an inappropriate diagnosis of ventricular tachycardia (TS) which initiated futile antitachycardia pacing (TP).

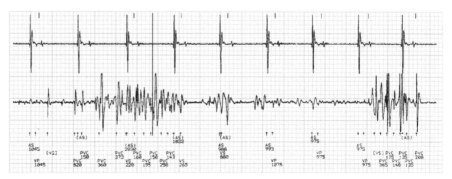

Figure 24.12 Electrical noise resulting from partial lead fracture registered on intraventricular electrogram (lower channel) that could lead to an incorrect diagnosis of ventricular tachycardia or fibrillation.

Minimising shock delivery

Shock delivery is unpleasant, can have psychological effects, increases battery drain and may disbar the patient from motor vehicle driving for up to two years. Measures should be taken, therefore, to avoid the patient receiving inappropriate or unnecessary shocks.

The commonest cause of an inappropriate shock is a fast ventricular response to atrial fibrillation. If the patient is or has been in atrial fibrillation, AV nodal blocking therapy (a beta-blocker or diltiazem) should be prescribed. If necessary, AV nodal ablation should be performed.

In some conditions such as the Brugada and long QT syndromes, monomorphic ventricular tachycardia requiring antitachycardia pacing is unlikely. The device should therefore be programmed not to provide antitachycardia pacing and only to deliver therapy in the ventricular fibrillation zone.

In patients with ischaemic ventricular damage or cardiomyopathy, consideration should be given to not delivering therapy in the slow ventricular tachycardia zone since it may accelerate the tachycardia and lead to shock delivery, whereas a relatively slow ventricular tachycardia is often well tolerated and may spontaneously stop. If therapy is programmed for this zone, there should be a long detection period before therapy is initiated – again because the arrhythmia may terminate spontaneously.

Sometimes, the T wave is of sufficiently large amplitude, or in the long QT syndrome relatively late, such that it is recognised as a separate ventricular complex and hence 'double-counting' occurs, resulting in inappropriate tachycardia diagnosis. Reduction of ventricular sensitivity and increasing the ventricular blanking period should obviate these problems.

Loose setscrews and partial lead fracture should be borne in mind as causes of inappropriate shocks.

ICD replacement

The batteries of ICD generators last 5–8 years, at which time generator replacement is clearly indicated provided the patient's overall medical condition has not changed significantly, and particularly if the ICD has delivered live-saving therapy.

However, some patients may have developed conditions such as dementia, cancer, renal and cardiac failure that will have a major impact on the patient's quantity and quality of life. Furthermore, there will be some ageing patients who had an ICD implanted for primary prevention purposes but who have not received appropriate therapy yet have been unfortunate enough to have experienced one or more ICD complications such as infection or inappropriate shock. In these circumstances, a patient may prefer not to have his or her ICD replaced. It is therefore important for a patient's medical condition to be assessed when battery depletion approaches and, where appropriate, for an informed discussion to take place regarding the benefits of ICD replacement rather than proceeding automatically to generator replacement.

Deactivation of device

Occasionally it is necessary to deactivate an ICD, either because it is delivering inappropriate shocks or because a patient has become terminally ill and resuscitation is no longer appropriate. The device can be deactivated using an external programmer. If not available, *deactivation can be achieved by placing a magnet over the generator and taping it in place*: the device will no longer deliver shocks or antitachycardia pacing but its pacemaker functions will continue.

Below are the recommendations of the UK Arrhythmia Alliance and British Heart Foundation with regard to patients with ICDs who are reaching the end of life:
• Health professionals working with dying patients should be made aware of the increasing number of patients who have an ICD implanted, particularly for the treatment of heart failure.

• Health professionals have a responsibility to ensure that the function of the ICD is optimised in the best interests of the patient, particularly for those close to the point of death.

• Open, sensitive communication with patients and their families is essential to ensure that their expectations are realistic and are compatible with the perceptions of the medical and nursing staff supervising their care.

• There should be close collaboration among medical staff, nursing staff and cardiac physiologists to facilitate timely device management in all care settings. Formal links with electrophysiologists and ICD/arrhythmia nurse specialists may be an advantage.

Hardware costs

In the United Kingdom, implantation costs are in the region of £16 000.

Precautions

ICDs are subject to electromagnetic interference in the same way as pacemakers are, as discussed in Chapter 23.

Clothing and accessories containing magnets should not be worn. An ICD should be inactivated during implantation or removal, otherwise the operator may possibly receive an electric shock. Like a pacemaker, an ICD must be removed before cremation. It is important that it is deactivated prior to removal.

People should be reassured that they will not be harmed if they touch a patient during shock delivery.

During surgery, an ICD should have its antitachycardia and shock functions temporarily deactivated by programming or by application of a magnet if surgical diathermy is to be used.

Driving

Discharge of an ICD during motor vehicle driving will at the very least cause distraction and will probably result in temporary incapacity. It might save the driver's life but could endanger others' lives. Furthermore, the device might be triggered to discharge therapy by ventricular arrhythmias that would not have otherwise caused collapse, and inappropriate discharge might result from supraventricular tachycardia or technical failure such as lead fracture.

Approaches to licensing drivers vary from country to country. The somewhat complex United Kingdom regulations, which have recently been revised, can be downloaded from www.dft.gov.uk/dvla/medical/ataglance.aspx, and the European guidelines can be found at http://europace.oxfordjournals.org/content/11/8/1097.full.pdf. The table summarises these UK and European guidelines.

Length of time for which a patient should not drive after common ICD events: UK guidelines (corresponding European guideline periods in brackets)

ICD implantation for secondary prevention: 6/12 *(3/12)*
ICD implantation for primary prevention: 1/12 *(4/52)*
Shock therapy or antitachycardia pacing (ATP) associated with incapacity where no measures to prevent recurrence undertaken: 2 years *(3/12)*
Shock therapy or ATP associated with incapacity after steps to prevent recurrence undertaken 6/12 *(3/12)*
Shock therapy or ATP associated with incapacity resulting from inappropriate shock, after appropriate measures undertaken 1/12 *(0/52)*
Shock therapy or ATP without incapacity 1/12 *(3/12)*
ICD generator change 1/52 *(1/52)*
Lead revision 1/12 *(4/52)*
Professional/vocational driving: permanent disbarment (permanent disbarment)

25

Catheter Ablation

Radiofrequency catheter ablation is a first-line treatment for supraventricular arrhythmias and for some ventricular tachycardias.

Atrioventricular (AV) nodal tachycardia is characterised by a very short ventriculoatrial conduction time: ablation of the AV nodal slow pathway is achieved by delivery of radiofrequency energy to a site close to the mouth of the coronary sinus. An accessory pathway, the cause of Wolff–Parkinson–White syndrome, is located by seeking the earliest site of ventricular activation during sinus rhythm or the earliest site of atrial activation during re-entrant tachycardia.

Pulmonary vein isolation techniques are effective at preventing paroxysmal atrial fibrillation. Atrial flutter is treated by ablating the isthmus of the right atrial re-entrant circuit that is located between the tricuspid valve and inferior vena cava. AV nodal ablation is effective in atrial arrhythmias that cannot be controlled: it necessitates pacemaker implantation.

Fascicular and right ventricular outflow tract ventricular tachycardias can be cured by ablation.

Radiofrequency catheter ablation has transformed the treatment of many rhythm disturbances, especially those of supraventricular origin. For many common arrhythmias it is not just another therapeutic option but first-line treatment, offering a cure and obviating the need for antiarrhythmic drugs. Success rates well over 90% are being widely achieved at very low risk. The purpose of this chapter is to illustrate briefly some of the main applications of catheter ablation and to provide an understanding, for those who refer patients for ablation, as to how sites for ablation are targeted.

Procedure

The procedure is usually carried out under local anaesthesia with intravenous sedation. The sequence of cardiac activation during normal and abnormal rhythms is studied by recording electrograms from various intracardiac sites using multipolar catheter electrodes introduced via percutaneous puncture of the femoral vein and, if necessary, the femoral artery. The electrodes also facilitate introduction of pacing stimuli that can initiate and terminate tachycardias.

Bennett's Cardiac Arrhythmias: Practical Notes on Interpretation and Treatment, Eighth Edition. David H. Bennett.
© 2013 John Wiley & Sons, Ltd. Published 2013 by John Wiley & Sons, Ltd.

Mapping the sequence of activation during normal, paced rhythms, and during tachycardia, enables location of the re-entrant circuit or focus causing the arrhythmia. Radiofrequency energy, which is high-frequency alternating current, is delivered via a special catheter electrode. This has a deflectable end, enabling the tip to be precisely positioned at the target site. Radiofrequency energy is delivered for 30–120 s. The endocardium in contact with the tip and the myocardium beneath is heated to 50–70 °C and is thereby coagulated. Surrounding myocardium is not damaged. Radiofrequency energy delivery via an electrode irrigated with saline can result in a larger, deeper lesion by preventing coagulum developing at the catheter tip and is useful in difficult cases and in ablation for atrial flutter.

Cryothermy is being evaluated as an alternative energy source.

Normal sinus rhythm

Figure 25.1 shows typical findings during normal sinus rhythm. Recordings are made at a paper speed of at least 100 mm/s. Below the six surface ECG leads are recordings from three intracardiac sites: high right atrium, tricuspid valve and the coronary sinus.

High right atrial electrogram

An electrode positioned in the high right atrium is close to the sinus node. It records the earliest atrial activity during each cardiac cycle. It coincides with the onset of the P wave seen on the surface ECG.

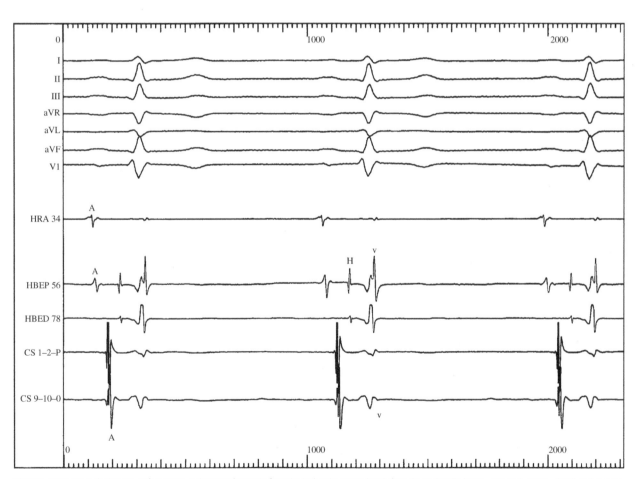

Figure 25.1 Sinus rhythm. Six surface ECGs, and intracardiac ECGs from the high right atrium (HRA), from the His bundle (HBEP = proximal, HBED = distal) and coronary sinus (CS P = proximal, CS D = distal). A, H and V = atrial, His bundle and ventricular electrograms, respectively).

His bundle electrogram

The His bundle electrogram is recorded by positioning an electrode across the tricuspid valve. Three waves can be seen:

- The A wave due to activation of the adjacent low right atrium.
- The H wave: the electrogram resulting from activation of the His bundle. The interval between A and H waves indicates the conduction time through the AV node.
- The V wave, which is the ventricular electrogram. It corresponds to the QRS complex on the surface ECG. The HV interval indicates the time of transmission by the His bundle and bundle branches from the AV node to the ventricular myocardium. It is normally 35–55 ms. Often, as in Figure 25.1, electrograms are recorded from two pairs of electrodes on the multipolar catheter across the tricuspid valve so that proximal and distal His bundle electrograms can be obtained.

Figure 25.2 shows a markedly prolonged HV interval in a patient with bifascicular block.

Coronary sinus electrograms

The coronary sinus runs in the groove between the left atrium and left ventricle. Activity from both left atrium and left ventricle can be recorded.

In Figure 25.1, a large left atrial electrogram can be seen, which is followed by a smaller wave resulting from left ventricular activity.

Mapping

Figure 25.1 provides a simple example of how the path of an activating impulse can be 'mapped'. During normal sinus rhythm, it shows how the atrial impulse originates in the high right atrium (i.e. close to the sinus node), passes to the low right atrium, near

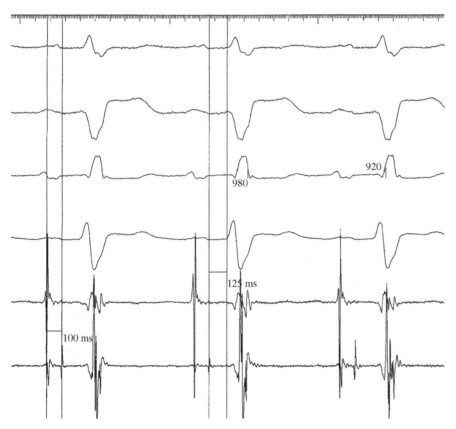

Figure 25.2 Surface leads I, II, V1 and V6 together with a bundle of His electrogram (bottom trace) in a patient with bifascicular block and a long PR interval. The AH interval (100 ms) is normal but the HV interval (125 ms) is markedly prolonged.

to the AV node, and then to the left atrium as recorded by the coronary sinus electrodes. Following atrial activation, His bundle and then ventricular activation occur.

Wolff–Parkinson–White syndrome

An accessory pathway is located by identifying the site of *earliest* ventricular activation during sinus rhythm, for that must be the site where the accessory pathway connects with ventricular myocardium. An electrogram at this site will precede the onset of the delta wave in the surface ECG (Figure 25.3). Sometimes, it is possible to actually demonstrate an accessory pathway potential (Figure 25.4).

Figure 25.5 shows how the surface ECG and electrogram at the site of radiofrequency delivery change as the accessory pathway is ablated by radiofrequency energy.

Left-sided pathways are ablated by introducing a catheter into the left ventricle via the femoral artery (Figure 25.6) or by transseptal puncture via the femoral vein, and positioning its tip across the mitral valve ring. Free right wall accessory pathways are ablated by introducing a catheter from the femoral vein and positioning across the tricuspid valve ring. Posteroseptal and anteroseptal pathways are also ablated by a

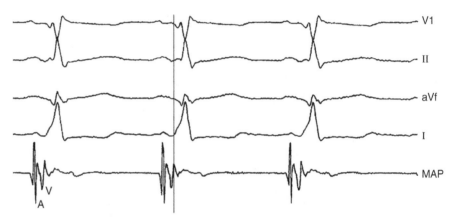

Figure 25.3 Wolff–Parkinson–White syndrome. The vertical line marks the onset of the delta wave on the surface ECG. The tip of the mapping electrode has been positioned at the site of successful ablation. Both A and V waves can be seen in the mapping electrogram. The V wave precedes the onset of the surface ECG delta wave by 25 ms.

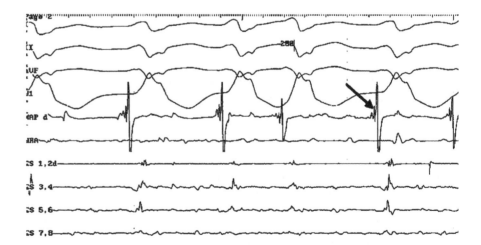

Figure 25.4 Wolff–Parkinson–White syndrome during atrial fibrillation. Surface leads I, II, AVF and V1. The arrow indicates a potential arising from an accessory pathway, recorded via the mapping electrode, which precedes the onset of the delta wave on the surface ECG.

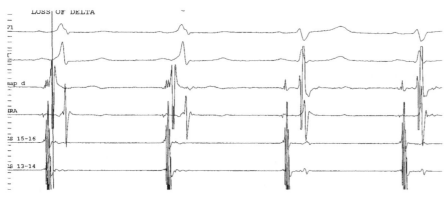

Figure 25.5 Wolff–Parkinson–White syndrome. The electrogram from the mapping electrode can be seen beneath two surface ECGs. The vertical line demonstrates that before ablation, ventricular activity recorded by the mapping electrode precedes the onset of the surface ECG delta wave. Radiofrequency energy is delivered after the first two beats and interrupts accessory pathway conduction. After ablation, the delta wave disappears and ventricular activity in the mapping electrogram succeeds rather than precedes the surface ECG QRS complex.

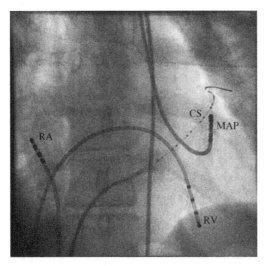

Figure 25.6 Ablation of left-sided accessory pathway. Electrodes are positioned in the right atrium (RA) and right ventricle (RV). There is a multipolar electrode in the coronary sinus (CS). The mapping electrode (MAP) has been introduced via the femoral artery, passed through the aortic valve and positioned across the mitral valve ring.

catheter in the right ventricle. Posteroseptal pathways are found near the mouth of the coronary sinus. Anteroseptal pathways are located close to the bundle of His.

There is a risk (1–4%) that anteroseptal and, to a lesser extent, posteroseptal accessory pathway ablation might cause complete heart block and the need for long-term pacing.

Sometimes, 'T wave memory' following successful posteroseptal ablation causes unnecessary concern (Figure 25.7).

Concealed accessory pathways

A concealed accessory pathway can transmit impulses from ventricles to atria and therefore facilitate AV junctional re-entrant tachycardia, but cannot conduct from atria to ventricles and thus there will be no delta wave during sinus rhythm.

Concealed pathways have to be located during AV re-entrant tachycardia (AVRT) or ventricular pacing. The site of earliest *atrial* activation will indicate the location of the accessory pathway.

For example, in Figure 25.8 electrograms are recorded from a multipolar electrode in the coronary sinus during AVRT. Earliest atrial activity is found in the mid coronary

(a)

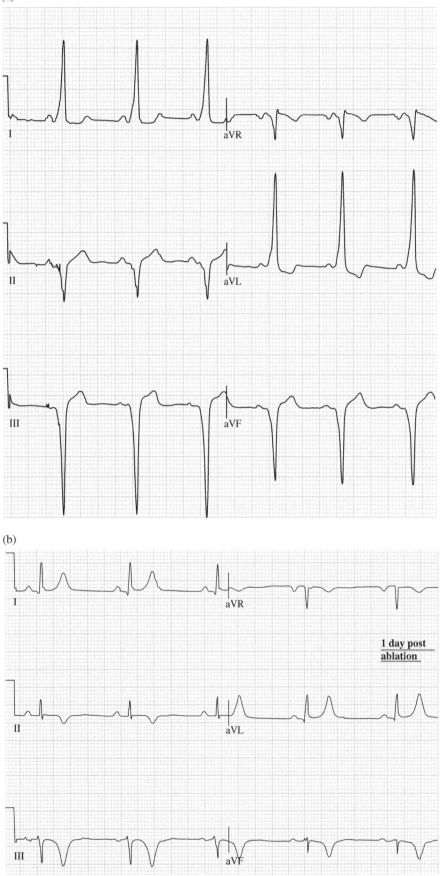

(b)

Figure 25.7 (a) ECG prior to successful ablation of posteroseptal accessory pathway. (b) ECG after ablation showed absence of pre-excitation, but deep T wave inversion in inferior leads caused concern about ischaemic damage. In fact it was due to 'T wave memory', i.e. the T wave continues in the same direction as the QRS complex in that lead prior to ablation (this phenomenon is not seen after ablation of concealed accessory pathways).

(c)

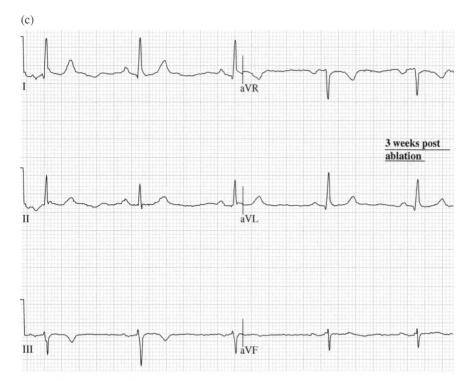

3 weeks post ablation

Figure 25.7(cont'd) (c) The ECG had returned to normal within two weeks.

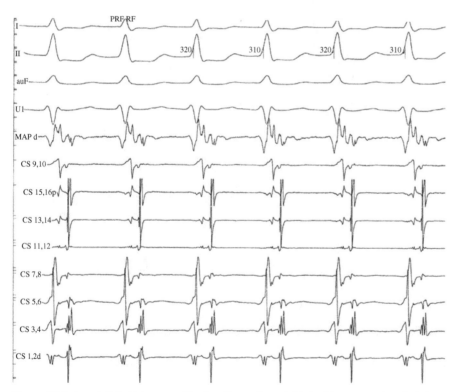

Figure 25.8 Concealed left-sided accessory AV pathway. The trace is recorded during AV re-entrant tachycardia. It shows four surface ECGs, electrograms from a mapping electrode (MAP) placed across the mitral valve, and a series of eight coronary sinus electrograms from proximal (CS 15, 16) to distal positions (CS 1, 2). The sequence of atrial electrograms from the coronary sinus indicates a left-sided free wall accessory pathway with earliest atrial activation recorded by electrodes CS 9,10.

sinus, thereby demonstrating a concealed left-sided free wall pathway. An electrode (MAP) positioned across the mitral valve close to coronary sinus electrode CS 9,10 showed even earlier atrial activity. Delivery of radiofrequency energy at that site blocked the accessory pathway.

Typical atrioventricular nodal re-entrant tachycardia

Because the length of the re-entrant circuit comprising slow and fast AV nodal pathways during typical AV nodal re-entrant tachycardia (AVNRT) is small, the conduction time from ventricles to atria via the fast pathway during tachycardia is very short (≤60 ms). Atrial activity coincides with, or just precedes or just follows, the ventricular complex. This is the hallmark of this arrhythmia (Figure 25.9).

'Slow pathway ablation' is the most common approach to AVNRT. The pathway is usually located just superior and anterior to the mouth of the coronary sinus. A typical slow pathway electrogram can be recorded (Figure 25.10). If successful, radiofrequency energy delivered to the site at which this electrogram is recorded will lead to a period of junctional rhythm, after which the tachycardia can no longer be induced and there will no longer be electrophysiological evidence of a slow pathway, or at least if the pathway remains its characteristics will have been markedly modified.

There is a risk (< 1%) of causing complete atrioventricular block when attempting slow pathway ablation. Patients should be informed of the small possibility that the procedure will lead to pacemaker implantation. This risk can be minimised by observing the heart rhythm during delivery of radiofrequency energy beat by beat and *immediately* stopping if a junctional tachycardia rather than junctional rhythm occurs,

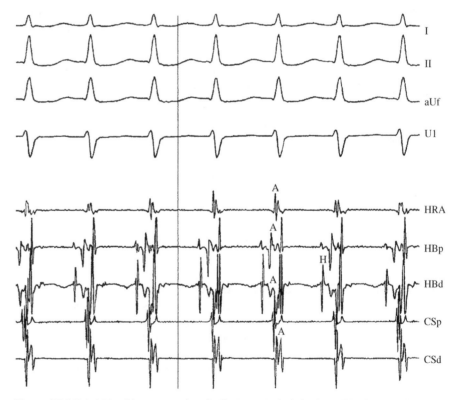

Figure 25.9 Typical AV nodal re-entrant tachycardia. The A waves in the high right atrial (HRA), His bundle (HB) and coronary sinus (CS) electrograms are almost coincident with ventricular activation. The His bundle electrogram (H) precedes the A and V waves.

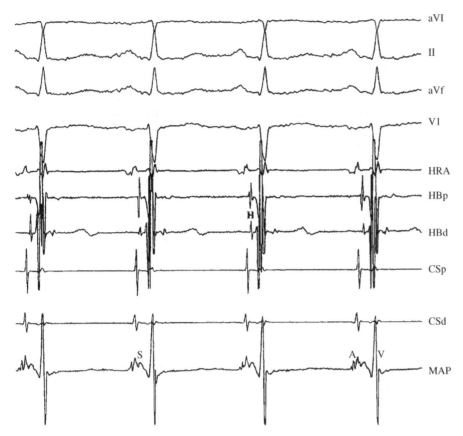

Figure 25.10 Recordings during sinus rhythm in a patient prone to AV nodal re-entrant tachycardia. The mapping electrode (MAP) is positioned just superior and anterior to the mouth of the coronary sinus. A typical slow pathway electrogram (S) has been recorded: a small A wave followed by continuous electrical activity and then a large V wave.

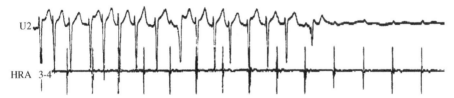

Figure 25.11 Slow pathway ablation. Trace shows surface lead V2 and high right atrial electrogram (HRA). Delivery of radiofrequency energy was not stopped in spite of junctional acceleration and loss of ventriculoatrial conduction. Complete heart block resulted. (Recording obtained from another cardiac unit!)

or if there is loss of ventriculoatrial conduction for even a single cardiac cycle during junctional rhythm (Figure 25.11).

Atypical atrioventricular nodal re-entrant tachycardia

In atypical AVNRT, the direction of the circuit is reversed so that conduction to the ventricles is via the fast AV nodal pathway and conduction from ventricles to the atria is via the slow pathway. This results in a long ventriculoatrial conduction time (Figure 25.12).

As a result of the long ventriculoatrial conduction time, the surface ECG will show that the interval between the QRS complex and the following retrograde P wave is longer than interval between the P wave and the subsequent QRS complex (Figure 25.13). Hence the term 'long RP–short PR tachycardia'. (For the record, there are three causes of a long RP–short PR tachycardia: atypical AVNRT, atrial tachycardia

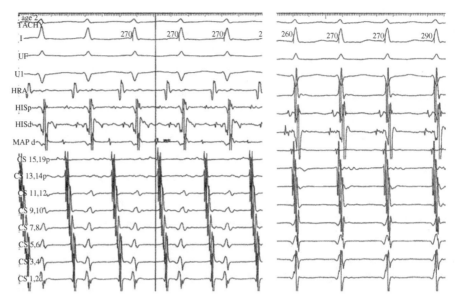

Figure 25.12 Atypical (left-hand panel) and typical (right-hand panel) AV nodal re-entrant tachycardia (AVNRT) recorded from the same patient. The traces show surface leads I, aVF and V1, high right atrial (HRA), His bundle and a series of coronary sinus (CS) electrograms. Ventriculoatrial conduction is very short during typical AVNRT but long during atypical AVNRT.

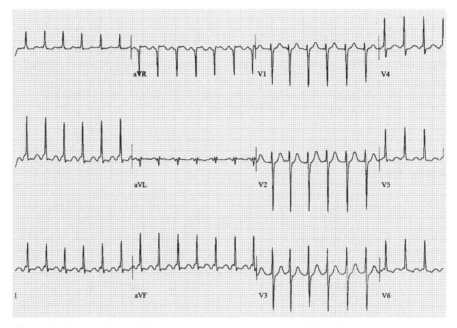

Figure 25.13 'Long RP–short PR' tachycardia. Inverted P waves precede each QRS complex.

with 1:1 AV conduction and AVRT with a slowly conducting accessory pathway (usually posteroseptal).)

Atrial tachycardia

The site of origin of atrial tachycardia is located by mapping of the right and, if necessary, left atrium to identify the point of earliest activation during tachycardia. This will precede the onset of the P wave in the surface ECG. Sometimes, a complex electrogram will be recorded at this site – a sign of myocardial damage (Figure 25.14).

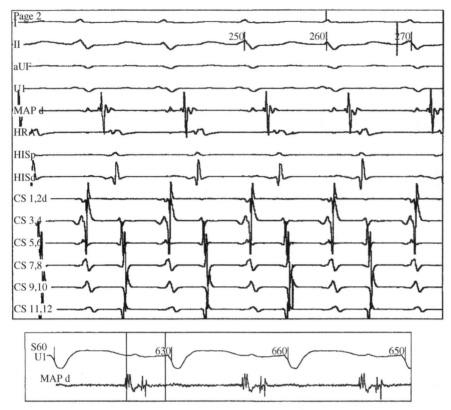

Figure 25.14 Atrial tachycardia. In the upper panel, atrial electrograms have been recorded from the high right atrium (HRA), region of the His bundle (HIS) and sites within the coronary sinus (CS). Earliest atrial activation was recorded by the mapping electrode (MAP) positioned on the lateral wall of the right atrium. The lower panel shows a fractionated, complex atrial electrogram (MAP) recorded from the site of origin of an atrial tachycardia. Its onset precedes the beginning of the P wave in surface lead V1.

Atrial flutter

Typical atrial flutter is caused by a re-entrant circuit in the right atrium (Chapter 7). The narrowest part of the circuit is between the inferior vena cava and the posterior part of the tricuspid valve and is termed the cavotricuspid isthmus. Radiofrequency energy is delivered to points along a line between these two sites in order to block isthmus conduction (Figure 25.15). Delivery of radiofrequency energy in the region of the inferior cava can sometimes be painful: generous analgesia may be required.

There is a small recurrence rate necessitating a repeat procedure, and atrial fibrillation sometimes develops after successful ablation. Nevertheless, ablation compares very favourably with medical treatment, drugs and/or cardioversions for atrial flutter.

Atrial fibrillation

In recent years, the application of catheter ablation to cure paroxysmal atrial fibrillation has become the subject of intense interest. It has been shown that the abnormal electrical activity that initiates atrial fibrillation usually arises from the junction of one or more of the pulmonary veins with the left atrium. Radiofrequency energy is delivered to the circumferences of the ostia of the pulmonary veins in order to electrically isolate them from the left atrium. Currently, success rates are moderately high but

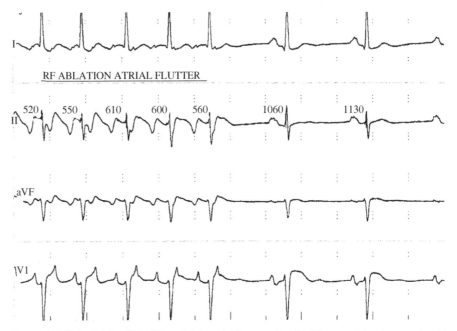

Figure 25.15 Leads I, II, aVF, V1 (100 mm/s) during atrial flutter as a line of radiofrequency lesions between tricuspid valve and inferior vena cava is completed: sinus rhythm returns.

antiarrhythmic drugs are still sometimes required, repeat procedures may be necessary and periods of *asymptomatic* atrial fibrillation have been shown to occur in some patients who have undergone apparently successful ablation.

The procedure involves transseptal catheterisation to gain access to the left atrium. There are small risks of stroke and atrial wall or aortic root perforation associated with this procedure. Furthermore, MR scanning has demonstrated that asymptomatic, small cerebral infarcts can result from pulmonary vein isolation, the incidence being higher if a multielectrode ablation catheter is used.

Compared with other widely performed forms of ablation, the success rates are lower and the risk of complication somewhat higher. At present, it would seem prudent to reserve this treatment for patients with troublesome symptoms from paroxysmal atrial fibrillation who have not responded to other forms of therapy. Success rates are lower when there is marked left atrial enlargement, structural heart disease or cardiac failure. It may well be that further developments will improve the effectiveness and reduce the risks of the procedure, allowing its application to become more widespread.

Ablation for persistent atrial fibrillation is more challenging. As well as electrical isolation of all four pulmonary veins, linear lesions are required to form anatomical barriers to conduction of electrical impulses within the left atrium. The lesions are delivered in lines to the roof of the left atrium connecting the two superior pulmonary veins, and also between the mitral valve and the left lower pulmonary vein. Often, in addition, fractionated atrial electrograms are sought and ablated. Success rates are lower when fibrillation has persisted for more than one year, and if the left atrium is significantly enlarged. Repeat procedures are often required.

Atrioventricular nodal ablation

In some patients, atrial arrhythmias cannot be controlled by medication, and ablation of the source of the arrhythmia either is not indicated or has failed. Radiofrequency

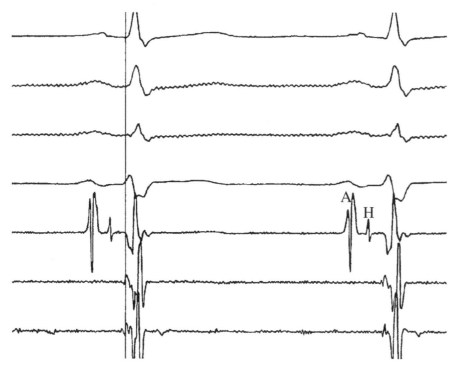

Figure 25.16 His bundle electrogram prior to AV nodal ablation, showing large A wave and smaller H wave.

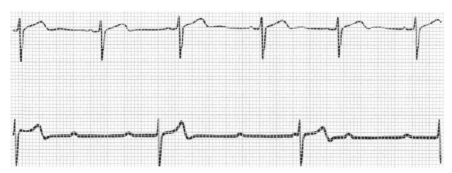

Figure 25.17 Patient with paroxysmal atrial fibrillation before (upper trace) and after (lower trace) AV node ablation.

energy can be used to ablate the AV node and to thus isolate the ventricles from the rapid atrial activity. AV node ablation will of course lead to complete heart block. In contrast to ablation for other arrhythmias, AV nodal ablation is palliative rather than curative, since the procedure necessitates pacemaker implantation.

Ablation of the AV node is usually easy, and failure is rare. The ablating electrode is positioned across the tricuspid valve to record a large His bundle electrogram. The tip of the electrode is then withdrawn slightly in order to record a large A wave with a smaller H wave (Figure 25.16). Delivery of radiofrequency energy usually first causes a junctional tachycardia and then complete AV block (Figure 25.17).

Occasionally, it is not possible to ablate the AV node via the right heart. In these cases, a left-sided approach via the femoral artery is invariably successful. The ablating electrode can be passed across the aortic valve. A large His bundle electrogram can be easily found below the aortic valve on the interventricular septum.

Cardiac pacing

Choice of appropriate pacing mode is important. The pacemaker must provide a chronotropic response. A VVIR pacemaker should be used in persistent atrial

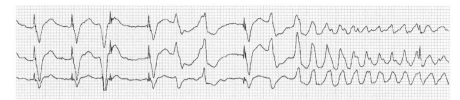

Figure 25.18 Patient with severe heart failure who had undergone AV nodal ablation a few hours earlier. After three ventricular ectopic beats, one of which was not sensed by the pacemaker, ventricular fibrillation occurred.

fibrillation or flutter. In patients with paroxysmal atrial arrhythmias, a DDDR pacemaker with mode-switching facility is required (Chapter 23).

Patients with poor ventricular function who had persistently rapid ventricular rates during their atrial arrhythmia are at a small risk of ventricular fibrillation within the first few days after ablation (Figure 25.18). This risk can be minimised by programming the lowest pacing rate to 80 beats/min for the first few weeks after ablation.

Heart failure has been reported to occur in some patients as a result of right ventricular apical pacing following AV nodal ablation. This complication may well be avoided by pacing the right ventricular outflow tract or by biventricular pacing (Chapter 23).

There are advantages in implanting the pacemaker prior to AV node ablation. One can ensure that there are no pacemaker complications before committing the patient to the need for a pacemaker. Furthermore, in some patients with paroxysmal atrial fibrillation, it has been found that pacing (plus or minus an antiarrhythmic drug) will prevent or markedly reduce the frequency of atrial fibrillation and thereby obviate the need for AV node ablation. Pacing the atrial septum appears to be more effective than pacing the atrial appendage.

Right ventricular outflow tract tachycardia

The origin of this tachycardia is just below the pulmonary valve. It can be located by seeking the earliest site of ventricular activation (Figure 25.19) and by pace-mapping (Figure 25.20).

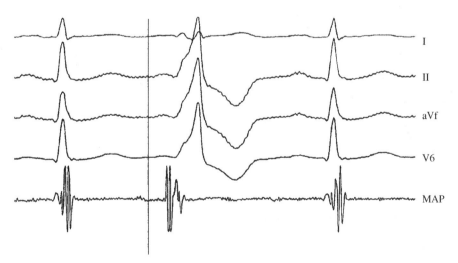

Figure 25.19 The second beat is a ventricular ectopic beat arising from the site of origin of right ventricular outflow tract tachycardia. In contrast to the normal sinus beats before and after, the mapping electrode positioned inferior to the pulmonary valve records ventricular activity earlier than seen on the surface ECGs.

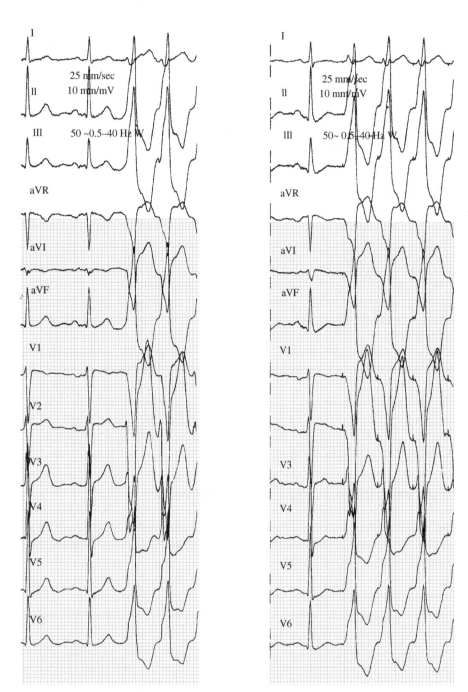

Figure 25.20 Pace-mapping. The left-hand panel shows two spontaneous beats arising from the right ventricular outflow tract. In the right-hand panel, pacing at a site just inferior to the pulmonary valve resulted in an almost identical configuration. Radiofrequency energy to that site abolished right ventricular outflow tract tachycardia.

Fascicular ventricular tachycardia

Fascicular tachycardia arises from the posterior fascicle or, rarely, anterior fascicle of the left bundle branch. The appropriate site for delivery of radiofrequency energy can be found by seeking the earliest area of left ventricular activation, and it is confirmed by the demonstration of a fascicular potential (Figure 25.21).

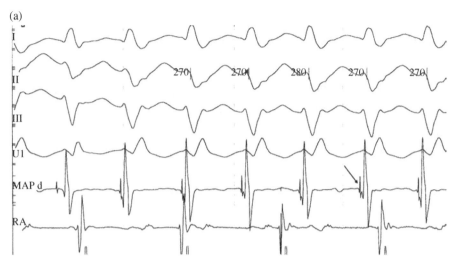

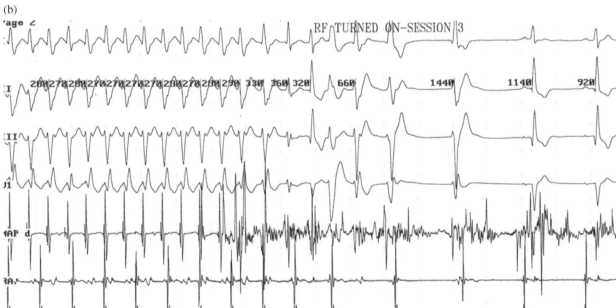

Figure 25.21 Left posterior fascicular tachycardia. (a) Early ventricular activation preceded by a fascicular potential (arrow) is recorded at a site in the posteroapical portion of the left interventricular septum (MAP). (b) Application of radiofrequency energy to site depicted in (a) terminates the arrhythmia, which could then no longer be initiated.

Ventricular tachycardia due to structural heart disease

Ablation of ventricular tachycardias due to myocardial infarction or cardiomyopathy is challenging. Success rates are lower and procedure times much longer than for ablation of other arrhythmias. Identification of the optimal ablation site is usually performed during tachycardia. Therefore, ablation is usually only attempted in patients with slower, well-tolerated tachycardias.

Bundle branch re-entry

This form of ventricular tachycardia typically occurs in patients with a dilated cardio-myopathy who have partial or complete bundle branch block during normal rhythm. During the arrhythmia, a circulating impulse is usually conducted from atria to ventricles via the right bundle and returns to the atria via the left bundle. Typically, the complexes during tachycardia are of left bundle branch block configuration. Each

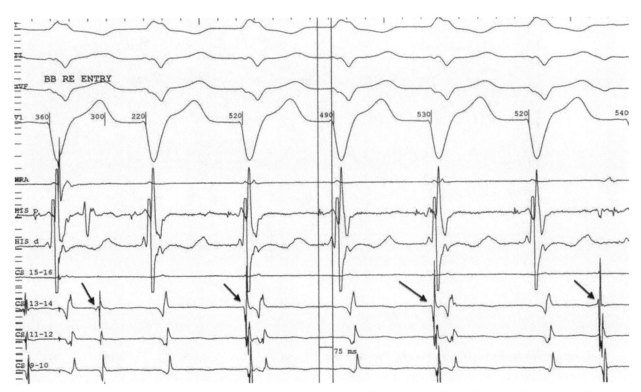

Figure 25.22 Ventricular tachycardia due to bundle branch re-entry. Each ventricular complex is of left bundle branch block configuration and is preceded by a His potential (HIS p). Independent atrial activity (arrows) is demonstrated in a series of coronary sinus (CS) electrograms.

is preceded by a His potential, but, in contrast to supraventricular tachycardias with bundle branch block, atrial activity is dissociated from ventricular activity (Figure 25.22).

Delivery of radiofrequency energy to the right bundle branch will prevent the arrhythmias, though sometimes heart block necessitating a pacemaker results.

Catheter ablation: what should the patient expect?

The patient should be reassured that a local anaesthetic and intravenous sedation will be administered and that little or no discomfort should be experienced. It should be emphasised that it is not possible to feel the electrodes as they are advanced from the femoral vein to the heart.

It should be explained that tachycardia will usually be initiated on one or more occasions during the procedure; that onset of tachycardia does not mean that anything is going wrong and that diagnostic information is being obtained; and that the tachycardia can be promptly terminated by an external pacemaker. A minority of patients, particularly those undergoing ablation for atrial flutter, will experience a feeling of 'heat' within the chest during delivery of radiofrequency energy, and they should be reassured that no harm is being done and that any discomfort will only last for short periods.

The patient should be given an estimate as to how long the procedure will last. For example, usually less than one hour for ablation of AVNRT, atrial flutter or straightforward accessory pathway, and approximately two hours for more complex arrhythmias.

Patients must be aware that ablation for some arrhythmias such as AVNRT and septal accessory pathways is associated with the small risk of heart block and the need for a pacemaker.

Sometimes patients do not appreciate that if anticoagulation was prescribed for an atrial arrhythmia it will still be indicated after AV nodal ablation.

Patients often experience ectopic beats ('as though my tachycardia is about to start') and sinus tachycardia in the weeks following ablation. They should be informed that these do not indicate that the procedure has failed: only a recurrence of the identical symptoms experienced prior to ablation would point to the procedure having been unsuccessful.

26

Arrhythmias for Interpretation

> One hundred and thirty ECGs are presented. Their interpretations, or in the case of questions asked, the answers, can be found at the end of the chapter. As is often the case in practice, there may be more than one observation to make about each example.

Questions

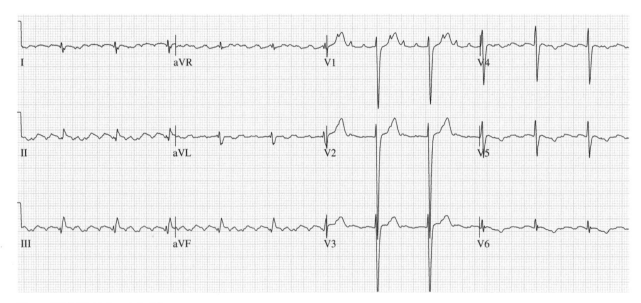

Figure 26.1 What is the arrhythmia?

Bennett's Cardiac Arrhythmias: Practical Notes on Interpretation and Treatment, Eighth Edition. David H. Bennett.
© 2013 John Wiley & Sons, Ltd. Published 2013 by John Wiley & Sons, Ltd.

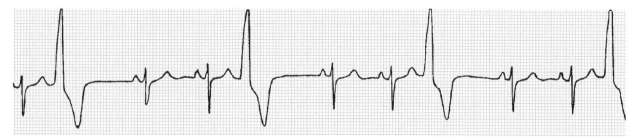

Figure 26.2 What is the arrhythmia?

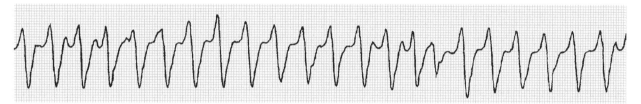

Figure 26.3 Adenosine or verapamil: which is indicated for tachycardia termination?

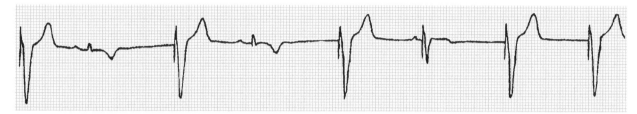

Figure 26.4 What is the pacing mode?

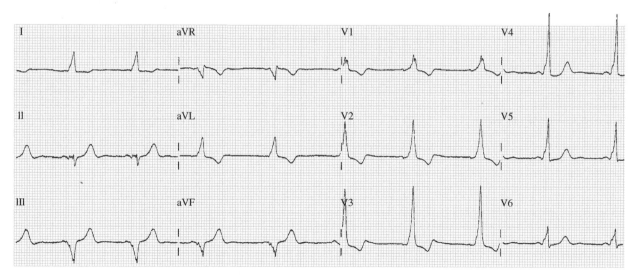

Figure 26.5 (a) Right bundle branch block? (b) Pre-excitation? (c) Right ventricular hypertrophy? (d) True posterior myocardial infarction?

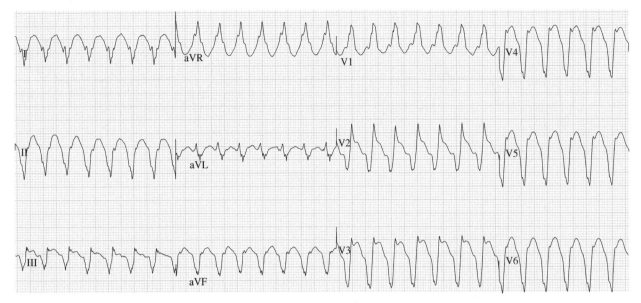

Figure 26.6 What is the arrhythmia?

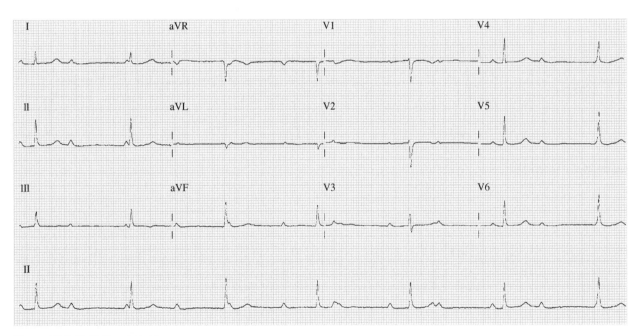

Figure 26.7 What is the arrhythmia?

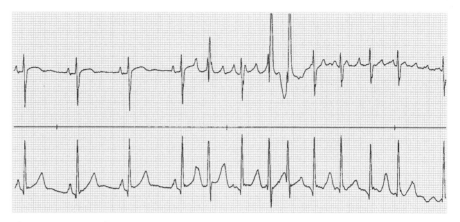

Figure 26.8 Two simultaneously recorded leads. What is the arrhythmia?

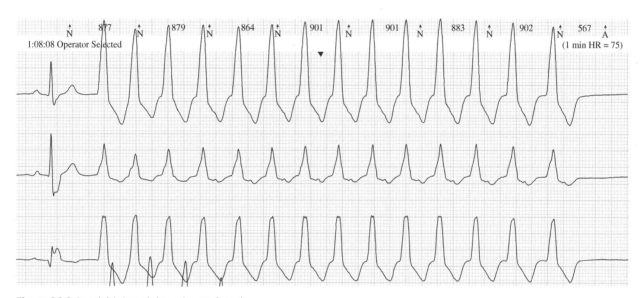

Figure 26.9 Recorded during ambulatory electrocardiography.

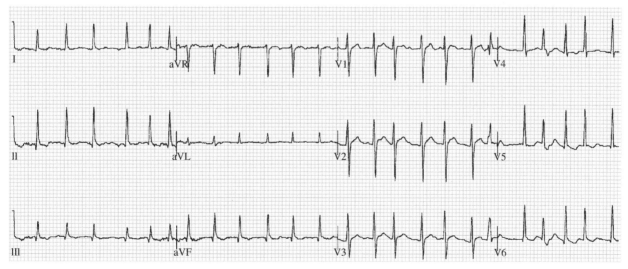

Figure 26.10 What is the arrhythmia?

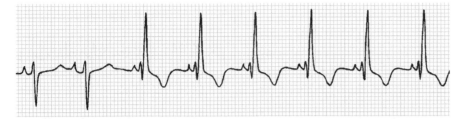

Figure 26.11 Lead V1. What is the arrhythmia?

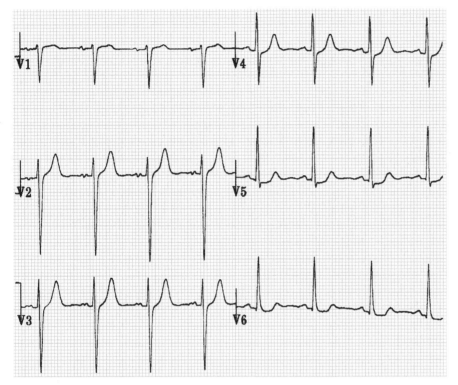

Figure 26.12 (a) and (b) What is the rhythm in each case? Both ECGs from same patient.

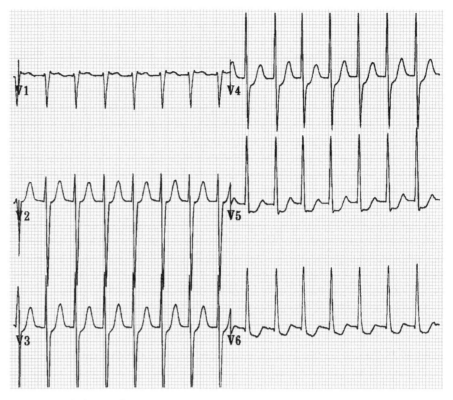

Figure 26.12b (Continued)

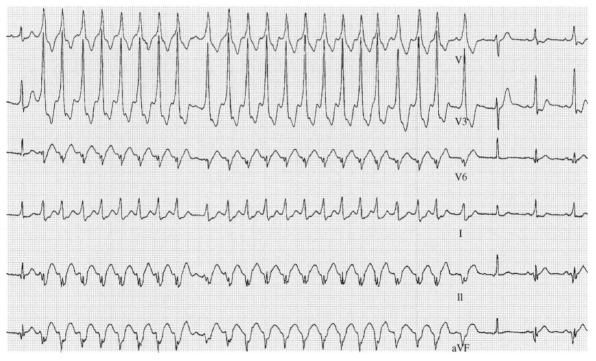

Figure 26.13 Which drug(s) might have been appropriately used? (a) Digoxin? (b) Flecainide? (c) Verapamil? (d) Sotalol? (e) Disopyramide

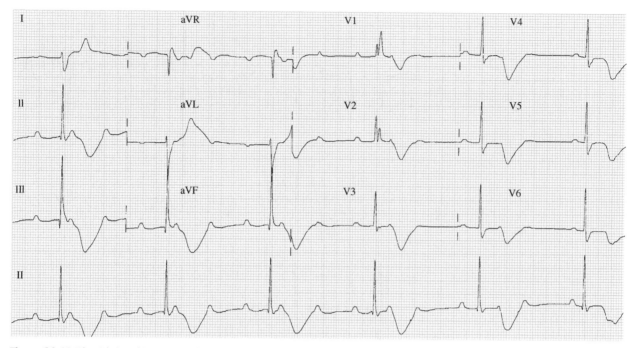

Figure 26.14 Why might have this patient complained of rapid heart beating preceding his 'dizzy attacks'?

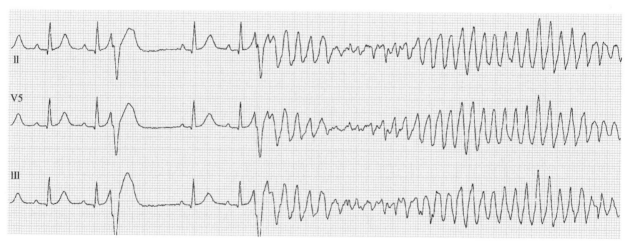

Figure 26.15 What is the arrhythmia?

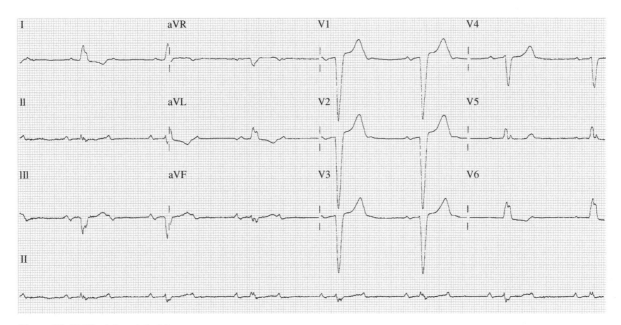

Figure 26.16 What is the arrhythmia?

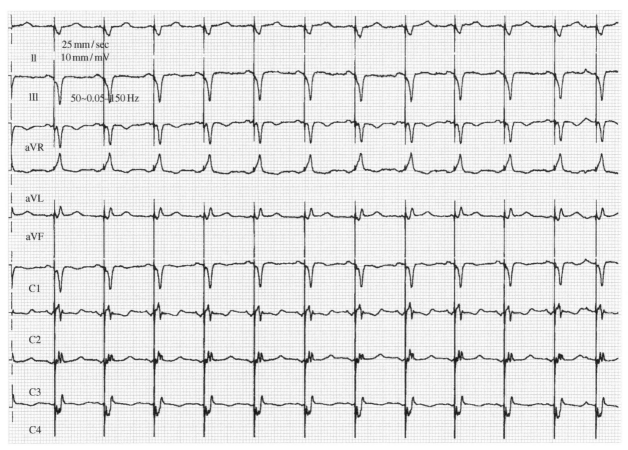

Figure 26.17 What type of pacemaker does this patient have?

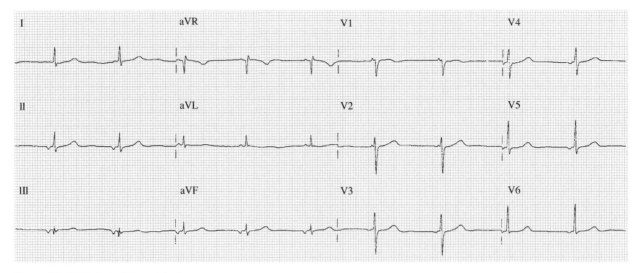

Figure 26.18 Why is the PR interval short?

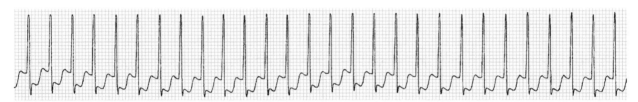

Figure 26.19 What is the arrhythmia?

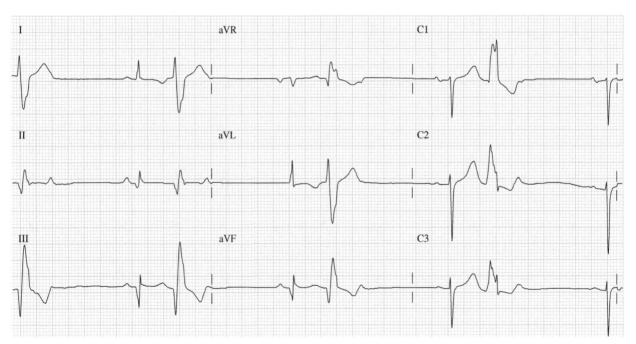

Figure 26.20 What is the arrhythmia? There are three observations to make about this ECG.

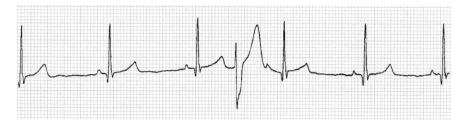

Figure 26.21 Why is the third PR interval prolonged?

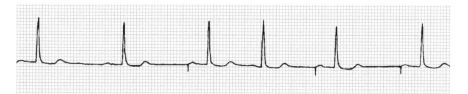

Figure 26.22 What type of pacemaker?

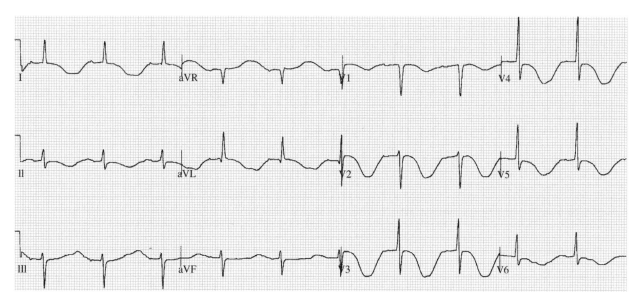

Figure 26.23 Which drug might the patient have been taking? (a) Flecainide? (b) Tetracycline? (c) Bisoprolol? (d) Clarithromycin? (e) Digoxin?

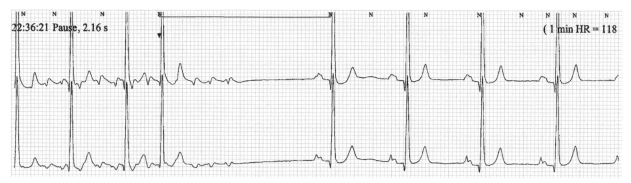

Figure 26.24 What is the arrhythmia?

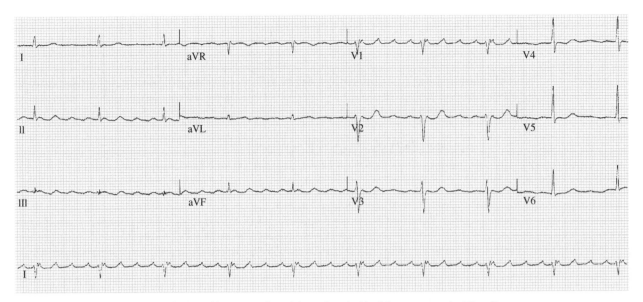

Figure 26.25 What is the arrhythmia? If catheter ablation were to be carried out, where should radiofrequency energy be delivered?

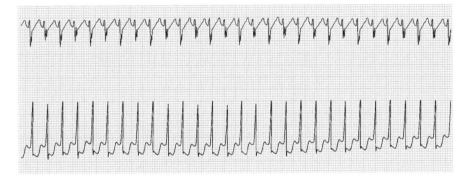

Figure 26.26 Leads V1 and V5. What is the arrhythmia? (Why is there changing morphology in lead V1?)

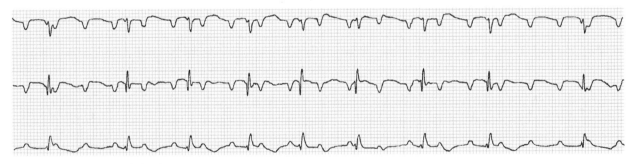

Figure 26.27 What is the arrhythmia?

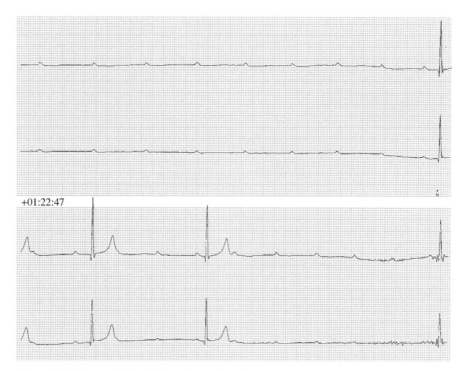

Figure 26.28 Syncope during ambulatory electrocardiography.

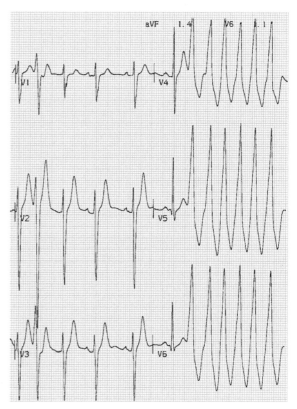

Figure 26.29 What is the arrhythmia?

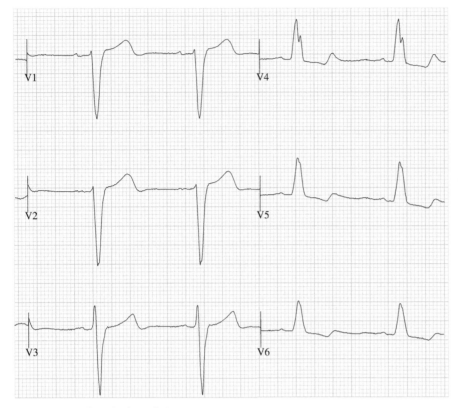

Figure 26.30 What is the abnormality?

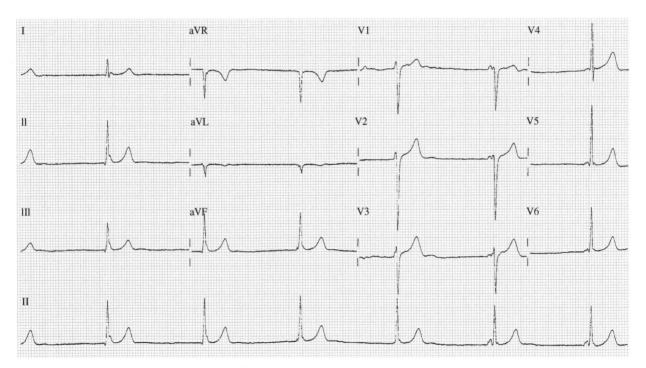

Figure 26.31 What type of pacemaker should this asymptomatic patient receive?

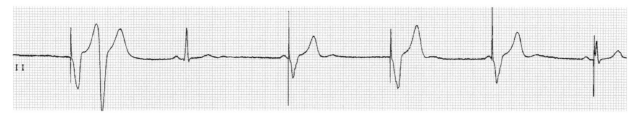

Figure 26.32 Why is the heart rate slow?

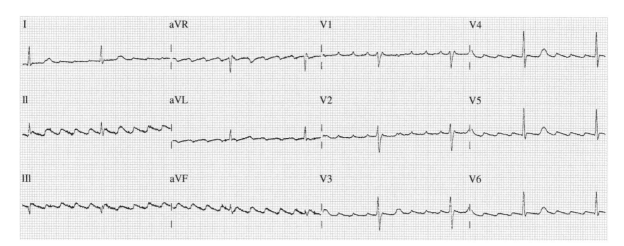

Figure 26.33 What is the arrhythmia?

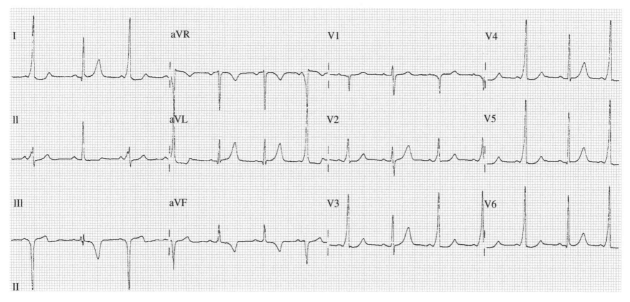

Figure 26.34 Should this outpatient be admitted to hospital?

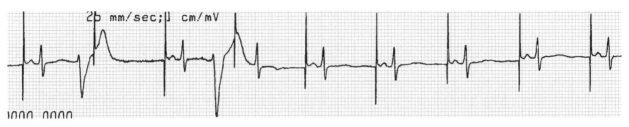

Figure 26.35 What is the pacing mode?

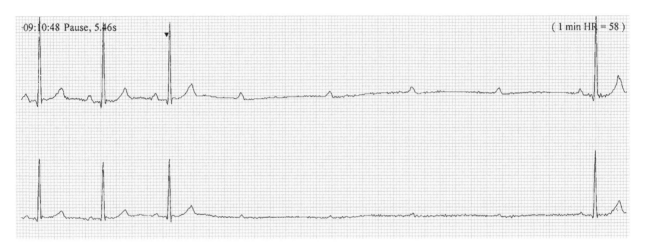

Figure 26.36 Ambulatory electrocardiography.

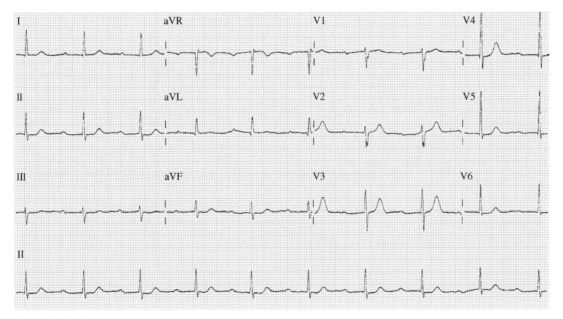

Figure 26.37 What antiarrhythmic drug in an excessive dose typically does this?

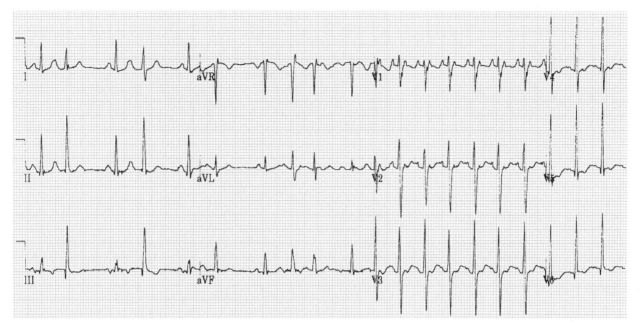

Figure 26.38 What is the arrhythmia?

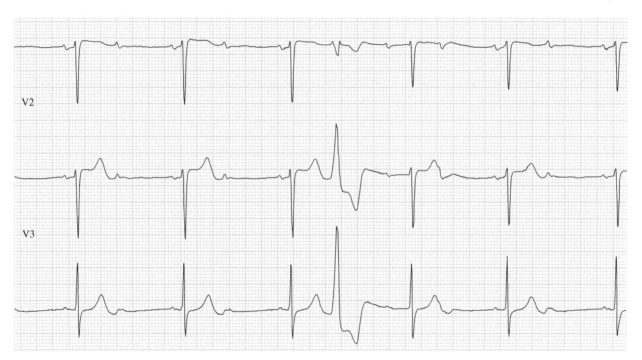

Figure 26.39 What is the arrhythmia?

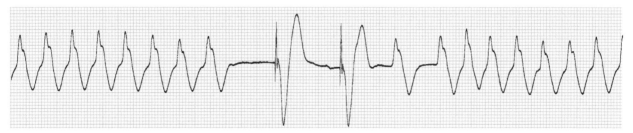

Figure 26.40 What are the rhythms?

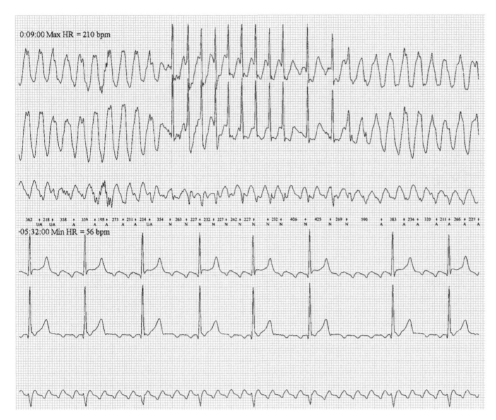

Figure 26.41 Ambulatory electrocardiography during karate when the patient felt faint, and at rest.

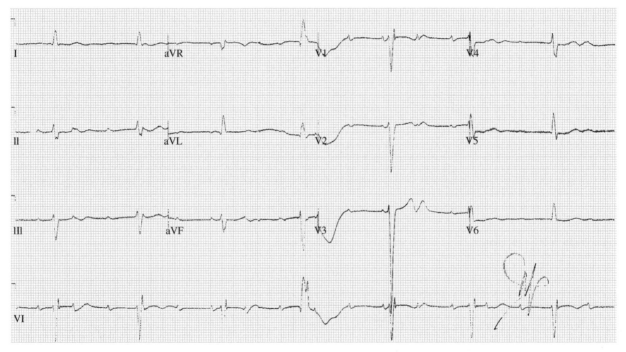

Figure 26.42 What is the arrhythmia? Any other observation?

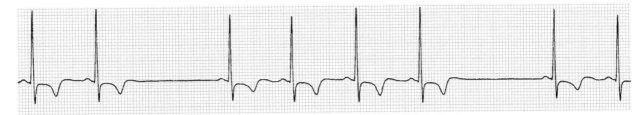

Figure 26.43 What is the arrhythmia?

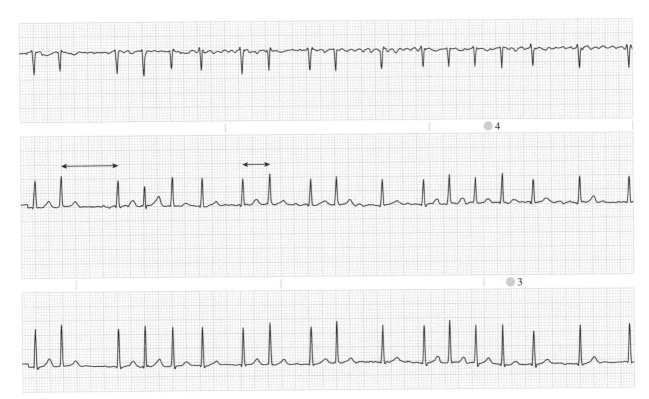

Figure 26.44 What is the arrhythmia?

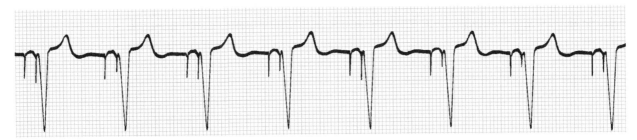

Figure 26.45 What does the ECG show?

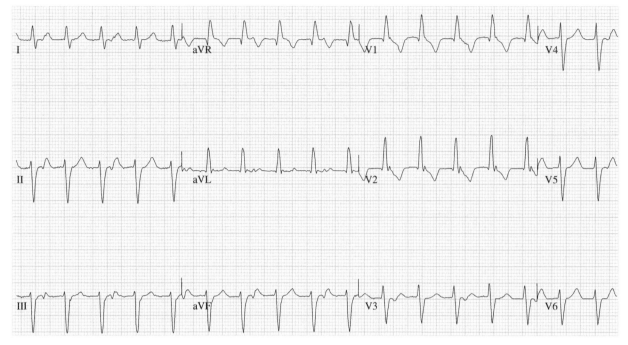

Figure 26.46 This arrhythmia could be terminated by (a) adenosine? (b) verapamil? (c) digoxin?

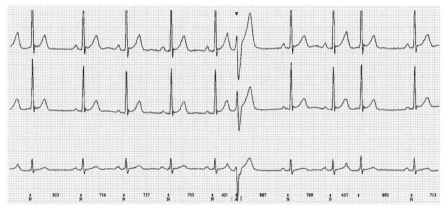

Figure 26.47 Ambulatory electrocardiography.

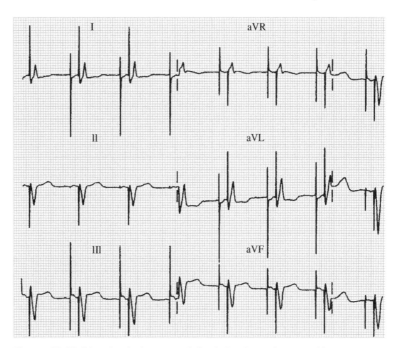

Figure 26.48 This patient had a very poorly functioning sinus node. How could an appropriate increase in heart rate during exercise be achieved?

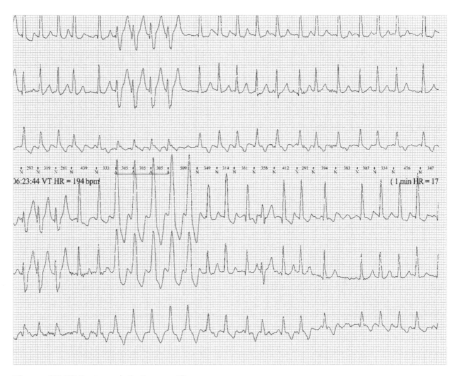

Figure 26.49 Are two arrhythmias present?

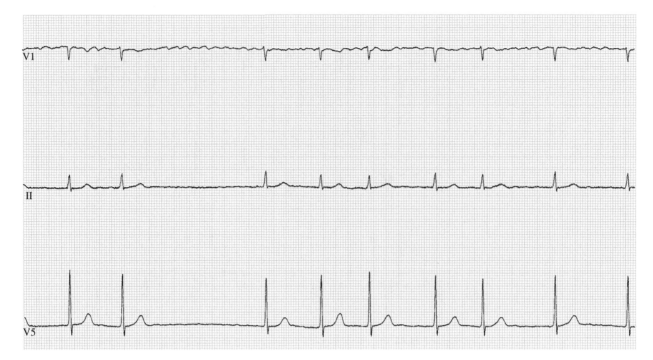

Figure 26.50 What is the arrhythmia?

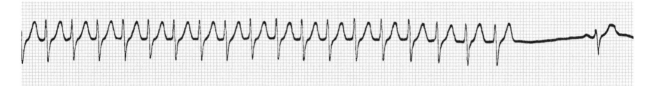

Figure 26.51 What is the arrhythmia?

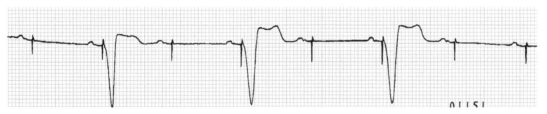

Figure 26.52 Why did this patient complain of blackouts?

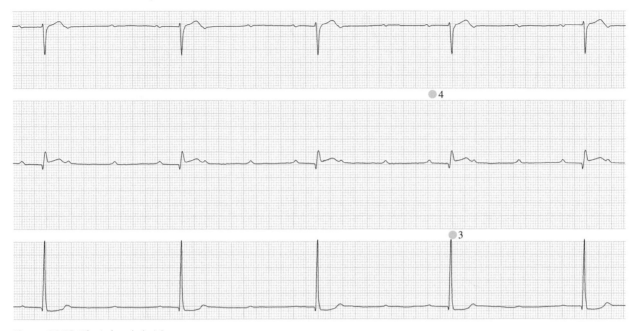

Figure 26.53 What is the arrhythmia?

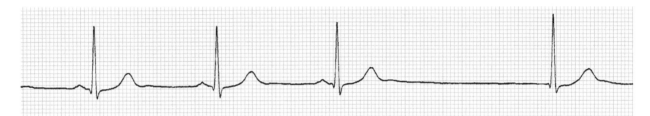

Figure 26.54 What is the arrhythmia?

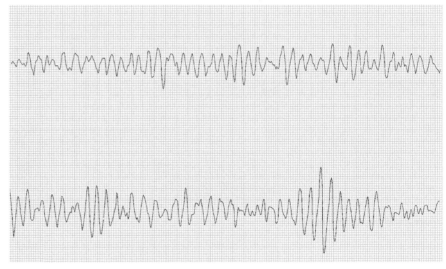

Figure 26.55 Recorded during ambulatory electrocardiography

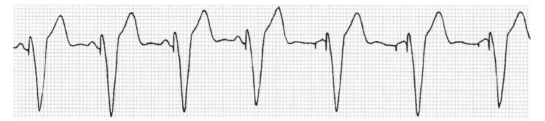

Figure 26.56 What is the pacing mode?

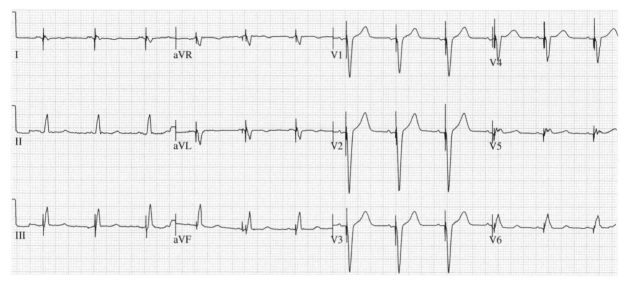

Figure 26.57 Is this pacemaker performing correctly?

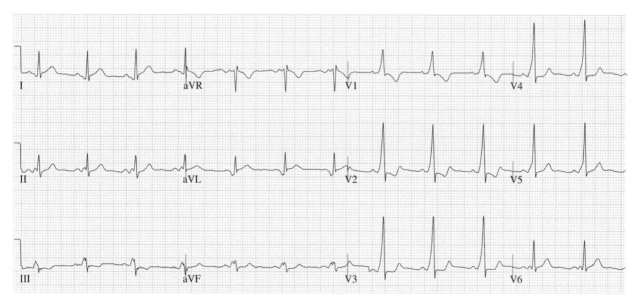

Figure 26.58 Where is the abnormal pathway?

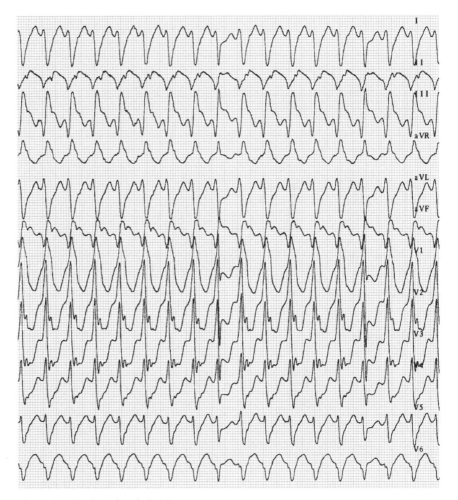

Figure 26.59 What is the arrhythmia?

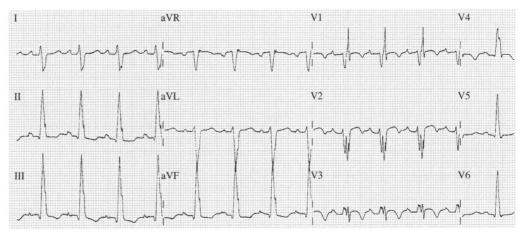

Figure 26.60 This patient experienced syncope but had a normal pulmonary artery pressure. What was the cause?

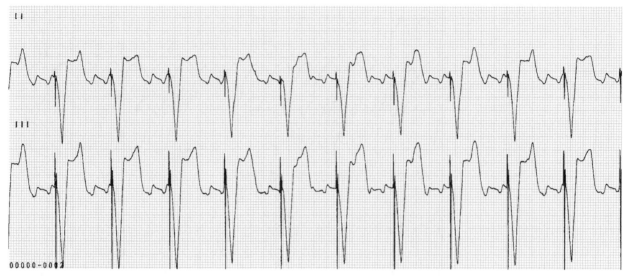

Figure 26.61 What observations can be made?

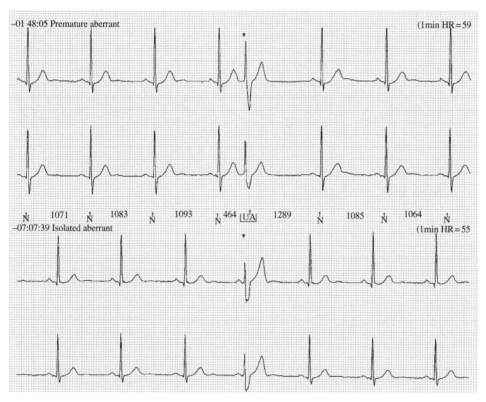

Figure 26.62 What are these minor events during ambulatory electrocardiography?

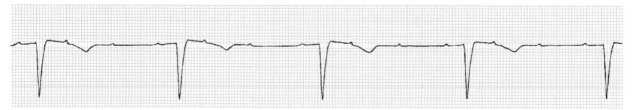

Figure 26.63 What is the arrhythmia?

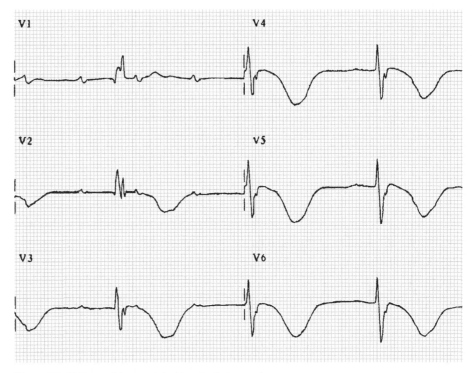

Figure 26.64 Two possible reasons why this patient had syncope?

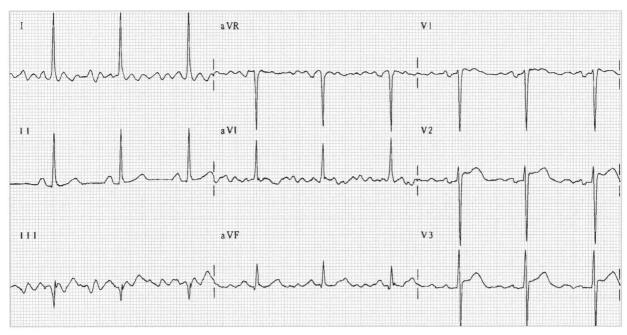

Figure 26.65 CHADS$_2$ score = 3. Aspirin, dabigatran or warfarin?

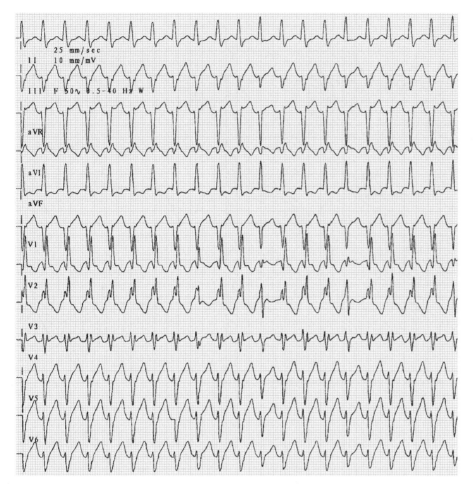

Figure 26.66 Is the arrhythmia due to impaired ventricular function (left or right)?

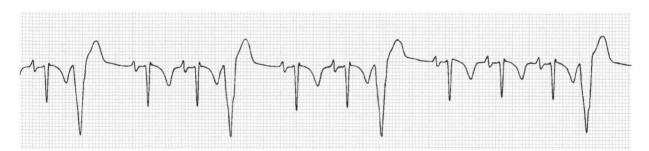

Figure 26.67 What is the arrhythmia?

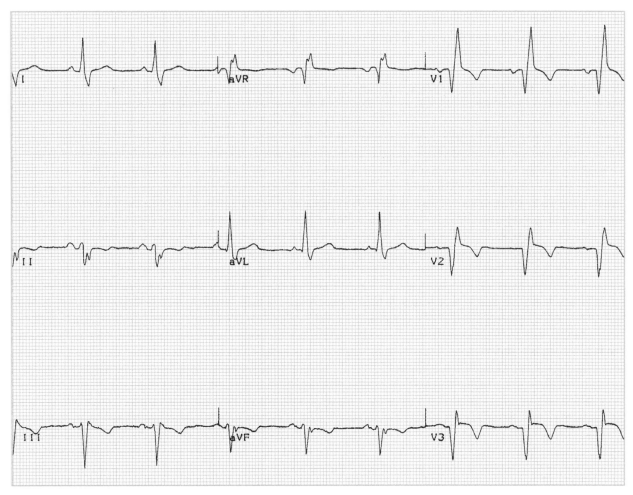

Figure 26.68 Interpretation?

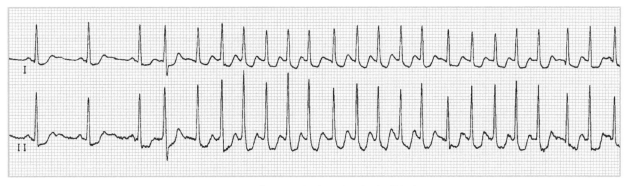

Figure 26.69 In spite of digoxin 0.125 mg daily with normal renal function and body weight. What should be done?

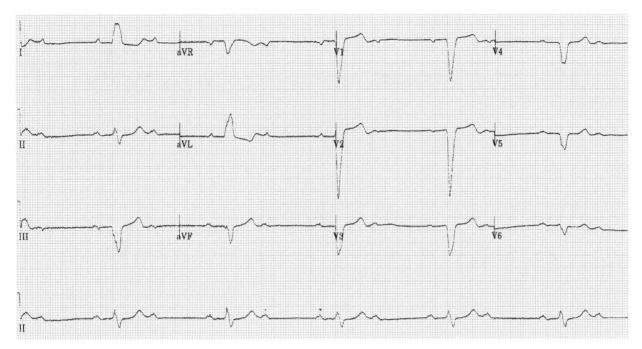

Figure 26.70 What is the arrhythmia?

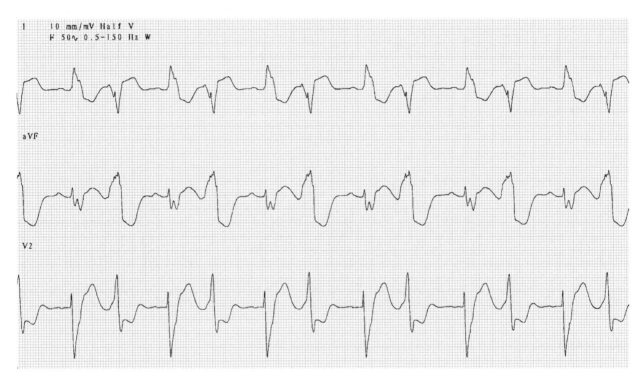

Figure 26.71 What is the arrhythmia?

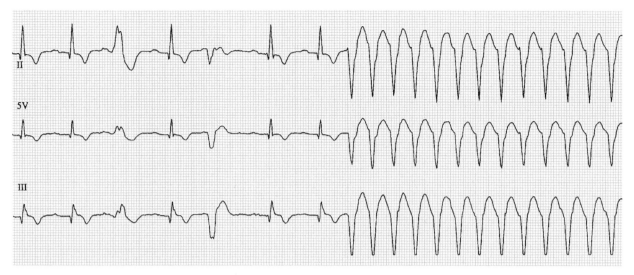

Figure 26.72 What is the arrhythmia?

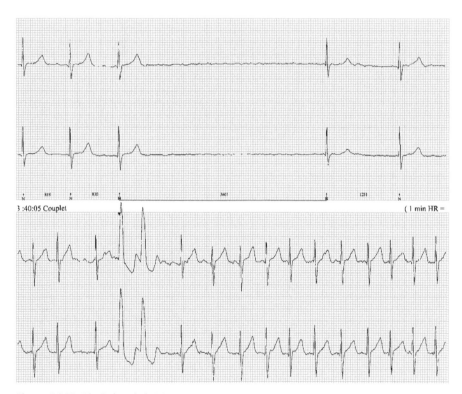

Figure 26.73 What is the arrhythmia?

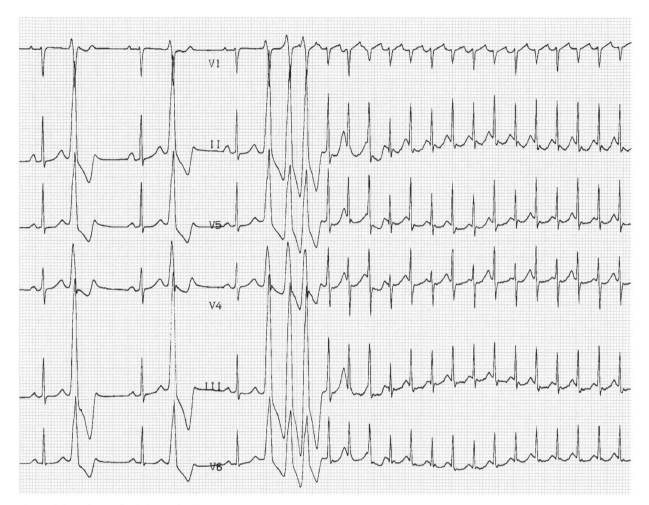

Figure 26.74 There are four findings in this ECG.

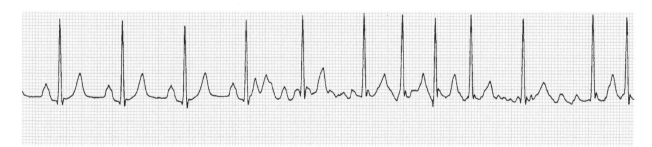

Figure 26.75 What is the arrhythmia?

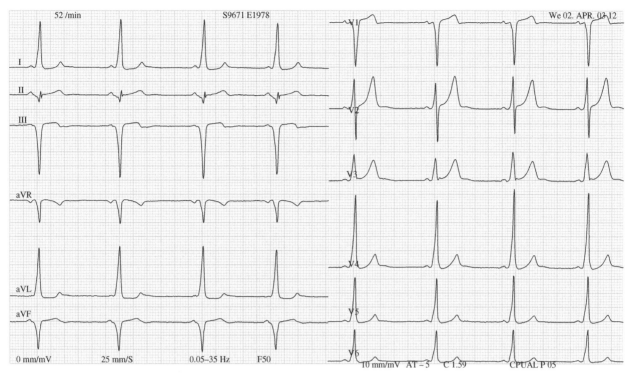

Figure 26.76 A or B?

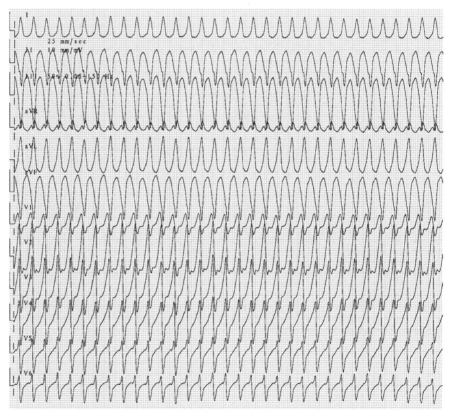

Figure 26.77 What is the arrhythmia?

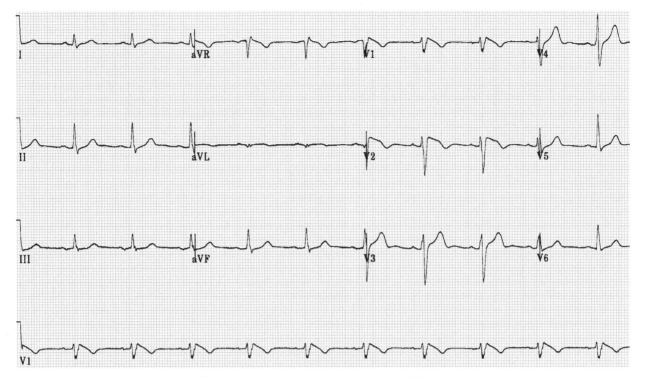

Figure 26.78 This patient had paroxysmal atrial fibrillation and good ventricular function and was prescribed flecainide.

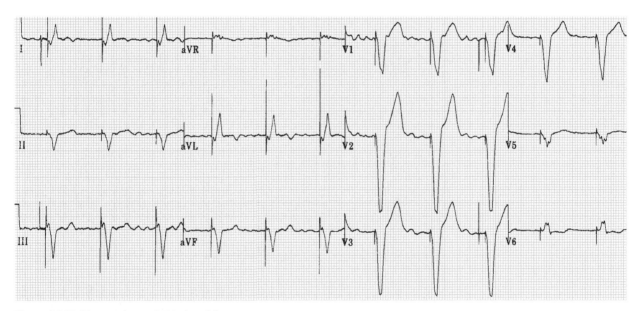

Figure 26.79 What type of pacemaker? Look carefully.

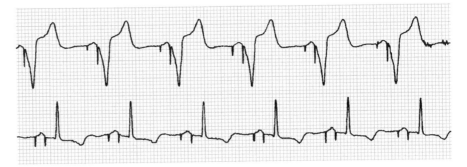

Figure 26.80 Why did this patient continue to have blackouts?

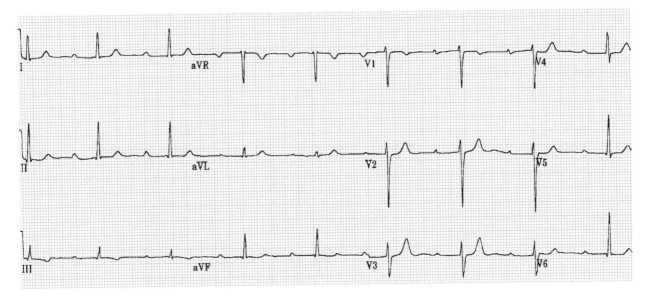

Figure 26.81 This patient complained of syncope. What action should be undertaken?

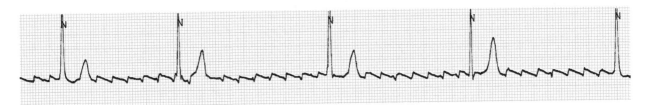

Figure 26.82 Referred for cardioversion. Proceed?

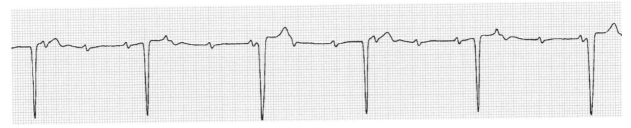

Figure 26.83 What is the arrhythmia?

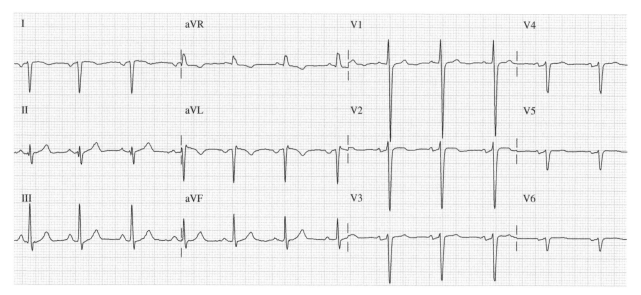

Figure 26.84 Inverted P wave in lead I. Why?

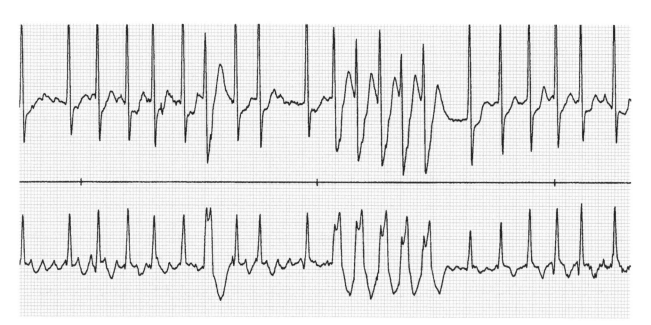

Figure 26.85 What is the arrhythmia?

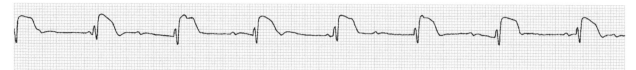

Figure 26.86 Lead aVF. Is action required to deal with the arrhythmia?

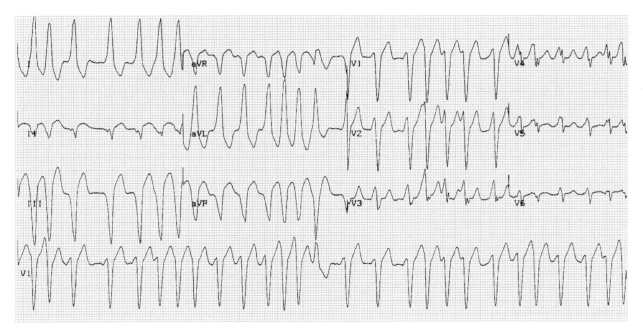

Figure 26.87 Digoxin should work?

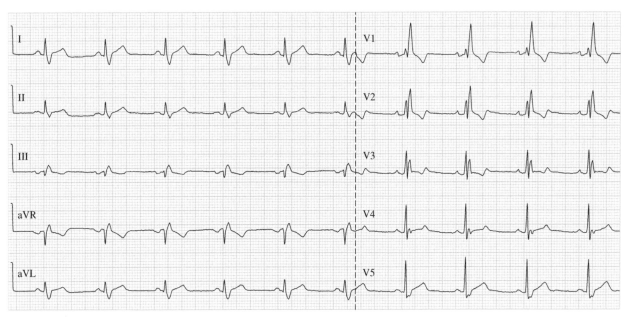

Figure 26.88 Interpretation?

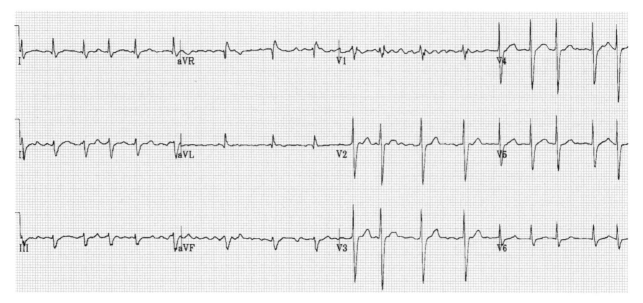

Figure 26.89 What is the arrhythmia?

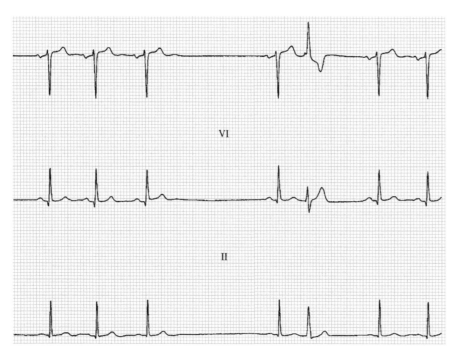

Figure 26.90 What are the rhythm disturbances?

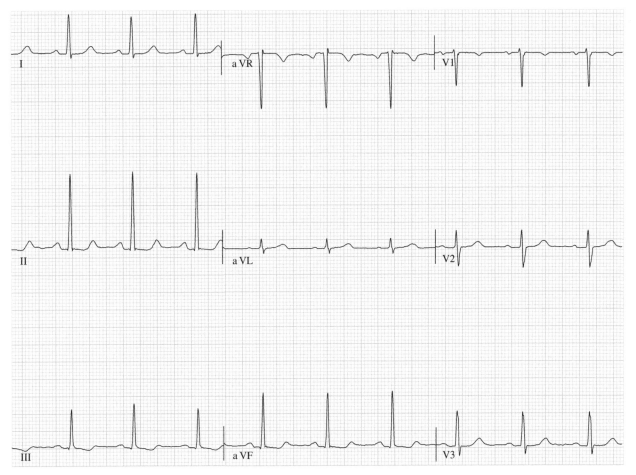

Figure 26.91 What is the abnormality?

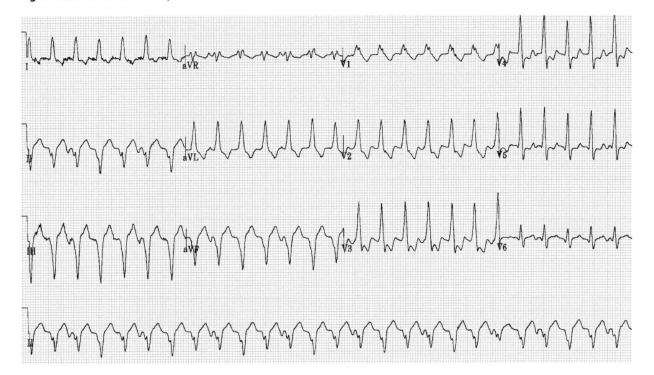

Figure 26.92 What is the arrhythmia?

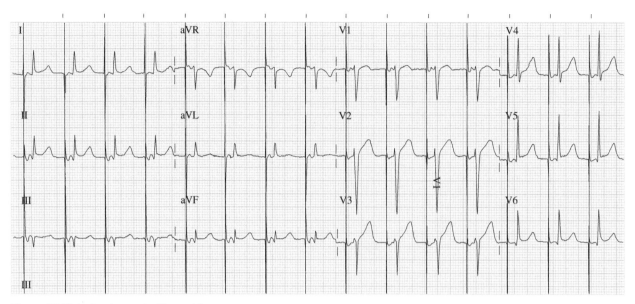

Figure 26.93 Implanted pacemaker. What mode?

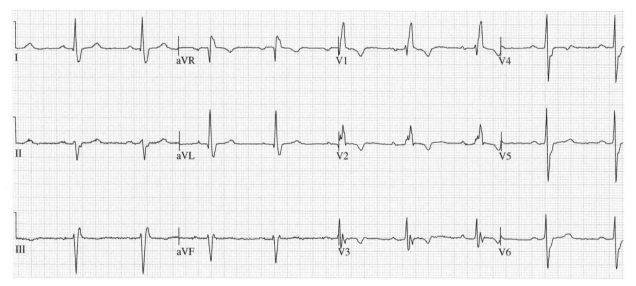

Figure 26.94 What is the likely cause of this patient's syncope?

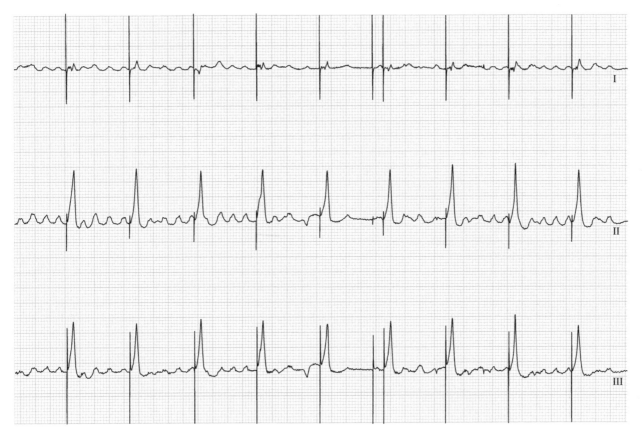

Figure 26.95 What type of pacemaker?

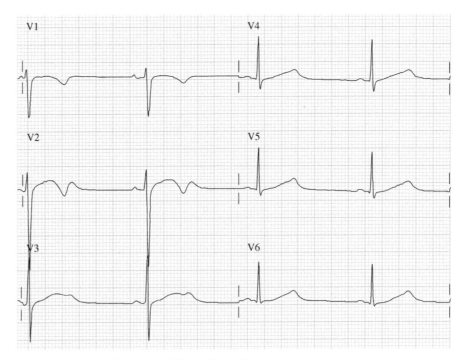

Figure 26.96 Does this hereditary condition ring alarm bells?

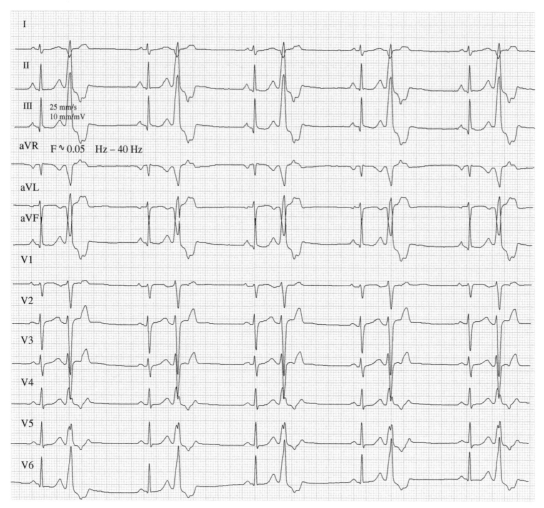

Figure 26.97 What is the arrhythmia?

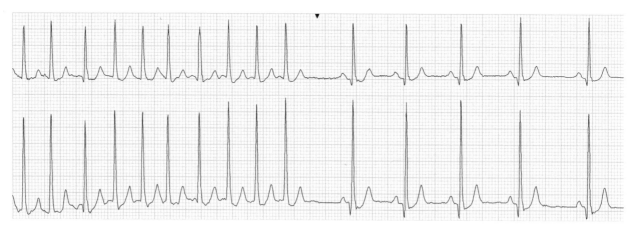

Figure 26.98 Ambulatory electrocardiography.

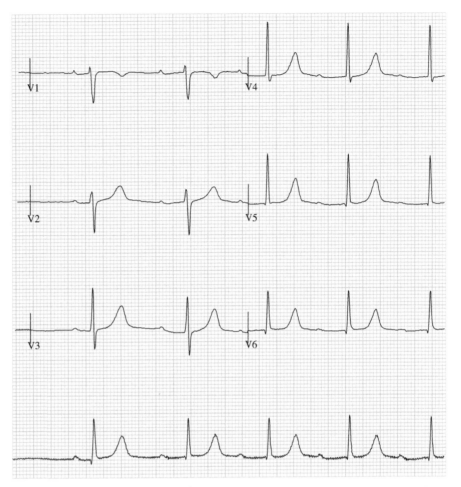

Figure 26.99 Look carefully at the PR interval.

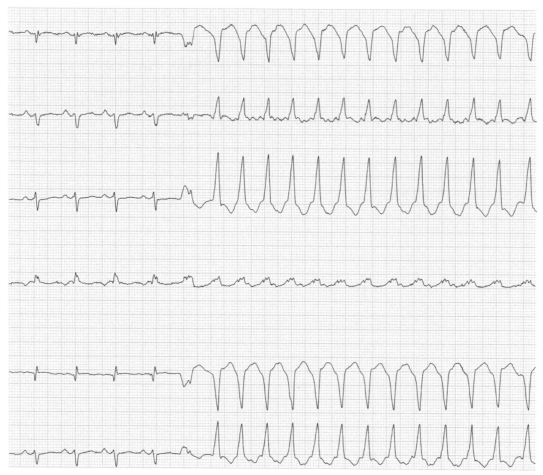

Figure 26.100 What is the arrhythmia?

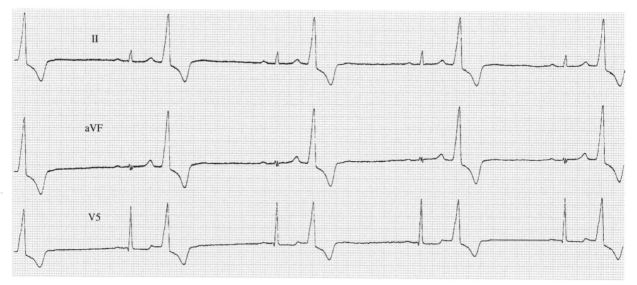

Figure 26.101 What is the arrhythmia?

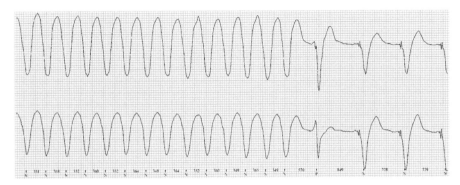

Figure 26.102 What is the arrhythmia?

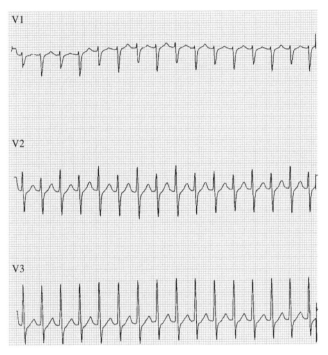

Figure 26.103 What is the arrhythmia?

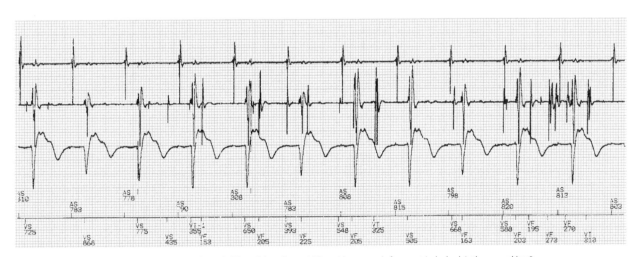

Figure 26.104 Telemetry from ICD: upper panel recorded from right atrium, middle and lower panels from ventricular lead. Is there a problem?

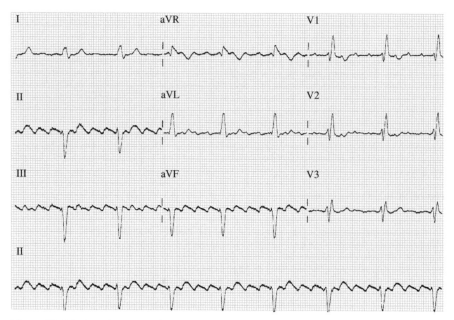

Figure 26.105 Three observations to be made.

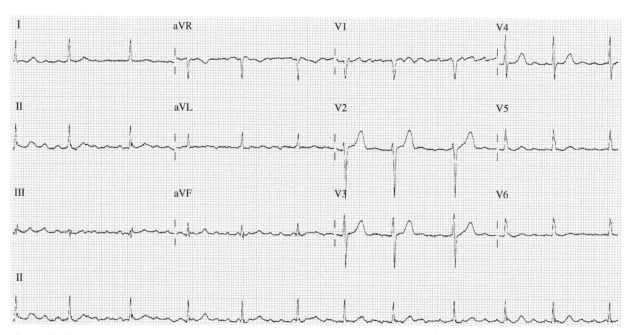

Figure 26.106 What is the arrhythmia?

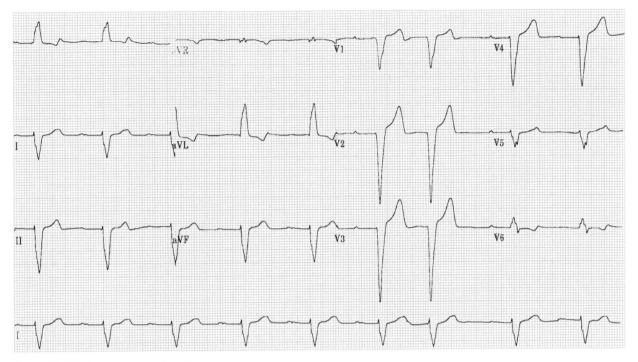

Figure 26.107 Three observations to be made.

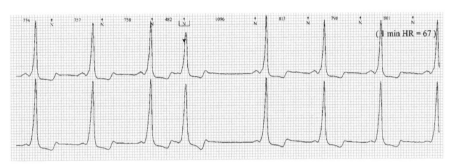

Figure 26.108 Ambulatory electrocardiography.

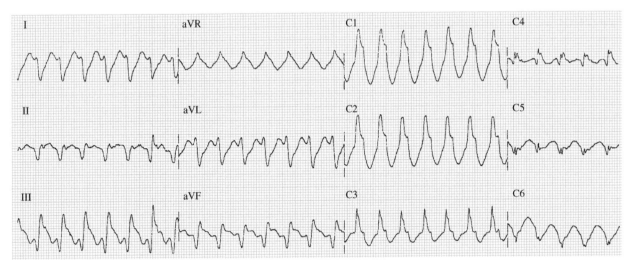

Figure 26.109 What is the arrhythmia?

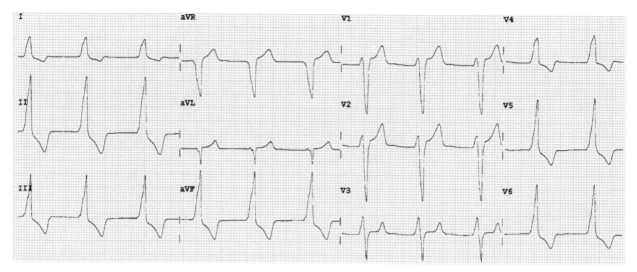

Figure 26.110 What is the arrhythmia?

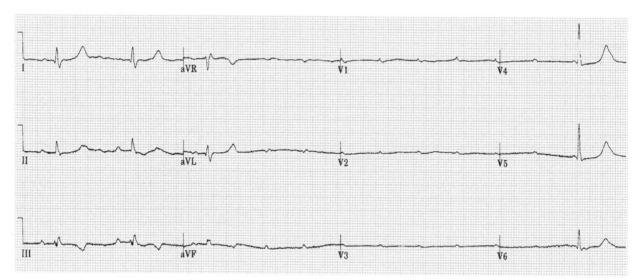

Figure 26.111 What symptom would you expect?

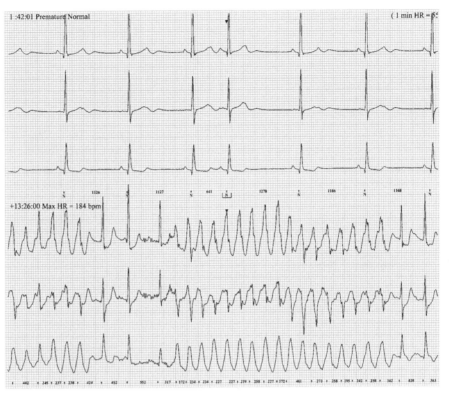

Figure 26.112 Ambulatory electrocardiography.

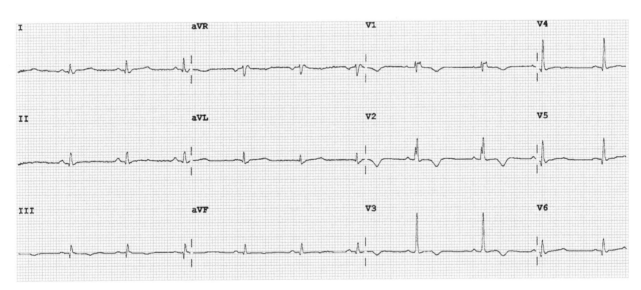

Figure 26.113 This patient experienced syncope while swimming. What is the diagnosis?

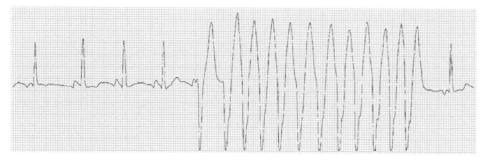

Figure 26.114 Ambulatory electrocardiography.

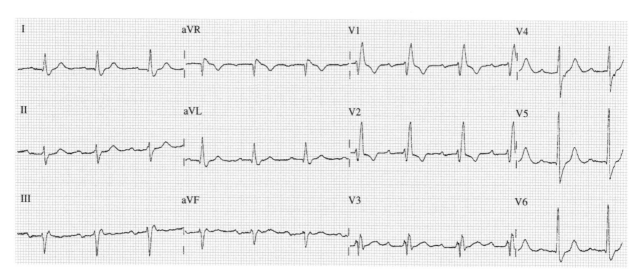

Figure 26.115 This patient had several unheralded brief syncopal episodes. What action is required?

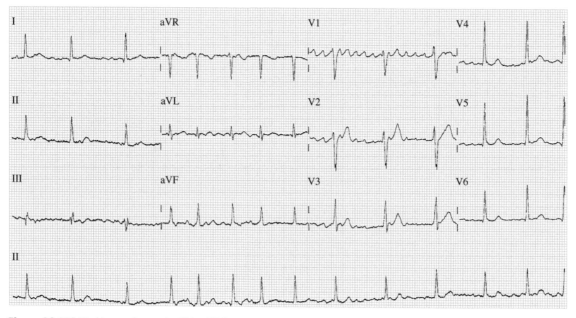

Figure 26.116 Would you cardiovert using 50 J or 150 J?

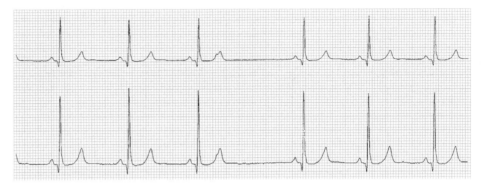

Figure 26.117 What is the arrhythmia?

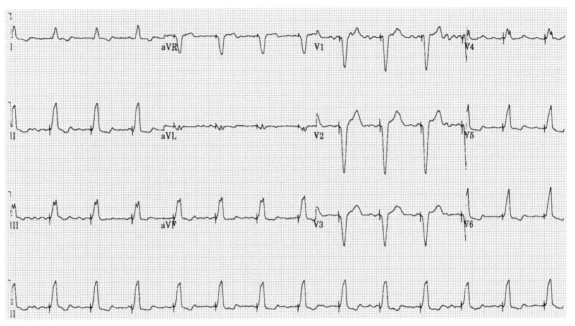

Figure 26.118 What are the rhythms?

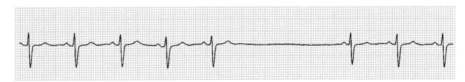

Figure 26.119 What is the arrhythmia?

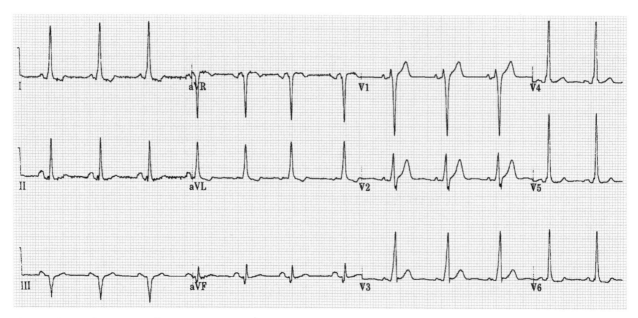

Figure 26.120 What is the cause of this patient's rapid heart beating and polyuria?

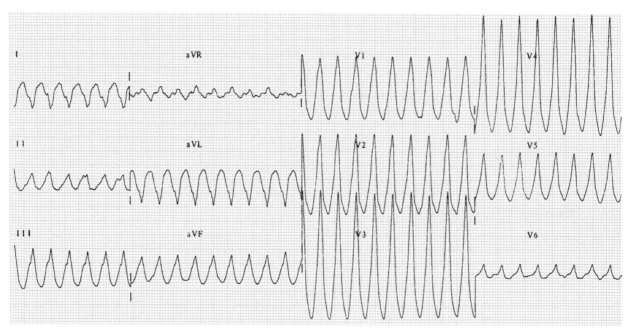

Figure 26.121 Origin of tachycardia in this patient with a dilated cardiomyopathy?

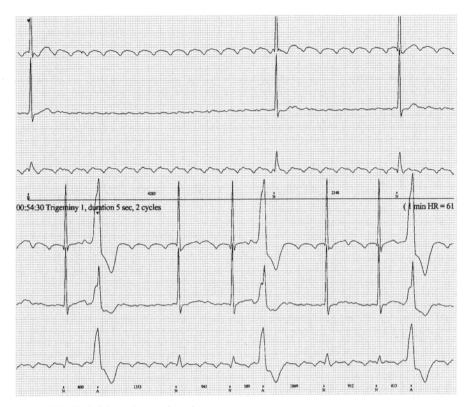

Figure 26.122 Ambulatory electrocardiography.

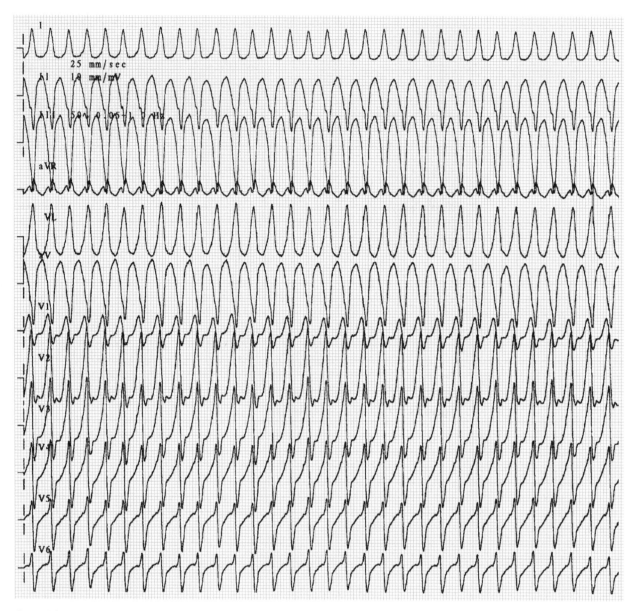

Figure 26.123 What is the arrhythmia?

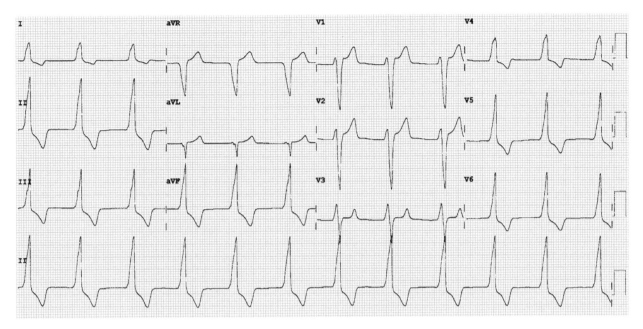

Figure 26.124 What is the arrhythmia?

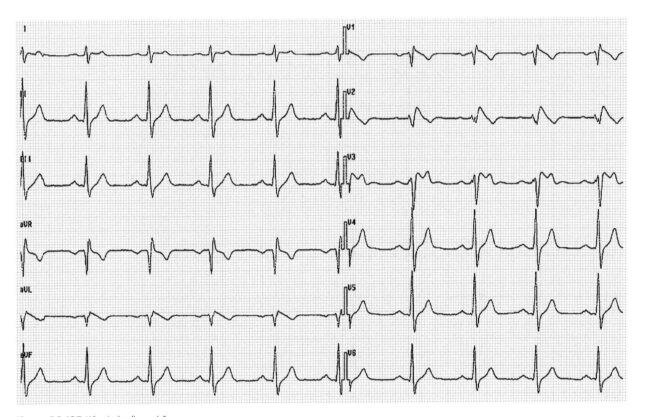

Figure 26.125 What is the diagnosis?

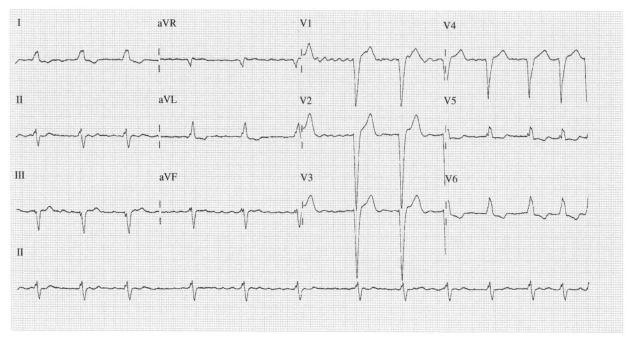

Figure 26.126 What is the arrhythmia?

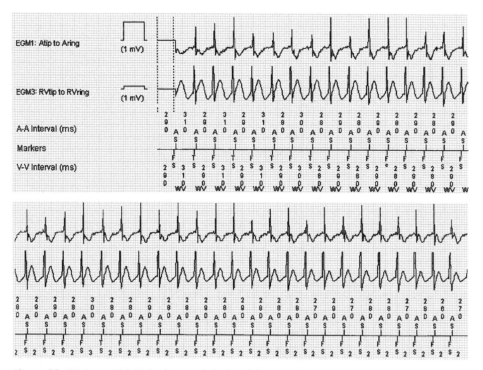

Figure 26.127 Intra-atrial (EGM1) and intraventricular (EGM3) electrograms from a patient with an ICD and HCM. The tachycardia led to shock delivery. Appropriate or not?

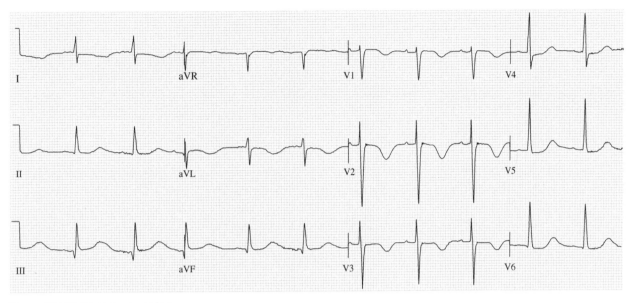

Figure 26.128 What is the abnormality?

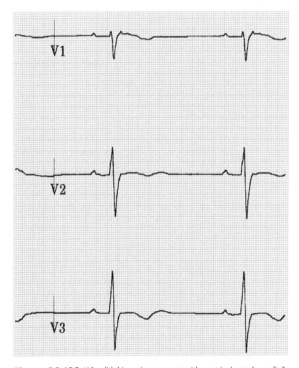

Figure 26.129 Why did this patient present with ventricular tachycardia?

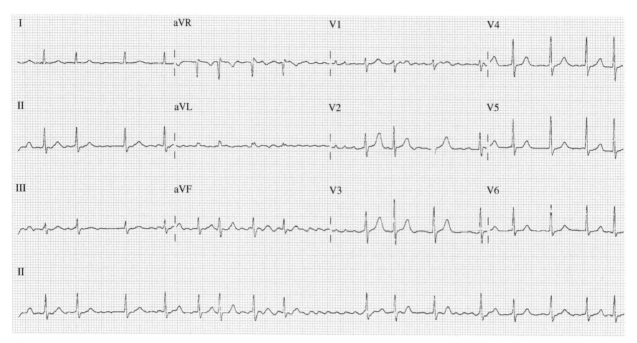

Figure 26.130 What is the arrhythmia?

Interpretations and answers

Figure 26.1 Typical atrial flutter: atrial rate 300 beats/min, atrial activity has sawtooth appearance in limb leads, discrete F waves in lead V1.

Figure 26.2 Sinus rhythm with ventricular trigeminy: after every second beat of sinus origin, there is a premature complex that is broad, abnormal in shape and not preceded by a premature P wave.

Figure 26.3 Neither! This is clearly a ventricular tachycardia (VT): a rapid succession of broad, bizarre complexes makes VT probable: the sixteenth complex is a fusion beat confirming the diagnosis. Adenosine is pointless and verapamil dangerous.

Figure 26.4 Ventricular demand pacemaker inhibited by sinus beats, i.e. VVI mode. Pacemaker stimuli are delivered following pauses in sinus node activity. They initiate broad complexes, indicating ventricular pacing. The paced ventricular complexes are not preceded by spontaneous or paced P waves, thus excluding a dual-chamber pacemaker. The sixth complex is a fusion beat.

Figure 26.5 (b) Pre-excitation: type A Wolff–Parkinson–White syndrome due to a left posterior accessory pathway. The PR interval is short and the ventricular complex is broadened and its upstroke is slurred due to the presence of a delta wave. The apparent Q wave in III and aVF is a negative delta wave.

Figure 26.6 Monomorphic ventricular tachycardia: regular tachycardia, QRS complexes > 140 ms. Though V1 has a right bundle branch block-like appearance which might be seen in a supraventricular tachycardia with aberration, the other chest leads look nothing like right bundle branch block.

Figure 26.7 Complete atrioventricular (AV) block with narrow ventricular complexes: atrial rate 60 beats/min, dissociated from slower ventricular rate of 40 beats/min.

Figure 26.8 An atrial ectopic beat superimposed on the T wave of the fourth ventricular complex initiates atrial flutter. The fifth, seventh and eighth ventricular complexes are broadened due to aberrant conduction.

Figure 26.9 After a single beat of sinus node origin, there is non-sustained monomorphic ventricular tachycardia (with ventriculoatrial conduction: a P wave can be seen superimposed on each T wave during tachycardia, best seen in middle trace).

Figure 26.10 Atrial fibrillation with a rapid ventricular response. The f waves are of low amplitude but the diagnosis is clear from the totally irregular ventricular rhythm.

Figure 26.11 There is no abnormality in rhythm. After two normally conducted sinus beats there is right bundle branch block: QRS > 0.12 s and an M-shaped complex in lead V1.

Figure 26.12 (a) Normal sinus rhythm. (b) Typical AV nodal re-entrant tachycardia. Compare leads V1 during sinus rhythm and during tachycardia. There is an apparent secondary r wave in V1 during tachycardia but this is not present during normal rhythm. It is due to retrograde atrial conduction. The very short ventriculoatrial conduction time indicates AV nodal re-entrant tachycardia.

Figure 26.13 The first, penultimate and last beats show sinus rhythm and Wolff–Parkinson–White syndrome, best seen in lead V3. After the first beat there is an episode of atrial fibrillation, resulting in a totally irregular rhythm, during which all complexes are pre-excited. Flecainide, sotalol and disopyramide would have been appropriate, but digoxin and verapamil might have increased the ventricular rate during atrial fibrillation and possibly caused ventricular fibrillation.

Figure 26.14 Complete AV block. P waves (70 beats/min) dissociated from slower QRS complexes (38 beats/min) with very marked QT prolongation indicating that the patient was prone to torsade de pointes tachycardia.

Figure 26.15 The second 'R on T' ventricular ectopic beat initiates ventricular fibrillation.

Figure 26.16 Mobitz II AV block: there is 2:1 AV block, best seen in lead II, and the QRS complexes are broad.

Figure 26.17 Correct if you said a DDD pacemaker (there is a ventricular stimulus after each spontaneous P wave) and full marks if you said a biventricular pacemaker, having noted that the ventricular complexes were narrow, not broad as is usually seen during ventricular pacing. The last paced complex is initiated by an atrial ectopic beat.

Figure 26.18 Junctional rhythm: the QRS complexes are preceded by a P wave which is negative in leads II, III and aVF.

Figure 26.19 AV junctional re-entrant tachycardia: a rapid, regular succession of narrow QRS complexes. Atrial activity is not apparent: the retrograde P waves are probably concealed by superimposed QRS complexes.

Figure 26.20 Ventricular bigeminy: premature broad, bizarre complexes not preceded by premature P waves. The Q wave in the inferior leads indicates past inferior myocardial infarction. There is a sinus bradycardia.

Figure 26.21 The fourth ventricular complex is an interpolated ventricular ectopic beat (normally an ectopic beat is followed by a pause); the PR interval after the ectopic is prolonged due to retrograde concealed conduction; the ectopic has partially penetrated the AV node, thereby slowing conduction of the next impulse from the sinus node.

Figure 26.22 Atrial demand pacing: there is a pacing stimulus prior to the P waves of the third, fifth and sixth complexes. The fourth complex is an atrial ectopic beat.

Figure 26.23 Major QT prolongation (QT = 0.6 s) caused by clarithromycin. The other drugs do not prolong the QT interval. There is also first-degree AV block.

Figure 26.24 Termination of atrial fibrillation followed by P waves that are notched and broad, suggesting an interatrial conduction delay.

Figure 26.25 Typical atrial flutter with 4:1 AV conduction. The target for ablation would be the isthmus between the tricuspid valve and the inferior vena cava, thereby breaking the right atrial re-entrant circuit that causes this arrhythmia.

Figure 26.26 AV junctional re-entrant tachycardia: lead V1 shows QRS alternans, i.e. alternation of the amplitude of the QRS complex. This phenomenon is seen with tachycardias caused by concealed pathways and also during very fast AVNRT.

Figure 26.27 Atrial tachycardia (atrial rate 160 beats/min) with varying AV block.

Figure 26.28 Complete AV block with long periods without a ventricular escape rhythm.

Figure 26.29 Second ventricular ectopic beat initiates monomorphic ventricular tachycardia: a rapid, regular succession of ventricular ectopic beats each with the same configuration.

Figure 26.30 Left bundle branch block: the QRS complexes are > 0.12 s, there is no M-shaped complex in V1, and V6 is 'notched'.

Figure 26.31 None! The atrial rate is fractionally slower that the ventricular rate: this is AV dissociation but not AV block.

Figure 26.32 The ventricular demand pacemaker has been set at 40 beats/min. There is a ventricular ectopic beat after the first paced complex. The last complex is a fusion beat: the ventricles have been simultaneously activated by a normal sinus beat and the pacemaker.

Figure 26.33 Atrial flutter with high-degree AV block. Typical sawtooth appearance in inferior leads, discrete F waves in V1.

Figure 26.34 No. The ECG shows intermittent pre-excitation and the morphology of the pre-excited beats indicate a posteroseptal pathway. The T inversion in the inferior leads in non-pre-excited beats is due to T wave memory, *not* myocardial ischaemia. Congratulations if you interpreted this ECG correctly!

Figure 26.35 Atrial pacing: each P wave is preceded by a pacing stimulus. There are two ventricular ectopic beats that are of course not sensed by the pacemaker since the pacing lead is in the right atrium, not the ventricle.

Figure 26.36 After three normal beats, there is complete AV block with ventricular asystole: normally timed P waves but no ventricular complexes.

Figure 26.37 There is marked first-degree AV block due to digoxin toxicity. Both the P waves and QRS complexes are normal but the PR interval is increased at 0.36 s.

Figure 26.38 Atrial tachycardia or possibly flutter with 2:1 AV block (best seen in lead V1) initiated after several atrial ectopic beats.

Figure 26.39 2:1 AV block. There is a single ventricular ectopic beat after the third ventricular complex leading to subsequent PR prolongation due to concealed AV conduction.

Figure 26.40 Two paced ventricular beats (a pacing stimulus can be seen initiating the two broad ventricular complex) preceded and succeeded by monomorphic ventricular tachycardia (a rapid, regular succession of broad, bizarre ventricular complexes).

Figure 26.41 The lower set of traces shows atrial flutter with varying degrees of AV block. The mid portion of the upper set of traces shows a narrow QRS complex tachycardia with a ventricular rate identical to the atrial rate in the lower traces, indicating atrial flutter with 1:1 AV conduction: an ample explanation for the patient's exertional symptoms. The broad complexes in the upper traces are due to aberrant conduction, which is often seen during flutter with 1:1 conduction: the appearance raises the possibility of multiform ventricular tachycardia but the ventricular rate is identical to the atrial rate, pointing to flutter with 1:1 conduction and aberrant intraventricular conduction.

Figure 26.42 Complete AV block with marked QT prolongation. The prolonged QT interval and notched T wave are best seen in leads V2 and V3.

Figure 26.43 Two episodes of second-degree sinoatrial block. There are two pauses without either P waves or QRS complexes. The interval between P waves encompassing a pause is twice the cycle length during the rest of the tracing, indicating that the sinus node has depolarised normally but that the impulses from the sinus node during two of the cycles have failed to activate the surrounding atria. Had there been sinus arrest, the subsequent pause would not have been a multiple of the sinus node discharge rate.

Figure 26.44 Atrial fibrillation with rapid ventricular response: f waves clearly seen in top lead (V1) but diagnosis can also be made from other leads because of the totally irregular ventricular rhythm.

Figure 26.45 AV sequential pacing: pacemaker stimuli precede both P waves and QRS complexes.

Figure 26.46 Verapamil. Left posterior fascicular ventricular tachycardia with independent atrial activity best seen in leads III and aVF. There is left axis deviation and right bundle branch block during the tachycardia. Fascicular tachycardia responds to verapamil but not adenosine. Shame on you if you diagnosed a supraventricular tachycardia!

Figure 26.47 Two atrial ectopic beats superimposed on preceding T waves; the first conducted with bundle branch block. Note that the superimposed P waves result in a 'pointed' appearance of the T waves.

Figure 26.48 AV sequential pacing: large-amplitude pacemaker stimuli. The patient had a DDDR pacemaker with a sensor that detected vibration and acceleration, thereby facilitating a chronotropic response to exercise.

Figure 26.49 No. There is atrial fibrillation with a rapid ventricular rate; some ventricular complexes are broad due to aberrant conduction, not ventricular tachycardia.

Figure 26.50 Atrial fibrillation with a slow ventricular rate: a totally irregular ventricular rhythm and f waves best seen in lead V1.

Figure 26.51 AV junctional re-entrant tachycardia: a rapid, regular succession of narrow QRS complexes, terminating into sinus rhythm.

Figure 26.52 There is complete AV block: several spontaneous P waves are not followed by QRS complexes. The P waves trigger pacemaker stimuli, indicating a dual-chamber pacemaker, but several stimuli are not followed by ventricular complexes, i.e. there is intermittent failure of ventricular capture.

Figure 26.53 Second-degree AV block with narrow ventricular complexes and 3:1 AV conduction: every third P wave is followed by a QRS complex.

Figure 26.54 After three normal beats there is a pause without P waves, indicating sinus arrest. The pause is terminated by an escape beat that has the same configuration as the ventricular complexes during normal rhythm, indicating a junctional origin.

Figure 26.55 Ventricular fibrillation.

Figure 26.56 Atrial synchronised and then AV sequential pacing, i.e. DDD pacemaker. The first four ventricular paced beats are triggered by spontaneous P waves, after which there is slowing of the spontaneous atrial rate leading to AV sequential pacing.

Figure 26.57 DDD pacing. The narrow QRS complexes are consistent with biventricular pacing. An atrial pacing stimulus is delivered in the fifth complex because of failure to sense the spontaneous P wave.

Figure 26.58 Type A Wolff–Parkinson–White syndrome: the QRS complex is positive in lead V1, indicating an accessory pathway on the left side of the heart.

Figure 26.59 Ventricular tachycardia. The ninth and fifteenth complexes are narrower: they are fusion beats (best seen in leads I and V5) indicating independent atrial activity during the tachycardia and thereby excluding any possibility of a supraventricular origin.

Figure 26.60 Right axis deviation (i.e. lead I predominantly negative and leads II and III predominantly positive) and right bundle branch block can be due to pulmonary hypertension but can also indicate widespread conduction tissue disease, as in this case: bifascicular block. Intermittent complete AV block was responsible for syncope.

Figure 26.61 The baseline sawtooth appearance indicates atrial flutter. Ventricular complexes, which are broad, are initiated by pacing stimuli, indicating ventricular pacing, and the negative complexes in leads II and III show left axis deviation, pointing to the pacing lead being positioned in the right ventricular apex.

Figure 26.62 The fourth beat (upper two panels) is an atrial ectopic beat (a premature P wave can be seen to be superimposed on the preceding T wave) and is conducted with bundle branch block (probably right bundle branch block). The fourth ventricular complex in the lower two panels is not an ectopic beat because it is not premature. It is an escape beat: it is preceded by a P wave but the PR interval is too short for AV conduction to have occurred.

Figure 26.63 Mobitz II AV block: there is 3:1 AV conduction and the QRS complexes are broad.

Figure 26.64 Complete AV block, best seen in V1, and marked QT prolongation: QT = 0.8s. (Patient presented with torsade de pointes tachycardia.)

Figure 26.65 None. There is normal sinus rhythm (see lead II). Apparent atrial fibrillation in some of limb leads is due to patient tremor.

Figure 26.66 Fusion and capture beats indicate ventricular tachycardia with independent atrial activity: the ninth complex is a fusion beat and the thirteenth and seventeenth complexes are capture beats. Relatively narrow QRS complexes together with right bundle branch block and left axis deviation indicate left posterior fascicular origin. This ventricular tachycardia is not due to impaired ventricular function; it has a good prognosis and is amenable to ablation.

Figure 26.67 Frequent unifocal ventricular ectopic beats during sinus tachycardia: the ectopics are broad and have an abnormal configuration and are not preceded by premature P waves.

Figure 26.68 Bifascicular block due to anterior myocardial infarction: there is left anterior fascicular block (lead I predominantly positive and leads II and III predominantly negative, together with an r wave in the inferior leads) and right bundle branch block. The Q wave in the anterior leads indicates septal infarction.

Figure 26.69 Paroxysmal atrial fibrillation. Digoxin even in therapeutic doses, e.g. 0.25–0.375 mg daily, will not prevent this arrhythmia. Appropriate first-line antiarrhythmic drugs include flecainide and propafenone, together with an AV nodal blocking drug, i.e. a beta blocker or calcium antagonist, to slow the ventricular rate should atrial tachycardia or flutter result.

Figure 26.70 Mobitz II AV block: 2:1 AV conduction together with a broad QRS complex.

Figure 26.71 Sinus rhythm, left bundle branch block (ventricular complexes which follow P waves are broad and notched in lead I) and ventricular bigeminy.

Figure 26.72 Multifocal ventricular ectopic beats: the third, fifth and eighth complexes, each with a different morphology. The first is an end-diastolic ectopic beat: it follows a normally timed P wave but it is slightly premature and the PR interval is very short, making it unlikely that it is the result of AV conduction. The third ectopic initiates monomorphic ventricular tachycardia. The Q wave and slight ST elevation in lead III raise the possibility of inferior myocardial infarction.

Figure 26.73 Atrial fibrillation with a very long pause followed by a rapid ventricular rate: the fourth and fifth ventricular complexes in the lower two panels are due to aberrant conduction.

Figure 26.74 Right ventricular outflow tract bigeminy: the complexes have a right axis and left bundle branch block configuration and are relatively narrow. Then a salvo of right ventricular outflow tract ectopics beats initiates AV re-entrant tachycardia. QRS alternans in lead V1.

Figure 26.75 Onset of atrial fibrillation after four sinus beats: atrial activity at times is coarse but the rhythm is atrial fibrillation not flutter.

Figure 26.76 Type B Wolff–Parkinson–White syndrome (negative complex in lead V1) due to posteroseptal accessory pathway characterised by negative delta waves or 'pseudo-inferior' infarction pattern in the inferior leads, and early transition in the chest leads, i.e. V2 is positive.

Figure 26.77 Monomorphic ventricular tachycardia: markedly broad, uniform complexes with a left axis configuration at a very fast rate.

Figure 26.78 Flecainide was contraindicated. The patient has Brugada syndrome: downsloping ST elevation in lead V1 and V2. Flecainide could have been arrhythmogenic.

Figure 26.79 Ventricular pacing during atrial fibrillation. The left axis configuration of the paced beats indicates that the pacing lead tip is at the right ventricular apex. After the eighth paced ventricular complex there are two, not one, pacing stimuli preceding the next complex (see leads V1 and V5). This indicates that the patient has a dual-chamber mode-switching pacemaker and for one cycle the pacemaker has failed to detect atrial fibrillation and therefore delivered an atrial stimulus.

Figure 26.80 Upper trace – normal AV sequential pacing. Lower trace – satisfactory atrial capture but failure of ventricular capture. At the time of this recording AV conduction was not impaired but syncope continued due to intermittent complete AV block.

Figure 26.81 There is marked first-degree AV block: PR = 0.36 s. This alone is not an indication for pacing: higher levels of AV block should be sought by ambulatory electrocardiography.

Figure 26.82 No! Atrial flutter with complete AV block: the sawtooth atrial activity typical of atrial flutter is dissociated from the slow, regular ventricular activity. A pacemaker is required.

Figure 26.83 Complete AV block: atrial rate approximately 75 beats/min dissociated from slower, regular ventricular rate 36 beats/min

Figure 26.84 Dextrocardia. The inverted but normally timed P wave in lead I indicates either arm lead reversal or dextrocardia: the latter is confirmed by the reversal of the normal chest lead sequence. Well done if you got the correct diagnosis.

Figure 26.85 Atrial fibrillation with a rapid ventricular rate; some broad QRS complexes due to aberrant conduction.

Figure 26.86 Complete AV block due to acute inferior infarction. Atrial rate 85 beats/min. Ventricular rate 50 beats/min. Marked ST elevation in lead aVF indicates acute inferior infarction. In complete AV block due to inferior infarction, temporary pacing is only required if there is marked hypotension, oliguria or syncope.

Figure 26.87 The totally irregular ventricular rhythm indicates atrial fibrillation. The QRS complex appearance suggests delta waves due to Wolff–Parkinson–White syndrome. Digoxin should be avoided: it could have accelerated the rate and caused ventricular fibrillation.

Figure 26.88 Right bundle branch block: sinus rhythm with QRS complexes >0.12s and an M-shaped ventricular complex in lead V1.

Figure 26.89 Left anterior fascicular block (lead I predominantly positive and leads II and III predominantly negative with an r wave in the inferior leads), and atrial fibrillation.

Figure 26.90 Sinus arrest after three normal beats. There is an ectopic beat after the fourth ventricular complex. It has a partial right bundle branch block configuration and may be due to an atrial extrasystole, but no premature P wave can be identified.

Figure 26.91 None! Normal ECG.

Figure 26.92 Monomorphic ventricular tachycardia with direct evidence of independent atrial activity. There are P waves at a rate of 75 beats/min dissociated from the rapid ventricular activity – best seen in the rhythm strip at the bottom of the trace.

Figure 26.93 Atrial pacing with large-amplitude pacing stimuli, suggesting unipolar pacing. The inverted P waves in the inferior leads are due to a pacing site low on the right atrial septum.

Figure 26.94 Left anterior fascicular and right bundle branch block, i.e. bifascicular block. Syncope probably due to intermittent trifascicular block, i.e. complete AV block.

Figure 26.95 Mode-switching, dual-chamber pacemaker. During atrial fibrillation there is ventricular demand pacing. There is termination of atrial fibrillation after the fifth ventricular complex that is followed by AV sequential pacing for one beat before atrial fibrillation returns and leads again to mode switching.

Figure 26.96 Marked QT prolongation. QT interval = 0.64 s. The notched T wave seen in lead V2 is typical of LQ2 hereditary long QT syndrome, in which sudden auditory stimuli can initiate a ventricular arrhythmia.

Figure 26.97 Right ventricular outflow tract ectopia: after each sinus beat there is a premature ventricular complex with a right axis and left bundle branch block configuration typical of a right ventricular outflow tract origin. There is a P wave in the ST segment of each ectopic resulting from retrograde AV conduction.

Figure 26.98 Paroxysmal atrial fibrillation: a rapid, totally irregular ventricular rhythm spontaneously terminates into sinus rhythm.

Figure 26.99 AV Wenckebach block: progressive PR prolongation.

Figure 26.100 Monomorphic ventricular tachycardia preceded by sinus rhythm. Close inspection reveals independent atrial activity.

Figure 26.101 Sinus bradycardia with ventricular bigeminy: after every beat arising from the sinus node there is a premature, broad bizarre complex not preceded by a premature P wave.

Figure 26.102 Spontaneous termination of ventricular tachycardia followed by ventricular pacing. During the tachycardia, there are very broad ventricular complexes, and dissociated P waves can be seen superimposed on the T waves of the second and tenth complexes in the upper trace. After tachycardia termination there are broad complexes preceded by small pacemaker stimuli.

Figure 26.103 AV junctional re-entrant tachycardia: a rapid, regular succession of narrow QRS complexes (with QRS alternans).

Figure 26.104 'Noise' from faulty ventricular lead can be seen in the middle trace, more frequent towards the end. The rapid signal rate was misinterpreted as ventricular fibrillation (see annotation – VF), resulting in inappropriate shock delivery.

Figure 26.105 There is typical atrial flutter. In addition there is right bundle branch block (V1 shows QRS > 0.12 s and M-shaped complex) and left anterior fascicular block (left axis deviation with lead I predominantly positive and leads II and III predominantly negative, with r wave in inferior leads), i.e. bifascicular block.

Figure 26.106 Atrial fibrillation. Totally irregular ventricular rhythm and f waves clearly seen in several leads.

Figure 26.107 There is first-degree AV block (PR = 0.36 s), left bundle branch block (QRS > 0.12 s during sinus rhythm but no M-shaped complex in V1): the seventh ventricular complex is a supraventricular ectopic beat: it is premature and has the same configuration as the normally timed complexes.

Figure 26.108 Ventricular pre-excitation. The fourth complex is caused by a supraventricular ectopic beat: it is premature and has the same configuration as the normally timed complexes.

Figure 26.109 Monomorphic ventricular tachycardia: a rapid, regular succession of very broad, bizarre ventricular complexes.

Figure 26.110 Idioventricular rhythm: has the characteristics of monomorphic ventricular tachycardia but the rate is only 75 beats/min.

Figure 26.111 Near-syncope: first-degree AV block, and then a succession of normally timed P waves not followed by QRS complexes, i.e. complete AV block with ventricular asystole.

Figure 26.112 Development of polymorphic ventricular tachycardia during ambulatory electrocardiography. There is an atrial ectopic beat in the upper trace. The T wave is either followed by a U wave, or is notched and hence the QT markedly prolonged.

Figure 26.113 Probable arrhythmogenic right ventricular cardiomyopathy: suggested by the epsilon wave in lead V1 and T inversion in right precordial leads. Congratulations if you interpreted the ECG correctly!

Figure 26.114 Non-sustained ventricular tachycardia.

Figure 26.115 Cardiac pacing. The ECG shows bifascicular block and first-degree AV block, i.e. trifascicular disease.

Figure 26.116 This is atrial fibrillation, not flutter: the rhythm is totally irregular, and though atrial activity in V1 is 'coarse', it is far too rapid and disorganised for atrial flutter. A low-energy shock is usually successful in atrial flutter but not fibrillation.

Figure 26.117 A non-conducted atrial ectopic beat is superimposed on the third T wave.

Figure 26.118 Ventricular pacing during atrial fibrillation. The normal QRS axis points towards a septal position for the lead, and certainly indicates that the lead is not in the right ventricular apex: had that been the case there would have been left axis deviation.

Figure 26.119 Sinus arrest terminated by a junctional escape beat which arises immediately after inscription of a P wave after a PR interval shorter than in other complexes and therefore making AV conduction unlikely.

Figure 26.120 Type B Wolff–Parkinson–White (WPW) syndrome: short PR interval and QRS complex broadened by a delta wave. Had V1 been positive there would have been type A WPW syndrome.

Figure 26.121 Ventricular tachycardia: regular broad complex tachycardia with a positive concordant pattern. (Antidromic tachycardia due to Wolff–Parkinson–White syndrome is a very unlikely alternative diagnosis: it is rare and this patient has a cardiomyopathy that commonly causes ventricular tachycardia.)

Figure 26.122 Atrial flutter with episode of high-degree AV block.

Figure 26.123 Very rapid monomorphic ventricular tachycardia.

Figure 26.124 Idioventricular rhythm.

Figure 26.125 Brugada syndrome: normal sinus rhythm with downsloping ST elevation in leads V1 and V2.

Figure 26.126 Atrial fibrillation and left bundle branch block.

Figure 26.127 Inappropriate shock. The atrial and ventricular electrograms are virtually synchronous: typical of AVNRT that was confirmed by electrophysiological study.

Figure 26.128 The QT interval is markedly prolonged (0.58 s). Remember, if the end of the T wave approaches the halfway point between QRS complexes, consider QT prolongation.

Figure 26.129 In lead V1, there is a small positive wave immediately after the QRS complex. It is an epsilon wave, pointing to a diagnosis of ARVC.

Figure 26.130 Yet another example of atrial fibrillation. If any other diagnosis was made, a career in dermatology beckons!

Index

Lightning Source UK Ltd.
Milton Keynes UK
UKOW06f0647051014

239606UK00002B/2/P